AN EMPOWERING LEADERSHIP GUIDE FOR EMERGING NURSES

AN EMPOWERING LEADERSHIP GUIDE FOR EMERGING NURSES

SURVIVING THE SHIFT

Linda Roney, Editor

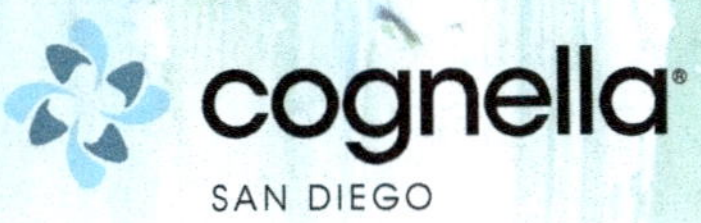

cognella® SAN DIEGO

Bassim Hamadeh, CEO and Publisher
Amanda Martin, Executive Publisher
Amy Smith, Associate Editorial Manager
Jeanine Rees, Production Editor
Jess Estrella, Senior Graphic Designer
Kylie Bartolome, Licensing Specialist
Natalie Piccotti, Director of Marketing
Kassie Graves, Senior Vice President, Editorial
Alia Bales, Director, Project Editorial and Production

This book is designed to provide educational information and motivation to our readers. It is sold with the understanding that the publisher is not engaged to render any type of psychological, legal, diet, health, exercise or any other kind of professional advice. The content of each chapter or reading is the sole expression and opinion of its author, and not necessarily that of the publisher. No warranties or guarantees are expressed or implied by the publisher's choice to include any of the content in this volume. Neither the publisher nor the individual author(s) shall be liable for any physical, psychological, emotional, financial, or commercial damages, including, but not limited to, special, incidental, consequential or other damages. Our views and rights are the same: You are responsible for your own choices, actions, and results and for seeking relevant topical advice from trained professionals.

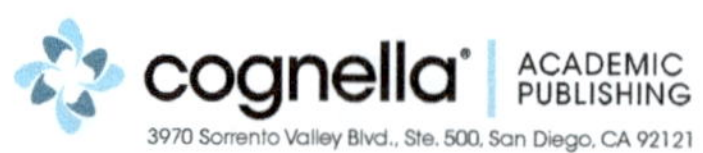

This book is dedicated to the nurses of today and tomorrow—
those who are living this work and those called to join our profession.
May this book honor your unseen work. You are never invisible among us.

*"You are braver than you believe,
stronger than you seem,
smarter than you think,
and loved more than you know."*

—Winnie the Pooh (*The House at Pooh Corner,*
A. A. Milne [1928])

BRIEF CONTENTS

DETAILED CONTENTS

CHAPTER 3   **THE IMPACT OF LEADERSHIP AND SUPPORT   47**

Lauren Jamieson, BSN, RN, RNC-NIC; Michelle M. Kelly, PhD, CRNP, CNE, FAANP, FAAN; and Linda Roney, EdD, RN-BC, CPEN, CNE, FAAN

PREFACE

Every two years, the National Council of State Boards of Nursing (NCBSN) and the National Forum of State Nursing Workforce Centers conduct the only nationally focused survey on the nursing workforce (NCBSN, 2024). In summer 2023, I read the newly published results of the 2022 National Nursing Workforce Survey (Smiley et al., 2023) and was heartbroken but unsurprised. In this survey of roughly 100,000 registered nurses (RNs) and 34,000 licensed practical and vocational nurses, half of the participants (45%–56%) reported feeling emotionally drained from a few times per week up to every day. More than one-quarter of all nurses in the study reported planning to leave nursing or retire in the next five years (Smiley et al., 2023). As we write this casebook for you, the 2024 National Nursing Workforce Survey is in progress (NCBSN, 2024). We do not know what those results will show, but we hope our profession is doing better than in 2022.

As nurses, we represent the United States' largest healthcare profession, with nearly 4.7 million RNs (NCSBN, 2024). We continue as the most trusted profession in the nation, with 78% of U.S. adults believing nurses have high honesty and ethical standards (Brennan & Jones, 2024). To say this plainly, if there are many of us and people seem to like us, why are we not on the national news every night until we fix "the problem?" I am not naïve enough to believe there is one solution to this problem, yet creating and leading this casebook project felt like one thing I could do now.

I have two aims for this casebook:

1. **My most important aim was to create a supportive resource for emerging and new nurses.**

Many of the themes addressed in this casebook are those that generations of nurses have faced, but a nurse with fewer than two years of experience when they encountered them will share their perspective. A nurse leader will then reflect on the new nurse's experience, sharing their experience, knowledge, and wisdom with you on addressing this situation if you find yourself in it, too. Finally, I will provide tactical tips and resources to help you develop self-efficacy in this area (the belief in yourself that you can do it, too).

I carefully assembled this team of 11 new nurses and 12 nursing leaders to work with me on this project. I am a full-time academic nurse educator in a BSN program, and each new nurse author is a former student. We remained in contact after graduation, and some shared their experiences navigating challenging situations as they transitioned into practice. They scattered around the country for their first jobs, working in various specialties. While their practice area is the setting of their story, there is value in what they share with you regardless of where you work as a nurse. As for the nurse leaders, they share in my love and concern for the future of our profession. Our past work together also represents different times in my nursing leadership journey. Most of the new nurses and nurse leaders did not know one another prior to this project. I picked a "super team" of hardworking, compassionate, innovative nurse leaders I have worked with in another capacity.

2.   **My second aim was to highlight the tremendous work of nurses.**
While we are highly regarded and trusted, many outside nursing do not know what we do. In preparing to write this casebook, I reviewed many new graduate nurse job postings, and most of them were centered on the American Nurses Association's *Scope and Standards of Practice* (2015a) and *Standards of Professional Performance* (2015b). Additionally, many of the postings required an employee to walk or stand for more than a half-day, potentially be exposed to infectious diseases and physical and mental illnesses. They put themselves at moderate risk of injury from patient care. Most job descriptions require the nurse to be able to move patients between 5 and 300 pounds. This is intellectually, physically, and emotionally demanding.

The job descriptions I reviewed did not discuss the "invisible work" of our jobs. *Invisible work* is the tasks, roles, and responsibilities essential to the functioning of a workplace but often go unnoticed, unrecognized, or undervalued (Kaplan Daniels, 1987). In addition to what you were trained to do in a health assessment or fundamentals of the nursing lab, there are many additional burdens and responsibilities on nurses today, including providing emotional support to patients, families, and colleagues; resolving conflicts among members of the healthcare team; offering mentorship and guidance; care planning for holistic patient care and work environments that is efficient and fiscally responsible; communicating and coordinating workflows and support with team members; and nurturing overall team dynamics (Kalita, 2023). Some of our work is intangible, meaning it cannot accurately be recorded or measured (Montañés Muro et al., 2023). No one will ever truly understand what it is like to be a nurse unless you are one. Yet, hopefully, this casebook will highlight some of the beauty and challenges we face daily. Feel free to share it with your loved ones who are not nurses.

Finally, if anyone out there believes that new nurses are less tough and resilient than previous generations, you are mistaken. As a doctorally prepared nurse who continues to work as a bedside nurse in the acute care setting, I can tell you that technology has advanced rapidly so that many of our sickest patients would not have been alive 27 years ago when I started my nursing career. The pace of nursing is too fast, and the patients are too sick for new nurses to develop the skills gradually that we did when we were starting our nursing careers. People have changed. I admire the grit of new nurses who enter our profession during these challenging times.

With experienced nurses leaving the bedside, newer nurses are sometimes prematurely forced into leadership positions, such as charge nurse, by being the most senior or only RNs in their clinical care due to staffing shortages, high unit turnover rates, and attrition of experienced nurses (Ting et al., 2024), we felt we needed to come together and do something. High workload and unprecedented levels of stress and burnout in this decade have already resulted in high turnover among younger, less experienced nurses (Martin et al., 2023). This book's nurse leader co-authors are pioneers in many professional organizations engaged in critical work to address many of these challenges nurses face on the aggregate level. We wanted to do something more personal, as if we had the chance to mentor you, *just you.*

On behalf of this 24-nurse author team, we see you. We hear you. We admire you. We are *with* you.

Final Notes That Are Essential for You to Remember

To illustrate the complexities of the case, some details in the story may be fictionalized to enhance the case narrative or to protect the identities of those involved. All characters, organizations, and other entities depicted in this work are fictitious. Any resemblance to real persons, living or dead, or actual events is purely coincidental. By using or referencing this casebook, readers acknowledge and agree that they cannot hold the authors, publishers, or any related parties liable for any legal claims arising from its content.

This casebook is intended solely as an educational resource to support your transition into registered nursing practice. It is not a substitute for guidance from your supervisor, organizational policies, or the relevant nurse practice act. The examples provided in this book are brief and serve as one of many tools to assist in developing clinical judgment in these areas. The co-authors of this casebook are not liable for any outcomes related to the use of this content.

At the end of every chapter, you will see a feature called "You Matter," an area that not only offers a brief summary of the content as it relates to your future nursing career but also reminds you that regardless of the situation you are in, you are important, and your concerns are significant. Many times, when we are in a new and challenging situation, it is easy to feel that we are alone, disregarded and marginalized. We will explain this more in Chapter 1. The co-authors of this book have collaborated to share their experiences and wisdom to help coach you through some of these new challenges you may face and help you feel supported and empowered.

Following the content of each chapter, you will find an area called "Book Club Questions." If you read this casebook as part of a cohort, such as at the end of your nursing program or during your new graduate orientation, you'll see that these questions are conversation starters for even more extensive discussions on these topics. If you are reading this independently, the questions offer prompts for discussion and may catalyze conversations with colleagues or mentors.

References

American Nurses Association. (2015a). *Nursing: Scope and standards of practice* (4th ed.).

American Nurses Association. (2015b). *Standards of professional performance* (3rd ed.).

Brenan, M., & Jones, J. (2025, February 26). Ethics ratings of nearly all professions down in U.S. Gallup.com.

https://news.gallup.com/poll/608903/ethics-ratings-nearly-professions-down.aspx

Kalita, S. M. (2023, September 26). How to end the unfairness of invisible work. *TIME.* https://time.com/charter/6317237/how-to-end-the-unfairness-of-invisible-work/

Kaplan Daniels, A. (1987). Invisible work. *Social Problems, 34*(5), 403–415. https://doi.org/10.2307/800538

Martin, B., Kaminski-Ozturk, N., O'Hara, C., & Smiley, R. (2023). Examining the impact of the COVID-19 pandemic on burnout and stress among U.S. nurses. *Journal of Nursing Regulation, 14*(1), 4–12. https://doi.org/10.1016/S2155-8256(23)00063-7

Montañés Muro, M. P., Ayala Calvo, J. C., & Manzano García, G. (2023). Burnout in nursing: A vision of gender and "invisible" unrecorded care. *Journal of Advanced Nursing, 79*(6), 2148–2154. https://doi.org/10.1111/jan.15523

National Council of State Boards of Nursing. (2024). *Active RN licenses.* https://www.ncsbn.org/active-rn-licenses

Smiley, R. A., Allgeyer, R. L., Shobo, Y., Lyons, K. C., Letourneau, R., Zhong, E., Kaminski-Ozturk, N., & Alexander, M. (2023). The 2022 national nursing workforce survey. *Journal of Nursing Regulation, 14*(1), S1–S90.

Ting, J. J., Babenko-Mould, Y., & Garnett, A. (2024). Early career nurses' experiences of engaging in a leadership role in hospital settings. *Canadian Journal of Nursing Research, 56*(3), 257–268. https://doi.org/10.1177/08445621241236666

ACKNOWLEDGMENTS

In reflecting on the past year since I committed to writing this casebook, I am grateful to many who supported this project. This casebook takes a different approach to supporting the transition of the emerging nurse to a practicing nurse from that of traditional textbooks. This casebook is based on years of informal data collection, including conversations behind medication and supply rooms' closed doors, empty patient rooms, and through heartfelt conversations and texts. The bond and camaraderie among nursing colleagues is a unique and profound connection, forged during long shifts filled with unexpected challenges and often, high emotion. We never forget how our nursing colleagues made us feel, and to those who were there for us, we can feel a sense of commitment to those special people no matter how many years go by. Thank you to all those whose paths have crossed mine in our nursing journeys. Your support and friendship have helped me become a better nurse and, more importantly, a better person.

I am grateful to the incredible team at Cognella Publishing for supporting my ideas, particularly *Amanda Martin* and *Amy Smith*, for helping me believe that anything was possible and that different is sometimes a really good thing. You helped me believe in myself and the dream of this project, and I am so grateful for your professionalism, connection, and support.

This project was possible only because of the 23 superstar nurses who joined me in this project.

To *Anabelle, Anna, Bridget, Grace, Iris, Janea, Lauren, Katie K., Katie M., Kayla,* and *Moira*: We met while you were on your nursing student journey, and from the first time I met each of you, I saw so many amazing things about you. Thank you for your generosity in meaningfully sharing your knowledge and wisdom with the next generation of nurses. You are the reason why the future of nursing is so bright.

To *Aaron, Danielle, Eileen, Erin, Kevin, Laura, Laurie, Maria, Michelle, Sarah, Sean,* and *Teresa*: We met on so many different parts of my nursing journey, and I knew in my heart that if we could create a super team of nurse leaders to show the world how much we cared about the next generation of nurses, we could do something amazing together. I appreciate each of you for not only your tremendous contributions to this project but also the role that you have played in my life.

To *Brian Ripley Crandall* and *Sonya Huber*: Thank you for your mentorship as I approached this project. You were generous with your time and support of me and the nurses.

To *Meredith*, *Diane*, *Vivian*, and *Dr. Westrick*: Thank you for always being there for me in too many ways to list. I am eternally grateful for your support that helped me get here.

To *Allie*, *Blakely*, *Carmela*, *Erica*, *Julia*, *Katherine*, *Kelly*, *Kenzie*, *Mekaylia*, *Michelle*, *Nicole*, *Teagan*, and *Reagan*: Thank you for generously offering your feedback and support for this project in so many ways. You will be nurses by the time this is published and I am excited for what is ahead for you.

To my husband, *John*: Thank you for being my greatest supporter. Few people have the chance to work with their spouse, and it was such a gift for me to have such direct insight into the talented provider you are. Thank you for understanding the time I poured into this project outside my regular work and helping our family in every way. I love you with all of my heart, and thank you for your support and always bringing fun into our lives.

To *Michael*: Thank you for always being the first to ask how my day went and for being patient with all of the dinner conversations about "the hospital" between Dad and me over the years. You will always be the best standardized patient in the nursing lab. You have such a big heart and will accomplish such great things. I am so proud to be your mom. I love you *more*.

To *Natalie*: I am excited to see what is ahead for you in your nursing career; you will accomplish such great things. You have such a big heart. I am so proud to be your mom. I have learned so many lessons and stories from my years as a nurse that I couldn't imagine a better way to share them with you other than within the pages of this book. I pushed forward with a tight timeline to finish this so you can read it before graduation. I love you *more*.

To all my colleagues, friends, and former students: This book is for and about us. Thank you to all of you who have been a part of my tremendous nursing journey. What we do is incredible, and it has been fantastic because of all of you. To my dear friends, especially Michele, Megan, Laura, Nancy, Julie, Carolyn, Brigitte, Kath and Chris—and my entire family who have patiently listened to my stories over the years, have kept me in check, and supported me in every way—thank you for the great memories filled with laughing and the day-to-day moral support.

Mom and Dad, I love you both, and thank you for instilling a love and appreciation for education and hard work. This accomplishment is as much yours as it is mine, as I could not have done any of this without both of you.

CHAPTER 1

Welcome to Your Nursing Career

Linda Roney, EdD, RN-BC, CPEN, CNE, FAAN

Learning Goals

1. Articulate the importance of leadership in the early stages of a nursing career.
2. Analyze external factors that affect the current nursing practice environment.
3. Examine the theory of marginalization and mattering and apply its concepts to the role of a new nurse.
4. Evaluate the relevance of domains 2 and 10 of the American Association of Colleges of Nursing (AACN) essentials to this casebook.
5. Value the importance of self-care for new nurses.

Welcome to your book, *An Empowering Leadership Guide for Emerging Nurses: Surviving the Shift*, written just for you. Congratulations on choosing nursing as your career. You are in a field that stands out as the most honest and ethical profession (Brenan & Jones, 2024). You have worked hard to reach this point today, as nursing programs are academically rigorous (American Nurses Association, 2023). You should be very proud of your hard work. It should be recognized that most of you decided to become a nurse during the COVID-19 pandemic or this global health event, which somehow affected your education. A recent study found that motives for nursing career choice include the desire to help others, diversity of work options, interest in working with others, and potential for promotion (Avraham et al., 2023). While each nurse has a unique story of how and why they selected nursing, each one is a member of the team of nearly 5.2 million nurses in the United States, the largest profession in health care (Smiley et al., 2023). Whether you went to nursing school immediately after high school or had a lifetime of experience before you started, you are vital to delivering safe, evidence-based health care in our communities. Our profession needs you to be a nursing leader.

Why Do You Need to Be a Leader When You Start Nursing?

While most nurses do not start their careers thinking about being leaders, we need these skills to collaborate as full partners with the interdisciplinary team of healthcare professionals (Institute of Medicine, 2011). Right now, you may ask yourself how to be a leader as you start your nursing journey. In your mind, mastery of tasks such as medication administration and documentation in an electronic health record is at the forefront of your mind. However, there is much more than you can imagine in your remarkable nursing career. Nursing is a community of leaders and learners who collaborate to support, treat, and care, and it is important to note that innovative leadership is often displayed by nurses who do not hold a formal management role (Quinn, 2020).

Our country needs you more than you could ever have imagined. You are joining as a team member of the U.S. healthcare system, which currently spends more than $4 trillion a year on health care, with the majority spent on medical interventions (Berwick & Williams, 2023). Compared with peer nations, the United States has the lowest life expectancy from birth, the highest death rate from avoidable or treatable causes, the highest rate of people with multiple chronic conditions, and the highest maternal and infant death rates (Commonwealth Fund, 2023). People who face all these situations will interact with healthcare providers. As nurses, we care for the individuals whose outcomes may become part of future reports about health care in our country. Research data support the association between higher nurse staffing levels and lower patient mortality (Haegdorens et al., 2019). You are entering a healthcare system inheriting many challenges, and it is essential to note that none of them are ones that you have created.

While the data support that having appropriate levels of nursing care is safer and better for patient and nurse satisfaction, this is not always possible as the total supply of nurses decreased by the most considerable amount in 40 years, with 100,000 fewer nurses from 2020 to 2021 (Buerhaus et al., 2022). The median age of U.S. nurses is 46, and more than one-quarter of registered nurses (RNs) report that they plan to retire or leave nursing in the next five years (Smiley et al., 2023). In one recent study, 93% of nurses reported that their hospital was currently experiencing a staffing shortage, with nearly 90% of respondents stating that this is a moderate-to-severe problem (American Association of International Healthcare Recruitment, 2022).

While some may think that this sounds like opportunities for job security for soon-to-be and new nurses, let us consider how this affects the healthcare work environment. Demanding workloads can increase stress and burnout (Shah et al., 2021). Unlike other occupational hazards, stress at work is not subject to oversight by organizations such as the Occupational Safety and Health Administration (OSHA), which ensures safe and healthy work environments (OSHA, n.d.). Stress at work is invisible and is often accepted as an inevitable part of contemporary workplaces. It is worsening everywhere, yet unhealthy work practices do not improve the performance or profitability of organizations as they decrease employee engagement, increase turnover, reduce job performance, and raise healthcare costs (Pfeffer, 2018).

The healthcare environment you enter is complex and, at times, intense. The volume of activity, the number of caregivers providing care with different yet often interdependent roles, and the high utilization of services contribute to the sophisticated tapestry of our modern healthcare system (Terry, 2022). As a new nurse, you will have many experiences that will challenge you. Sometimes you will feel that so many things are hard in your day, and the cumulative stress can add up. The result can be negative responses to caring, which include burnout and compassion fatigue. At this point, you might ask yourself why this casebook starts with so much information about the challenges facing nursing and health care. Newly graduated nurses are not always prepared for the challenges of the chaotic clinical environment. As leaders in nursing, we have an opportunity and professional obligation to support your transition as competent leaders in health care (Stubin, 2021).

We hope to offer proactive strategies in this book to implement into your personal and work life to help you feel centered and valued. While some employee wellness programs focused on the individual (e.g., employee assistance programs and counseling) are well designed and appreciated by staff, there is also strong support for the effectiveness of organizational change and work redesign on improving worker well-being (Fleming, 2023; Fox et al., 2022; Lovejoy et al., 2021; National Institute for Health and Care Excellence, 2022). While we cannot directly control our work environment and the resources that our employer offers, there are opportunities to share feedback in ways such as an employee engagement survey that may help influence our working environments (Fleming, 2023). Together, we will explore strategies that will empower you to amplify your impact in today's practice environment.

You worked too hard in nursing school not to feel valued in your work. Some nurses have compounding challenges at work and "quietly quit their jobs" (Galanis et al., 2024, p. 1). The term *quiet quitting* refers to detaching (quitting) from activities perceived as above and beyond a basic job description (Krueger, 2022). Those who feel their work has purpose are less likely to quit quietly and are more engaged (Ellis & Yang, 2022). An alternative to actual job resignation, for some, this type of limit setting relates to work-life balance choices that have been influenced by a variety of situations, such as generational priorities, income shortfalls, and the COVID-19 pandemic experience that have encouraged workers to hold back from the overly demanding needs of work (Zuzelo, 2023).

In a recent Gallup poll of American workers in all areas, not just health care, as of 2023, employees felt more detached from their employers, with less clear job expectations and lower levels of satisfaction with their organization (Harter, 2024). Nurses quietly quit their jobs more frequently than other healthcare workers (Galanis et al., 2024). As a collective of nurses, the authors of this casebook felt called to action to share our experiences and support with you, the reader, as you prepare to begin your nursing career. Most people would agree that the nursing school experience does not allow students to limit their work effort without dramatically impacting their performance and progression in the program. You are entering the profession with the preparation and enthusiasm that our healthcare system needs for change.

Empowering the New Nurse as a Leader

Closely connected with the caring process in nursing, empathy is a clinical indicator of high-quality nursing care characterized by nurses' ability to understand their patients' feelings, experiences, and psychosocial ability (Wu, 2021). Empathy toward coworkers contributes to positive relationships and workplace organizational cultures (Brower, 2021). Individuals who work in helping professions that tend to share in the positive emotions of others, such as with positive empathy, were associated with having lower levels of burnout (Stosic et al., 2022). Establishing empathy toward patients and colleagues as a social norm in the interdisciplinary workplace sounds like a great idea to support a positive work environment. However, a complex tapestry of personal and professional factors can influence how we show up to work each day.

Through a phenomenon known as *emotional contagion*, employees continuously spread their moods and receive and are influenced by others' moods, which can happen when people are physically together but can also be spread through social media and email (Barsade, 2022). Unlike fields outside of helping professions, nurses cannot take a break from their work and put off what is stressing them for another day when they feel better equipped to address the problem. This casebook will discuss strategies for nurses to promote their workplace well-being and career commitment and lower their susceptibility to negative emotional contagion (Liu et al., 2021).

Chances are that before this moment, you have had the opportunity to develop some leadership skills at school, at work, or in your community. In nursing, you will demonstrate leadership by promoting quality nursing care, inspiring your team to accept innovation and transformation action, and positively influencing your work environment (Menezes et al., 2023). This casebook is centered on supporting your development as you progress toward your role as a professional nurse and leader. Our dedicated team of nurse authors has contributed to writing this book to create an environment of support for you as you prepare and enter practice.

This book is formatted as a casebook, an educational tool designed to provide real-life examples of implementing strategies to improve the quality of care and professional experiences of nurses (Anderson & Gagliardi, 2021). Chapters 2 through 12 begin with a composite story written by a newer nurse about an encounter they faced with fewer than two years of nursing experience. These brave nurses share an experience that challenged them or their peers. To illustrate the complexities of the case, the details in the story are fictionalized to enhance the case narrative or to protect the identities of those involved. All characters, organizations, and other entities depicted in this work are fictitious. Any resemblance to real persons, living or dead, or actual events is purely coincidental. It must be highlighted how much these authors are committed to sharing their knowledge with you in this book. The authenticity and vulnerability they share with us through their writing is a testament to their passion for the future of nursing and how much they want to support you.

The second part of chapters 2 through 12 will be a response to the case by an experienced nurse leader whose passion for supporting you and your new nursing colleagues is palpable. After identifying the main issues in the case, the nurse leader will offer a reflection on the challenges the nurse bravely faced. Because they have had a variety of professional positions culminating in their current professional role, they will share wisdom and their unique vantage points to offer tactical advice should you ever face this type of challenge in the workplace. We share a passion for empowering the next generation of nurses by developing the leadership tools you will need as the foundation of your professional nursing career. The nurse leaders will describe tactical suggestions of what can be done if a nurse faces these challenges, works in a supportive organization, and—perhaps at times even more importantly—if they do not. The final part of each chapter will provide additional information on topics related to the theme of the chapter, as well as resources and activities that can help advance your professional development in each thematic area. The last chapter of this casebook is about what happens next. Whether you are reading this casebook as you are about to graduate from your nursing program or after your graduation as you start working in professional nursing practice, we hope that you feel the support of your colleagues in our nursing profession, as we will all serve as your coaches in this book. In this book, the term *coaching* refers to the "empowering partnership that is thought-provoking and creative in the process, inspiring individuals to maximize their personal and professional potential, with a positive performance outcome, that is time-limited and focused on specific areas of development through action-oriented goals" (Richardson et al., 2023, p. 6636). Leadership coaching has been noted to have positive outcomes for nurses (Menezes et al., 2023).

Framework: Theory of Marginalization and Mattering

Because we have written this book with you in mind and with an appreciation of this particularly challenging moment in nursing practice, we mindfully selected the *Theory of Marginalization and Mattering* (Schlossberg, 1989) as the theoretical implementation framework for this book. You may recall the term *theoretical framework* from your research and evidence-based practice class. A theoretical framework is a foundation from which all knowledge is constructed and is typically used to ground the design of a research study (Grant & Osanloo, 2016). The term *theoretical implementation framework* is meant to be used prospectively to guide nurse leaders through the implementation process of a change in complex environments in such a way that might enhance implementation success (Barnden et al., 2023).

Can New Nurses Be Marginalized?

Marginalized means "casting aside of groups that are considered 'other' within society" (Pratt & Fowler, 2022, para. 2). In contrast, *mattering* is the opposite, or "the feeling that people are important in the world and make a difference in the lives of others" (Mohamed et al., 2022). Schlossberg (1989) described the theory of mattering and marginalization in relationship to the experiences of college students. In this case, marginality can be a temporary condition, such as how a first-year student feels when they first set foot on campus versus how they feel when fully integrated into the community and about to complete their program.

While much attention thoroughly scholarly activities should be paid to groups of nursing students who experience marginalization, such as nontraditional students (Englund, 2019), male students in a female-dominated profession (Englund et al., 2023; Sedgwick & Kellett, 2015; Taylor et al., 2022), and underrepresented groups (Englund & Basler, 2020; Englund & Lancaster, 2022; Lancaster & Englund, 2022), for this casebook, we will consider the aggregate of new nurses and their experiences with mattering and marginalization. We must note that we strongly believe in creating a nursing workforce that advances equity, diversity, and inclusivity and works intentionally to dismantle racism, build a diverse workforce, and promote inclusive patient care (American Nurses Association, 2018). This casebook's stories, strategies, and resources have been selected with that goal in mind.

The idea that new nurses experience marginalization is not new. Duchscher and Cowin (2004) described the new nursing nurse as a "marginalized person" (p. 290), and more than 20 years later, the idea still resonates with the experience. When nursing students graduate, they are no longer part of the academic institution where they studied to become nurses. However, they may perceive a lack of acceptance by their new professional colleagues—the feeling of not belonging anywhere and finding themselves at the intersection between two cultures. The new nurse:

> may experience inherent value discrepancies between the academic environment where they were raised and the industry into which they are being initiated. At the same time, these nursing professionals are being recruited into practice areas where unprecedented workload expectations commonly occur in work environments with critically high stress levels. (Duchscher & Cowin, 2004, p. 290)

There are many ways in which marginalization and the idea that one does not matter can be conveyed. Flett (2018) describes this through actions, such as treating people in an impersonal way, not remembering someone when they should be acknowledged, or talking over another person. If they are experienced in the workplace, these negative behaviors can significantly affect how a nurse feels about their role and job. Because of the complexities of the modern nursing work environment, it is possible to feel *intradisciplinary marginalization* (among nurses) and *interdisciplinary marginalization* (among the other disciplines that nursing works with).

Marginalization of nurses has also been explored among those who experience moral distress in response to caring for people in challenging situations (Fourie & Campelia, 2024).

Moral distress often occurs with a moral failure in patient care and can be associated with institutional constraints, such as cost-cutting measures, understaffing, and power imbalances among team members. If it is determined that the actions taken by the patient care team are indeed morally justifiable, it is also possible that the nurse has been marginalized. Nurses who spend many hours with patients and their families may unintentionally be excluded from critical conversations with the care team and family members, making them feel marginalized. Those who work during the off shift or are too busy with patient care to attend long discussions about the best course of action for their patients may feel disregarded (Fourie & Campelia, 2024). The nurse's voice is central to these conversations due to our capacity as "knowers" (Morley et al., 2022, p. 1315).

New Nurses: People Who Matter

Rosenberg and McCullough (1981) introduced the concept of mattering as being a person's need to feel that they are significant to others, and, over time, the definition evolved to include seven components that include the following: *attention, importance, dependence, ego extension, noted absence, appreciation, and individuation* (Flett, 2018). Consider each of these components and an example related to nursing practice. *Attention* is a person's feeling when others notice them and their actions (Flett, 2018). An example is when a nurse receives feedback from their manager that a patient identified them in a patient satisfaction survey and described the nurse's positive impact on their patient care experience. *Importance* is the feeling of being significant and cared for by others (Flett, 2018). When coworkers text a new nurse who calls out sick from work for several days to check how he is feeling, the nurse who is ill may feel important.

Dependence is the feeling of importance as others count on you (Flett, 2018). It is an example of dependence if a nurse comes in for overtime to cover a staffing need because they know that their coworkers have been working short and would appreciate their help. *Ego extension* happens when an individual sees another person emotionally invested in you (Flett, 2018). This might be a nurse who shares with a coworker that they are happy when they see their name on the schedule as working a shift together and know that no matter what happens at work, they will have a great day and get through it together.

Noted absence is when an individual is missed by another (Flett, 2018). At work, a patient comes in for their weekly infusion and asks if their favorite nurse is working today when they do not see them at their regular location. When the nurse returns to work, a coworker tells the nurse that the patient has been in and asked for them. *Appreciation* is the feeling that you and your actions are valued and matter to someone else (Flett, 2018). An example that might contribute to this feeling might be receiving a thank-you text from the nurse manager who sees that the nurse stayed late to help her coworkers with two admissions who arrived on the floor at shift change. Finally, *individuation* is made to feel special based on how someone regards you (Flett, 2018). Perhaps a nurse is working on their birthday, and their coworkers all sign a card with thoughtful messages sharing their positive feelings about that individual that may not have been shared. Considering these components of mattering and the examples provided, they all contribute to a positive work environment and a place where you might like to work.

Mattering Is a Psychological Need

Feeling that you matter in life is a psychological need that includes feeling valued and that you add value (Prilleltensky, 2020). People who feel like they matter have higher levels of self-compassion, relationship satisfaction, and a greater belief in their ability to achieve their goals (Flett, 2022). The idea of mattering as it relates to how one sees one's value is seldom mentioned in textbooks. While there are many possible reasons that this construct has received limited attention in scholarly literature, it is essential for human flourishing (Cornwall, 2023). Think about a time when you showed up for others, and your talents were vital to the positive outcome of the situation. It could be when you scored the winning point in the state championship soccer game. Or it could have been when you drove by a friend with a flat tire and stopped to help them. Sometimes we have these moments of mattering when we least expect them.

Christina had just graduated from her nursing program and was waiting to take her National Council Licensure Examination for Registered Nurses (NCLEX-RN). Frustrated that her school did not send her transcript to the state for processing until the end of the month, Christina had to select an NCLEX-RN date a few weeks later than she had hoped. For two months, she studied during the day and worked as a waitress at a casual dining restaurant in the evening. Christina had worked at the restaurant since she was a senior in high school and could not wait to move on and start her nursing career. She felt that every minute she spent working at the restaurant wasted her time. One of Christina's coworkers called her to another restaurant section on the night of her last waitressing shift. A customer was choking on a chicken bone, hands clutched to the throat, and was starting to have circumoral cyanosis. After asking the customer if he was choking, Christina swiftly ran behind, wrapping her arms around his abdomen. *One, two, three, four, and five* inward and upward thrusts, and the bone came up. His airway was now clear. His color improved. His wife was in tears and hugged Christina, saying, *"You saved my husband's life. I could have lost him if it was not for you. How do I even begin to thank you?"* It was at that moment that Christina realized that **she mattered**.

Considering things from a new perspective and, in this casebook, exploring challenges as told by nurses who are only a few steps ahead of you will bring to light real-world challenges encountered by our newest generation of bedside leaders. We will be sharing stories and experiences that can help you develop new strategies to bring to practice. The insight and reflection of nurse leaders committed to supporting you as a coach in this casebook will help you think of things differently and empower you with new tools to add to your personal and professional nursing toolkit.

Nursing Curricula Designed to Support Your Leadership Development

Tremendous thought and care have ensured that prelicensure nursing curricula are responsive to preparing the next generation of nurses for this complex healthcare setting. Assembling a task force of academic and clinical leaders, the AACN, responsible for establishing quality standards in nursing education and influencing the nursing profession to improve health care, has reimagined nursing education. In its publication *The Essentials: Core Competencies for Nursing Education* (AACN, 2021), 10 domains (content areas) and competencies (knowledge, attitudes, motivations, self-perceptions, and skills) that nursing students should demonstrate upon completion of a nursing program that prepares them to take the NCLEX (AACN, n.d.). The domains include the following: Domain 1: Knowledge for Nursing Practice; Domain 2: Person-Centered Care; Domain 3: Population Health; Domain 4: Scholarship for Nursing Discipline; Domain 5: Quality and Safety; Domain 6:

Interprofessional Partnerships; Domain 7: Systems-Based Practice; Domain 8: Informatics and Healthcare Technologies; Domain 9: Professionalism; and Domain 10: Personal, Professional, and Leadership Development (AACN, 2021, pp. 10–11).

While elements of many of these domains will be threaded in the voices, stories, and insights shared in this book, the primary focus of this casebook is on Domain 2: Person-Centered Care and Domain 10: Personal, Professional, and Leadership Development. At the core of nursing's values, Domain 2 focuses on the "individual within multiple contexts to ensure person-centered care that is holistic, individualized, just, respectful, compassionate, coordinated, evidence-based, and developmentally appropriate" (AACN, 2021, p. 10). Our focus on Domain 2 in this casebook provides examples and strategies to engage and communicate with individuals to create a caring relationship (AACN, 2021, p. 32). This includes your patients, their families, and support persons as well as your colleagues.

Domain 10 focuses on the development of the individual, nurse, and nurse leader through "participation in activities and self-reflection that foster personal health, resilience, and well-being; contribute to lifelong learning; and support the acquisition of nursing expertise and the asser-tion of leadership" (AACN, 2021, pp. 10–11). There are three specific competencies, or professional expectations, that are related to entry-level nurses regarding the concepts of Domain 10: Personal, Professional, and Leadership Development. They include the following: Demonstrate a commitment to personal health and well-being, nurture a spirit of inquiry that fosters flexibility and professional maturity, and develop leadership capacity (AACN, 2021, p. 54). Throughout your nursing career, you will grow deeper in your knowledge and experience in these and many other areas of practice. So much of your nursing education has been focused on helping you develop the knowledge, skills, and attitudes necessary for patient care. It is now time to focus on your personal, professional, and leadership development (AACN, 2021). Throughout each chapter, we will provide resources and activities to help advance your development as a person, nurse, and leader.

Engage With the Individual in Establishing a Caring Relationship (AACN, 2021)

Nurses care for patients and their families through empathy, compassion, and mutual respect. While this is at the heart of nursing practice and does not need to be said loudly as a competency for the entry-level (new) nurse, many challenges must be considered. I like to think that I always bring these to my professional nursing practice, but through reflection, I know that can be off-balanced and negatively affect me.

As a pediatric nurse, not all my caring relationships can be based on mutual respect, as some of my patients do not have the capacity due to their developmental age. I cannot hold them responsible for something they are incapable of doing. I keep this same viewpoint in mind when I care for others who do not have the capacity at the moment of my care to show me mutual respect, such as those who are under the influence of drugs and other substances as well as those experiencing a psychiatric emergency. This is not to say that I allow these individuals to emotionally or physically harm me. However, I know that at the moment of our encounter, due to their situation, they cannot show me the level of respect that I would typically expect from a patient or family member. As someone who feels deeply, I have had to work hard to develop strategies for caring in these situations focused on empathy, compassion, and respect for the patient and myself as a professional nurse. These interactions can weigh heavily on nurses; we will discuss them more in upcoming chapters. Sometimes, as nurses, we care too deeply and have negative responses to our role as caregivers that carry over into our personal lives. While much attention has been paid in the scientific literature to describing nurses experiences with compassion satisfaction (the positive reactions to caring) and compassion fatigue (the negative responses to caring), made up of burnout and secondary traumatic stress (Stamm, 2010), not as much of the tactical strategies to mitigate the negative responses to caring reaches those who need it the most. We will try to share some ideas with you throughout this book to help you reach this goal.

Communicate Effectively With Individuals (AACN, 2021)

The average adult says about 16,000 words daily (Curcic, 2023), but that does not guarantee that they communicate effectively. As a nurse, it is vital to demonstrate emotional intelligence and respect when communicating with patients, families, and colleagues. While many of you have navigated the challenges of exchanging ideas with a patient using an interpreter to communicate with a patient who does not speak English, there is so much more to our communication, including our tone, nonverbal communication, and ability to listen to others (Emerson, 2021). We are not expected to be experts in every cultural tradition but rather to develop a sense of cultural humility, a process of self-reflection where individuals gain a more profound respect for cultural differences, reflection, openness to establishing power-balanced relationships, and appreciation of another's community expertise on the social and cultural context of their lived experience (Lekas, Pahl, & Fuller Lewis, 2020).

Commitment to Personal Health and Well-Being (AACN, 2021)

To be a team player and be there for everyone else who depends on you, you need to start by showing up for yourself (Horowitz, 2020). Nursing is a demanding job requiring you to care for others, often meaning you put others' needs over your own. Consider the following example. Due to an unforeseen circumstance with your patients, you realize that you have not had a sip of water several hours into your shift and now missed your lunch break. At the same time, you feel the frequent vibration of your cell phone in your pocket as family members are texting you with an update about a sick family member, which you are too busy to check. Worried about your family member and the stresses of your personal life, you did not sleep well last night. Already overwhelmed and exhausted, your charge nurse now comes to you to tell you that you will be getting an admission. You are too upset to have a response, so you storm away and run to the nurses' station to catch up on charting before your admission arrives on the floor. Big tears stream down your cheeks, and you pull your facemask over your nose and mouth, hoping that no one will notice.

Nurses are excellent at identifying and meeting their patients' physical and mental health needs but may not be as good at applying the same skills to themselves (Croston & Rutter, 2023). While it may seem as if there is no alternative to the situation, the negative impacts are significant for those who do not exercise regular self-care to promote their wellness. It is important to remember that our work as nurses is remarkable in every way. In our day-to-day work as nurses, we commonly witness the extremes of human lived experience, substantially more so than the average person may see throughout their lifetime (Roney & Acri, 2018). Challenges in our personal and professional lives may force us to cope by functioning in "survival mode." This involves going through the motions of life to do what is necessary (Turmaud, 2020). People are sometimes led to function in survival mode when they are forced to cope with difficult personal frustrations and system failures (Grissinger, 2017). While traumatic experiences can bring on survival mode, they can also creep into a nurse's life through high levels of constant stress (Meehan, n.d.). Prolonged periods of living in survival mode can trigger unhealthy coping and declines in mental health (Marson, 2022).

Special efforts must be incorporated into our daily routines and rituals to mitigate the adverse effects of this hard work. Unfortunately, *self-care* has recently received backlash as some negative stereotypes are associated with the word that conjures images of indulgent or selfish behavior (Boyes, 2020). The demands of your personal and professional life may make it seem as if it is impossible to integrate any self-care into your day; we will reexamine this concept as it may look differently than you may have previously thought. Self-care is about setting priorities, setting boundaries, and finding purpose (Parker-Pope, 2021). With all that you may have going on in your life, you may feel like a decision to make a significant shift to prioritize behaviors that promote wellness in your life is overwhelming. Throughout this book, we will share many examples of tiny steps that you can take toward these goals. Your life is not one major decision but millions of small ones (Clear, 2018).

Nurture a Spirit of Inquiry That Fosters Flexibility and Professional Maturity (AACN, 2021)

Julia was a nursing student ready to graduate from her prelicensure program in May 2020. She went to nursing school with the dream of becoming an oncology nurse. In February 2020, Julia was thrilled when she was offered an RN position after graduation on her first-choice unit at a hospital close to her home. During the first week of March 2020, she and several friends from school went away for spring break. At the end of their trip, they received an email from the university that classes would pivot to remote instruction through the end of March, when students and faculty would return to campus to resume traditional modalities. As the COVID-19 pandemic accelerated in virulence and spread, Julia's school and others across the country did not resume in-person instruction for the rest of the spring 2020 semester. Not only were clinical hours and classroom instruction virtual, but so were celebrations, such as pinning and graduation. While she was disappointed that the end of her nursing school experience was not as she had imagined, Julia kept a positive attitude as she studied for and successfully passed the NCLEX-RN.

Julia was excited about something finally going as planned when she arrived for her first day of hospital orientation in June 2020. During one of the breaks, one of the nursing education staff asked her to be open-minded and flexible as they gave her some news: She would not be starting on the oncology unit, but rather, at least for the foreseeable future, she would be part of the resource pool of nurses deployed to take care of COVID-19 patients throughout the hospital. Donning a gown, gloves, goggles, a face shield, an N95 mask, and double masks over the N95, Julia had an abbreviated orientation, and each shift went from unit to unit to wherever the greatest staffing need was. Under all the personal protective equipment, most of her new coworkers had no idea that she was a new graduate. Julia was very disappointed to have a delay in starting her career in oncology nursing. Still, she knew that her community needed her to be flexible and resilient and display professional maturity during this global pandemic.

We cannot prepare for every possible event that could affect our nursing practice. However, adapting well to significant stressors, also known as *resilience*, has been consistently linked to cognitive flexibility, or the ability to adjust behavior to changing situation demands (Rademacher et al., 2023). Strategies to enhance our skills in this area exist, and we will discuss them later in this book.

We often think about our days and experiences, where we analyze information and arrive at conclusions that are different from reflection, yet the deliberate introspective process of self-evaluation that helps us gain a deeper understanding of ourselves (Manaher, 2023). Seeking, reflecting on, and integrating feedback to improve performance is essential for the new nurse (AACN, 2021). Together, in this casebook, we will explore and practice strategies to develop these critical skills in your nursing toolkit. Developing a strategic network of colleagues, role models, and mentors can help support your professional development (American Management Association, n.d.). It might sound like activities that a business professional would engage in rather than a nurse. By the end of this casebook, you will appreciate how vital this is to your professional growth. We will also discuss how openness to change through ongoing learning is critical to your personal and professional satisfaction.

Capacity for Leadership (AACN, 2021)

Through the tapestry of stories and reflections from the nurse authors of this casebook, you will become better acquainted with examples and styles of leadership behaviors in the professional work environment. The first two competencies, commitment to personal health and well-being and a spirit of inquiry that fosters flexibility and professional maturity (AACN, 2021), are the foundation that we build our capacity as nursing leaders. As you read the stories and reflections introducing each chapter, you can identify which attributes resonate with you and which feel less familiar as you formulate your leadership style (AACN, 2021). As mentioned earlier, we strongly believe in creating a nursing workforce that advances equity, diversity, and inclusivity and works intentionally to dismantle racism, build a diverse workforce, and promote inclusive patient care (ANA, 2018). The stories, strategies, and resources shared within this casebook have been selected with that goal as we all strive to become more self-aware of our implicit biases and how they affect our role as people, nurses, and leaders.

Later in this casebook, we will discuss Team Strategies and Tools to Enhance Performance and Patient Safety (TeamSTEPPS®), the evidence-based tools that healthcare teams can use to improve communication and teamwork (American Hospital Association, 2019). TeamSTEPPS 3.0 was developed by experts in teamwork and team training, including patients, families, and caregivers, to impact how to clearly communicate with all types of teams in stressful situations (Agency for Healthcare Research and Quality, 2024). You may have received part of this training as part of your prelicensure education, or you may have received this training from your employer.

YOU MATTER: EMPOWERING YOUR NURSING CAREER

We are excited to inspire you to maximize your personal and professional potential as a nurse leader. We wrote this book for you. Are you ready to join us? Let's go!

Book Club Questions

1. How do you define the word *leader*? Who are some examples of leaders you admire? What qualities do they have that you value?
2. What concerns you the most about the current healthcare climate as you start your nursing practice?
3. Have you ever felt marginalized? When do you feel like you matter?
4. What self-care practices do you incorporate into your daily routine? Is there anything you wish you could add?

References

Agency for Healthcare Research and Quality. (2024). *TeamSTEPPS 3.0 welcome guides.* https://www.ahrq.gov/teamstepps-program/welcome-guides/index.html

American Association of Colleges of Nursing. (n.d.). *What is competency-based education?* https://www.aacnnursing.org/essentials/tool-kit/competency-based-education

American Association of Colleges of Nursing. (2021). *The essentials: Core competencies for professional nursing education.* https://www.aacnnursing.org/Portals/0/PDFs/Publications/Essentials-2021.pdf

American Association of International Healthcare Recruitment. (2023, January 19). *Nurse survey results: Staffing crisis worse than ever.* http://www.aaihr.org/2023-national-nurse-survey-results/

American Hospital Association. (2019, February). TeamSTEPPS. Understanding Team STEPPS. https://www.aha.org/system/files/2019-02/TeamSTEPPS_guide_final.pdf

American Management Association. (n.d.). *Create a plan to develop your strategic network.* https://www.amanet.org/assets/1/6/2565.pdf

American Nurses Association. (2018). *ANA position statement: The nurse's role in addressing discrimination: Protecting and promoting inclusive strategies in practice settings, policy, and advocacy.* https://ojin.nursingworld.org/table-of-contents/volume-24-2019/number-3-september-2019/nurses-role-in-addressing-discrimination/

Anderson, N. N., & Gagliardi, A. R. (2021). Development, characteristics, and impact of quality improvement casebooks: A scoping review. *Health Research Policy and Systems, 19*(1), 123. https://doi.org/10.1186/s12961-021-00777-z

Avraham, R., Wacht, O., Yaffe, E., & Grinstein-Cohen, O. (2023). Choosing a nursing career during a global health event: A repeated cross-sectional study. *Nurse Educator, 48*(4), E116–E121. https://doi.org/10.1097/NNE.0000000000001392

Barnden, R., Snowdon, D. A., Lannin, N. A., Lynch, E., Srikanth, V., & Andrew, N. E. (2023). Prospective application of theoretical implementation frameworks to improve health care in hospitals a systematic review. *BMC Health Services Research, 23*(1), 607. https://doi.org/10.1186/s12913-023-09609-y

Barsade, S. (2022, February 21). *Leadership influence: Controlling emotional contagion.* Wharton @ Work Nano Tools for Leadership. https://executiveeducation.wharton.upenn.edu/thought-leadership/wharton-at-work/2022/03/controlling-emotional-contagion/

Berwick, D., & Williams, M. (2023, May 24). Hospitals need to focus on social drivers of American health. *TIME*. https://time.com/6281957/american-health-care-is-broken-major-hospitals-solution/

Boyes, A. (2020, January 20). *5 things people get wrong about self-care*. Psychology Today. https://www.psychologytoday.com/us/blog/in-practice/202001/5-things-people-get-wrong-about-self-care

Brenan, M., & Jones, J. (2024, January 25). *Ethics ratings of nearly all professions down in U.S. Gallup.com.* https://news.gallup.com/poll/608903/ethics-ratings-nearly-professions-down.aspx

Brower, T. (2024, June 3). Empathy is the most important leadership skill according to research. Forbes. https://www.forbes.com/sites/tracybrower/2021/09/19/empathy-is-the-most-important-leadership-skill-according-to-research/

Buerhaus, P., Staiger, D., Auerbach, D., Yates, M., & Donelan, K. (2022, January). Nurse employment during the first fifteen months of the COVID-19 pandemic. *Health Affairs, 41*(1). https://doi.org/10.1377/hlthaff.2021.01289

Clear, J. (2018). *Atomic habits: Tiny changes, remarkable results: An easy and proven way to build good habits and break bad ones.* Avery.

Commonwealth Fund. (2023, January 31). *U.S. health care from a global perspective, 2022: Accelerating spending, worsening outcomes.* https://www.commonwealthfund.org/publications/issuebriefs/2023/jan/us-health-care-global-perspective-2022

Cornwall, G. (2023, September 27). Want to believe in yourself? "mattering" is key. *The New York Times.* https://www.nytimes.com/2023/09/27/well/mind/mental-health-mattering-self-esteem.html

Croston, M., & Rutter, S. (2023). Becoming an inner ally: The compassionate minds approach to self-compassion—An online programme. *British Journal of Nursing, 32*(1), S20–S23. https://doi.org/10.12968/bjon.2023.32.1.S20

Curcic, D. (2023). *How many words does the average person say a day?* Words Rated. https://wordsrated.com/how-many-words-does-the-average-person-say-a-day/

Duchscher, J., & Cowin, L. (2004). The experience of marginalization in new nursing graduates. *Nursing Outlook, 52*(6), 289–296.

Ellis, L., & Yang, A. (2022, August 12). *If your co-workers are 'quiet quitting,' here's what that means. The Wall Street Journal.* https://www.wsj.com/articles/if-your-gen-z-co-workers-are-quiet-quitting-heres-what-that-means-11660260608

Emerson, M. S. (2021). *8 ways you can improve your communication skills.* Harvard Division of Continuing Education. https://professional.dce.harvard.edu/blog/8-ways-you-can-improve-your-communication-skills/

Englund, H. M. (2019). Nontraditional students' perceptions of marginalization in baccalaureate nursing education: Pushed to the periphery. *Nurse Educator, 44*(3), 164–169. https://doi.org/10.1097/nne.0000000000000581

Englund, H., & Basler, J. (2020). Life at the margins: Marginality and race in undergraduate students and faculty. *Western Journal of Nursing Research, 42*(6), 415–422. https://doi.org/10.1177/0193945919865737

Englund, H. M., & Lancaster, R. J. (2022). Differences in marginality between nursing students with and without disabilities. *Journal of Nursing Education, 61*(8), 429–438. https://doi.org/10.3928/01484834-20220602-03

Englund, H. M., Mott, J., & MacWilliams, B. (2023). Experiences of undergraduate male students in nursing: On the outside looking in. *Nurse Educator, 49*(2), 61–66.

Fleming, W. J. (2023). Employee well-being outcomes from individual-level mental health interventions: Cross-sectional evidence from the United Kingdom. *Industrial Relations Journal, 55*(2), 162–182. https://doi.org/10.1111/irj.12418

Flett, G. L. (2018). *The psychology of mattering: Understanding the human need to be significant.* Elsevier Academic Press.

Flett, G. L. (2022). An introduction, review, and conceptual analysis of mattering as an essential construct and an essential way of life. *Journal of Psychoeducational Assessment, 40*(1), 3–36. https://doi.org/10.1177/07342829211057640

Fourie, C., & Campelia, G. (2024). Moral distress and the marginalization of nurses. *American Journal of Bioethics, 24*(1), 132–134. https://doi.org/10.1080/15265161.2023.2278555

Fox, K. E., Johnson, S. T., Berkman, L. F., Sianoja, M., Soh, Y., Kubzansky, L. D., & Kelly, E. L. (2022). Organisational- and group-level workplace interventions and their effect on multiple domains of worker well-being: A systematic review. *Work & Stress, 36*(1), 30–59.

Galanis, P., Katsiroumpa, A., Vraka, I., Siskou, O., Konstantakopoulou, O., Katsoulas, T., Moisoglou, I., Gallos, P., & Kaitelidou, D. (2024). Nurses quietly quit their jobs more often than other healthcare workers: An alarming issue for healthcare services. *International Nursing Review, 71*(4), 850–859. https://doi.org/10.1111/inr.12931

Grant, C., & Osanloo, A. F. (2016). Understanding, selecting, and integrating a theoretical framework in dissertation research: Creating the blueprint for your 'house.' *Administrative Issues Journal, 4*, 12–26.

Grissinger, M. (2017). Disrespectful behavior in health care: Its impact, why it arises and persists, and how to address it—Part 2. *Pharmacy and Therapeutics, 42*(2), 74–75, 77.

Haegdorens, F., Van Bogaert, P., De Meester, K., & Monsieurs, K. G. (2019). The impact of nurse staffing levels and nurses' education on patient mortality in medical and surgical wards: An observational multicentre study. *BMC Health Services Research, 19*(1), 864. https://doi.org/10.1186/s12913-019-4688-7

Harter, J. (2024, January 23). *In new workplace, U.S. employee engagement stagnates.* Gallup.com. https://www.gallup.com/workplace/608675/new-workplace-employee-engagement-stagnates.aspx

Horowitz, D. (2020, June 9). *Council post: Leaders: Put your own oxygen mask on first. Forbes.* https://www.forbes.com/sites/forbescoachescouncil/2020/06/09/leaders-put-your-own-oxygen-mask-on-first/?sh=5fa641fc77ad

Institute of Medicine. (2011). *The future of nursing: Leading change, advancing health.* National Academies Press.

Krueger, A. (2022, August 23). *Who is quiet quitting for? For those not ready to make a grand exit, a softer approach may work. The New York Times.* https://www.nytimes.com/2022/08/23/style/quiet-quitting-tiktok.html

Lancaster, R. J., & Englund, H. (2022). Perceived marginality in veteran and nonveteran nursing students in baccalaureate programs. *Nursing Forum, 57*(2), 219–224. https://doi.org/10.1111/nuf.12666

Lekas, H. M., Pahl, K., & Fuller Lewis, C. (2020). Rethinking Cultural Competence: Shifting to Cultural Humility. Health services insights, 13, 1178632920970580. https://doi.org/10.1177/1178632920970580

Lovejoy, M., Kelly, E., Kubzansky, L. D., & Berkman, L. F. (2021). Work redesign for the 21st century: Promising strategies for enhancing worker well-being. *American Journal of Public Health, 111*(10), 1787–1795.

Liu, B., Zhu, N., Wang, H., Li, F., & Men, C. (2021). Protecting nurses from mistreatment by patients: A cross-sectional study on the roles of emotional contagion susceptibility and emotional regulation ability. *International Journal of Environmental Research and Public Health, 18*(12), 6331. https://doi.org/10.3390/ijerph18126331

Manaher, S. (2023, August 10). *Thought vs reflection: Differences and uses for each one.* The Content Authority. https://thecontentauthority.com/blog/thought-vs-reflection

Marson, G. (2022, April 19). *The negative impact of prolonged survival mode: What can you do to thrive?* https://drgiamarson.com/the-negative-impact-of-prolonged-survival-mode-what-can-you-do-to-thrive/

Meehan, J. (n.d.). *Coping skills to overcome survival mode.* Restorative Counseling. https://rcchicago.org/coping-skills-to-overcome-survival-mode/

Menezes, H., Bernardes, A., Amestoy, S., Cunha, I., Cardoso, M., & Balsanelli, A. P. (2023). Relationship between leadership coaching and nurses' resilience in hospital environments. *Revista da Escola de Enfermagem da U S P, 56*, e20220265. https://doi.org/10.1590/1980-220X-REEUSP-2022-0265en

Mohamed, S. A., Hendy, A., Mahmoud, O. E., & Mohamed, S. M. (2022). Mattering perception, work engagement and its relation to burnout amongst nurses during coronavirus outbreak. *Nursing Open, 9*(1), 377–384. https://doi.org/10.1002/nop2.1075

Morley, G., Bradbury-Jones, C., & Ives, J. (2022). The moral distress model: An empirically informed guide for moral distress interventions. *Journal of Clinical Nursing, 31*(9–10), 1309–1326. https://doi.org/10.1111/jocn.15988

National Institute for Health and Care Excellence. (2022). *Mental well-being at work.* NICE Guideline (NG212). https://www.nice.org.uk/guidance/ng212/chapter/Recommendations

Occupational Safety and Health Administration. (n.d.). *About OSHA.* https://www.osha.gov/aboutosha.

Parker-Pope, T. (2021, January 6). *Why self-care isn't selfish. The New York Times.* https://www.nytimes.com/2021/01/06/well/live/why-self-care-isnt-selfish.html

Pfeffer, J. (2018). *Dying for a paycheck: How modern management harms employee health and company performance—and what we can do about it.* HarperCollins Publishers.

Pratt, A., & Fowler, T. (2022, June). *Deconstructing bias: Marginalization—NICHD connection—science@nichd.* Eunice Kennedy Shriver National Institute of Child Health and Human Development. https://science.nichd.nih.gov/confluence/pages/viewpage.action? pageId=242975243

Prilleltensky, I. (2020). Mattering at the intersection of psychology, philosophy, and politics. *American Journal of Community Psychology, 65*(1–2), 16–34. https://doi.org/10.1002/ajcp.12368

Quinn, B. (2020). Using Benner's model of clinical competency to promote nursing leadership. *Nursing Management, 27*(2), 33–41. https://doi.org/10.7748/nm.2020.e1911

Rademacher, L., Kraft, D., Eckart, C., & Fiebach, C. J. (2023). Individual differences in resilience to stress are associated with affective flexibility. *Psychological Research, 87*(6), 1862–1879. https://doi.org/10.1007/s00426-022-01779-4

Richardson, C., Wicking, K., Biedermann, N., & Langtree, T. (2023). Coaching in nursing: An integrative literature review. *Nursing Open, 10*(10), 6635–6649. https://doi.org/10.1002/nop2.1925

Roney, L., & Acri, M. (2018). The cost of caring: An exploration of compassion fatigue, compassion satisfaction and job satisfaction in pediatric nurses. *Journal of Pediatric Nursing, 70,* 74–80. https://doi.org/10.1016/j.pedn.2018.01.016

Schlossberg, N. K. (1989). Marginality and mattering: Key issues in building community. *New Directions for Student Services, 48,* 5–15. https://doi.org/10.1002/ss.37119894803

Sedgwick, M. G. & Kellett, P. (2015). Exploring masculinity and marginalization of male undergraduate nursing students' experience of belonging during clinical experiences. *Journal of Nursing Education, 54*(3), 121–129.

Shah, M. K., Gandrakota, N., Cimiotti, J. P., Ghose, N., Moore, M., & Ali, M. K. (2021). Prevalence of and factors associated with nurse burnout in the US. *JAMA Network Open, 4*(2), e2036469. https://doi.org/10.1001/jamanetworkopen.2020.36469

Smiley, R. A., Allgeyer, R. L., Shobo, Y., Lyons, K.- C., Letourneau, R., Zhong, E., Kaminski-Ozturk, N., & Alexander, M. (2023). The 2022 national nursing workforce survey. *Journal of Nursing Regulation, 14*(1), Supplement (S1–S90).

Stamm, B. H. (2010). The concise ProQOL manual. Pocatello, ID: ProQOL.org; Retrieved from http://ProQOL.org/uploads/ProQOL_Concise_2ndEd_12-2010.pdf

Stosic, M. D., Blanch-Hartigan, D., Aleksanyan, T., Duenas, J., & Ruben, M. A. (2022). Empathy, friend or foe? Untangling the relationship between empathy and burnout in helping professions. *Journal of Social Psychology, 162*(1), 89–108. https://doi.org/10.1080/00224545.2021.1991259

Stubin, C. (2021). Igniting the leadership spark in nursing students: Leading the way. *International Journal of Nursing Education Scholarship, 18*(1), 20210087. https://doi.org/10.1515/ijnes-2021-0087

Taylor, J., Marland, G., Whitford, H., Carson, M., & Leece, R. (2022). Isolation and marginalization: Exploring attrition of men in preregistration nursing programs. *Journal of Nursing Education, 61*(4), 179–186. https://doi.org/10.3928/01484834-20220209-02

Terry, J. (2022, January 26). *Why is hospital care so complex, and what is being done about it? Newsweek.* https://www.newsweek.com/why-hospital-care-so-complex-what-being-done-about-it-1672213

Turmaud, D. (2020, June 30). *Why survival mode isn't the best way to live. Psychology Today.* https://www.psychologytoday.com/us/blog/lifting-the-veil-trauma/202006/why-survival-mode-isnt-the-best-way-live

Wu, Y. (2021). Empathy in nurse-patient interaction: a conversation analysis. *BMC Nursing, 20*(1), 18. https://doi.org/10.1186/s12912-021-00535-0

Zuzelo, P. R. (2023). Discouraging quiet quitting: Potential strategies for nurses. *Holistic Nursing Practice, 37*(3), 174–175. https://doi.org/10.1097/HNP.0000000000000583

CHAPTER 2

Your First Nursing Position

Moira Dougherty, BSN, RN, and Linda Roney, EdD, RN-BC, CPEN, CNE, FAAN

Learning Goals

1. Describe Moira's strengths and challenges in caring for a critically ill patient in the emergency department (ED) after resuscitation as a new-graduate nurse.
2. Value the role of the team in supporting Moira's care of the patient in the trauma bay and the other eight patients on her assignment.
3. Reflect on personal beliefs and attitudes that affect one's decision to pursue specialty nursing practice as a new-graduate nurse.
4. Design your approach to your job search using the seven steps of the New Nurse's Career Toolkit.

'You Could Hear a Pin Drop.'

By Moira Dougherty, BSN, RN

My first job out of nursing school was in an ED in New York City. While it is not a level-one trauma center, we saw our fair share of traumas due to the nature of New York City. As a new-graduate nurse choosing to work in such a fast-paced environment, I knew that there would be new challenges to face almost every, if not every, shift. I decided to work here due to my passion for emergency nursing, caring for individuals, and being part of the treatment team for individuals and their families during some of the most challenging times of their lives.

It was a day shift like any other in an ED. I promptly left my apartment at 6:40 a.m. to catch the bus to work—a warm October morning walk from the bus to the hospital. The streets were filled with the sounds of the city: car horns, whistles, and steam from the subway grates and commuters hustling to work. Entering the hospital through the ED doors, I could sense it was already busy, chaotic, and loud. On this particular day, I saw the charge nurse first and learned that we needed to be fully staffed.

Midway through my shift in the ED, I was already at eight patients, as were the rest of my coworkers. This was not an atypical day for us, as we only had enough staff to have five sections open in the main bay of the ED. Additionally, this day was one with high census and high acuity. This is something you learn to accept fast in an ED. An emergency medical services (EMS) crew who had transported a patient told us, "*We heard over the radio that there is a cardiac arrest in progress nearby; he jumped.*" The EMS radio looks like a walkie-talkie that each crew member carries on their person to audibly hear the calls that come in over dispatch. Each radio station covers a specific area, and certain EMS crews cover those designated areas to be able to respond to those calls.

Everyone in the near vicinity of hearing this news stopped what they were doing as we knew this patient would likely have no airway in place and be receiving bag-mask-valve ventilation. If they were nearby, this patient would arrive at our ED shortly. Due to the nature of a witnessed cardiac arrest, we knew this patient would not be pronounced dead on the scene. Additionally, if EMS "rules" do not allow for the placement of an advanced airway, such as a king tube or an endotracheal tube, the patient will be transported to the nearest hospital—not necessarily the appropriate designated trauma hospital. However, we all had to continue to our next task or assess the next patient until we knew that this patient was coming to us.

On this shift, I was assigned to be the fourth nurse in the round-robin rotation to receive a critical patient. I knew it was my turn if this patient was to be received by our ED. At our ED, before a critical patient arrives, EMS calls ahead on a special phone. This red phone hangs on the wall near the charge nurse's station, and it has the most distinct telephone ring, almost like the ring of an old rotary phone. It's one you can hear from almost anywhere in the ED. I heard the phone ring and instantly froze while the charge nurse took a brief report from the operator. I knew that this was going to be a critical patient, possibly and most likely the person in cardiac arrest. In addition, this would now be my ninth patient of the day. When I heard my coworker tell me that the prenotification we received was five minutes out from the hospital, an unknown man who had jumped into the East River of Manhattan and was in cardiac arrest. I knew we all had to prepare quickly.

As I could feel my heart racing, almost beating out of my chest, I assigned roles to my team members who arrived at the resuscitation bay, which went from an empty room to one filled with numerous nurses, doctors, pharmacists, and a respiratory therapist, ready to jump into action to save a life. Almost in unison, everyone donned yellow personal protective equipment gowns with goggles, shoe covers, and double gloves in preparation for the unknown. We all waited for what seemed the longest five minutes. The entire team stood in silence; I remember it like it was yesterday. You could hear a pin drop. The sounds of other monitors, intravenous (IV) pumps, and various other sounds were muffled while everyone was standing in their designated positions for the patient to arrive. Although this was not my first cardiac arrest patient as the primary nurse, this one felt different. I was nervous, unsure, and afraid of the patient's state. Would we even have a chance at the return of spontaneous circulation (ROSC), meaning the restart of a sustainable cardiac rhythm, given the situation? Who would be watching my other patients? Typically, the charge nurse or your other coworkers would carry out orders for your other patients while you handle your critical patient. However, due to the high census and high acuity, I did not know if this would be remotely possible on this day. How could I possibly keep up with my orders for my other patients? Would I continue to get more patients? How long would my coworkers be able to help me?

Upon arrival, the patient was receiving cardiopulmonary resuscitation (CPR) with the Lucas device (a machine that performs CPR) and only had one intraosseous (IO) needle placed. Providing only a singular venous access line for necessary medications, which unfortunately was lost on the way to our hospital. As chaotic as it felt, I knew I could trust my team members to support my patients and carry out their roles. Everyone worked rapidly to try to save this patient's life. The nurse whom I had delegated to secure vascular access and drill a new IO needle into the bone with a hollow needle used during emergencies then immediately gave epinephrine, which is the first line drug that we use for a patient in cardiac arrest. Two minutes later, at the next pulse check, the patient had a pulse. To everyone's shock, *we got the patient back!* As a nurse of less than one year, this was the first patient of mine ever to receive ROSC. A rush of emotions followed as I knew this patient was now my sole priority because the larger group would leave once this happened.

IV drip after IV drip was hung to keep this patient alive. This is followed by warming with the bear hugger (a noninvasive device that looks like a vacuum cleaner hose that forces warm air through disposable blankets), measuring and trending core temperature with a temperature probe foley (a special type of indwelling catheter often used on critically ill patients), and maintaining a mean arterial pressure of or equal to 65. There were countless other additional nursing orders and tasks, all at the top of my priorities. The intensive care unit (ICU) team was consulted and assessed and accepted my patient to their unit. The typical flow is for the patient to go upstairs shortly after it's been decided to accept them to the ICU. Yet, due to the high census in the ICU, I was told that "it could be a few hours" before they could take him upstairs.

I was terrified. I could feel my fight-or-flight response ramp up as the adrenalin circulated through my body. All my muscles were tense, and I remember feeling sweat roll down my back. All I wanted to be able to do was safely care for every one of my patients while making sure this patient did not code again. For the next three hours, not only was I tasked with what should be a one-to-one nurse-to-patient ratio, but I also had eight other patients to care for. At this time, I knew I could not leave this patient's room; therefore, I had to lean on my coworkers even though they all had the same number of patients, if not more than I did. I honestly do not know how they kept up with all my orders and tasks, but they did. That is one of the most beautiful things about nursing: No matter the task, no matter how short-staffed or up-staffed, if supportive coworkers surround you, they go to any lengths to support and help you and one another.

When I came home from work that evening, I opened my journal—something I had not done since my first months of nursing orientation. I was extremely moved by this nursing experience, not only from the standpoint of patient care but also because of the support of those with whom I work. I often go back and read that journal entry on bad and good days to remind myself of our impact as nurses—the impact on our patients, their families, and our coworkers. It is easy to forget this, and it's important to take the time to reflect on the important work that we do.

'I Took Only Some of My Advice ... and Almost Left Nursing.'

By Linda Roney, EdD, RN-BC, CNE, CPEN, FAAN

Reading Moira's story, I wonder, after having had many days like she shares with us throughout my career, how it is possible that we, as nurses, seamlessly transition from the intense adrenaline-rushing, never-done-before experiences of our professional life to our regular day-to-day personal lives? It is as if Moira is the main character in a superhero movie; somehow, she found superpowers that she did not know she had until she needed them the most in this situation. How do we (as nurses) do it? How did Moira do it this early in her ED nursing career? She is amazing, isn't she?

Even in this new challenge, Moira demonstrates aptitude in the American Association of Colleges of Nursing (AACN) essentials' (2021) domains 2 and 10 competencies and subcompetencies.

TABLE 2.1 Examples of Domain 2: Person-Centered Care and Domain 10: Personal, Professional, and Leadership Development in This Exemplar

Domain 2: Person-Centered Care	
2.2 Communicate effectively with individuals.	Moira worked very hard to communicate effectively with the team in this challenging new clinical situation as the primary nurse caring for this complex trauma patient.
2.3 Integrate assessment skills in practice.	Moira performed a clinically relevant trauma assessment on her patient, distinguishing between normal and abnormal findings in her patient.
2.6 Demonstrate accountability for care delivery.	Moira demonstrated accountability not only for her trauma patient but also the needs of her other seven patients whom she could not see when she was one on one with this patient.
Domain 10: Personal, Professional, and Leadership Development	
10.1 Demonstrate a commitment to personal health and well-being.	Moira took time to reflect and journal after her shift.
10.3 Develop capacity for leadership.	Moira accessed her resources when dealing with the challenge of caring for the critically ill trauma patient for a prolonged period of time. She demonstrated leadership behaviors in working with her team.

I have been working with new nurses and supporting them through their transition into practice since I oriented my first coworker in the pediatric ED. As a faculty member and clinical nurse at a children's hospital, I have witnessed the transition of countless new graduates and nurses in changing clinical work environments. Many of my students feel pressure to work in certain areas immediately following graduation due to their perception of the prestige of one specialty over another. I felt compelled in some ways to do the same when I graduated from nursing school. Moira had experience as a student nurse in a community ED, which affirmed her passion for this specialty. As described in the story she shares, she has a very supportive team. Sometimes, this is a rare combination, but as we can sense from this story, this makes Moira feel empowered and believe she can face new challenges.

I share this advice when working with emerging nurses as they begin their job searches, but please know that *I took only some of my advice*, and choosing to follow only some of it almost led me to leave nursing. For anyone who knows me well, this statement almost seems incomprehensible. I love nursing, and the thought that I would be at a point where I would consider leaving the profession does not seem like something I would do, but I can assure you that it almost happened to me in my first year of nursing practice.

During my last semester of nursing school, I applied to nearly every hospital in my state for almost any open position. I was fortunate to have four job interviews and subsequent job offers at three hospitals. The positions were in labor and delivery (per diem), pediatrics (part-time), adult orthopedics (full-time), and adult urology (full-time). My favorite interview and shadow experience was on the adult urology floor. The manager was warm and welcoming, and the staff entered our meeting to greet her and me. They genuinely seemed happy to meet me and asked me routine questions (where I went to nursing school, where I was from, and what I was doing in their manager's office). They told me they had the "best team" and "best boss" and asked me if I had any questions. I had one: *What made their boss "the best"?* The manager sat with me as the staff responded, and she seemed curious, almost amused, as she waited for their answer.

The three nurses described their care of a patient who had multiple admissions over many months to their unit. Before his last admission, he decided to transition to comfort measures from curative ones. According to the nurses, it was clear from his state of health on this admission that he would not return home. When the nurse manager found out that his favorite football team, the Green Bay Packers, had made it to the Super Bowl, she started to organize a surprise Super Bowl party in his room. She figured out ways to get him out of his room so that staff could come in, decorate, and set up refreshments. Staff changed into dark green and gold T-shirts and sweatshirts (the Green Bay Packers colors). They wheeled in a big-screen television so that he did not have to watch the game alone; he watched it with his hospital team in his room. The nurses told me that the energy in his room was joyous and energetic, with the patient at the center of the happiness. The nurse manager worked on the unit, covering the nurses so that they could be with their Super Bowl patient. Sadly, the patient died the next day, but as a team, they knew that they had collaborated to provide the patient with a fantastic experience. After this conversation with the nurses, the manager gave me a tour of the unit, and I spent some time with a nurse shadowing her. The experience was very positive, and I felt welcomed.

Later that same week, I met with the co-nurse managers of the pediatric unit to which I had applied for an interview. They seemed very friendly, and they shared responsibility for managing two units. I was applying for a position on a unit that cared for children with medical-surgical diagnoses between ages 5 and 12 and from birth to age 12 with hematological-oncological diagnoses. One of the managers gave me a unit tour, but I did not have opportunity to speak with the staff. As the manager walked me off the unit, she offered me a 24-hour position. I thanked her and asked her for a few days to consider the offer.

I took the pediatric position despite my need for a full-time position and loving the urology unit's manager and staff. The children's hospital building was only a few years old, and while the pediatric unit I was hired for was not in this new space, I was excited about being part of something new. I also felt that, as a high-achieving student, I had earned this pediatrics position at a time when new-graduate nurses were not often hired into a specialty. A few days before I started my first nursing position, a co-manager called me and offered to increase my hours to a full-time position. I was grateful and excited to begin. I had a six-week orientation to the unit with a great preceptor who was in the final weeks of her pediatric nurse practitioner program and was excited to impart her knowledge to me.

During my first year as a new nurse, there was still a large population of children whose mothers had not received perinatal antiretrovirals and often were admitted to our unit for health conditions related to their disease state. Often predeceased by their mothers, the children with HIV/ AIDS frequently became wards of the state. This group of patients quickly became my favorite patient population on the unit. I was surprised by the number of my coworkers who did not want to care for these patients, such as one colleague who asked me to switch patient assignments, saying, "*I am a mom now … I cannot take any chances, you know?*" No, I disagreed with my coworker. As a highly vulnerable population, these children needed our care and not our judgment. Many of these kids were too young to know their diagnosis or what it meant to them or society at large to have AIDS. They knew they came to our unit and had some semblance of consistency and "family." I often took care of children and their families with psychosocial complexity that was beyond my comprehension and skill as a new nurse. My first year as a pediatric nurse took an emotional toll on me after I attended the funerals of eight infants and children, all of whom were my primary patients.

Slowly, my entire personal wardrobe consisted of only black clothes. I started to isolate myself from friends and family. I found myself sleeping long hours most of my days off. My mother called out my outward behaviors as being consistent with depression, which I vehemently denied. Looking back with a lens of more life experience, why would I think it is necessary to deny my reactions to such significant losses of patients at work? How could I possibly quickly move on from (*try to forget*) the trauma of losing these patients whom I cared so much about? Reacting emotionally to such significant professional trauma in such a short time was not a sign of weakness but was, instead, a sign that these experiences truly mattered and that I am, in fact, human. We will explore the negative responses to caring more in Chapter 8.

I left the unit after less than a year. On one of my last days as a full-time nurse on the floor, one of the nurses who was the least supportive of me on the unit made me feel very uncomfortable when she asked me if I had "used" the opportunity to work on this floor to get my one year of experience before going to the pediatric ED. These words hurt me and I did not know what to say. For the 10 months I had not developed the skills that demonstrated a commitment to my personal health and well-being (AACN, 2021, Domain 10.1). I was struggling with my reactions to caring.

Why do I share this with you? It is because I picked the wrong first nursing job. I chose a specialty when I thought that was what I should do, as if it was not enough to take the position on a med-surg unit. I should have spent time meeting my colleagues on the pediatric unit before I accepted the offer to see if they made me feel as supported as the nurses who had the Super Bowl party for their patient. When a shadow experience on the unit and meeting with the nursing staff was not offered to me on the pediatric unit, I should have asked for it as part of my decision-making process. Since then, I have coached hundreds of emerging nurses in their final year of nursing school as they try to secure their dream job and have often been asked how someone can get their "dream job" after graduation. After you read Moira's and my stories, I challenge you to reimagine your expectations of your dream job. Moira shared with us that *if supportive coworkers surround you, they go to any lengths to support and help you and one another.* This is critical in your nursing career, especially in your transition to practice as a new-graduate nurse. To be clear, many of the nurses I worked with in that first position were among the nicest and most caring nurses I have ever known. Yet without the resources and supports for all of us to deal with our own reactions to caring for this very challenging population, there were not many opportunities to support one another or for my coworkers to see me as struggling with my work. I hid my reactions from them and when I could not take it anymore, I transferred out of the unit.

You are reading this book as an emerging nurse or new nurse. Consider a few things as you interview for positions, or if you are reading this in your first position, and wondering if it is a right fit. Church et al. (2023) shared the top five reasons that new nurses leave their first position, which include (1) inadequate staffing, (2) better pay/benefits, (3) lack of good management/ leadership, (4) stressful work environment, and (5) burnout, noting that more than one-third of nurses leave their position in the first two years in the role. Having supportive coworkers can help partially mitigate this risk, but there are other things to consider.

Applying for Your First Job: Different From Applying to Nursing School

I have worked with hundreds of nursing students as they prepare to find their first job after graduation. Many put considerable pressure on themselves to enter their "dream specialty" when they graduate. When you applied to your nursing program, data determined the number of students that could be accepted, such as how many faculty were available to teach in the program, the availability of clinical sites, and the physical space of the buildings that house the programs. Data also determine the number of nursing positions available in any given unit or healthcare organization at any given time. The number of nurses working in a unit on a particular shift is based on the number of patients, their acuity, and the amount of work anticipated to provide nursing care. According to the American Nurses Association's (ANA) *Principles for Nurse Staffing* (ANA, 2019), addressing nurse staffing challenges supports our nurses, patients, and the nation's health and well-being. Published literature supports the critical role of appropriate nursing staffing levels in preventing falls, medication errors, pressure ulcers, infections, and readmissions (Uchmanowicz et al., 2024).

Some emerging and new nurses need to realize that, unlike when applying to a nursing program, many human factors also determine the number of positions available in any unit when they choose to apply. If you graduate in May, but two positions were open on a specific unit in which you would like to work due to resignations in February, and they were already filled before you graduate, a position will not be posted for you to apply to on that unit. If another student completes their final nursing capstone clinical on a unit and makes a strong in-person impression, you might not even be interviewed for an open position. This has nothing to do with you; however, sometimes factors outside your control can be frustrating.

I have already shared with you that I am a nurse who has only worked in pediatrics my entire career. Throughout this casebook, you will hear stories from other nurses about their first nursing experiences. Some will offer their thoughts regarding their entry into nursing through specialty practice. I commonly receive the question *"Do you think I need one year of med-surg before I pursue specialty nursing practice?"* Here is my answer: Your patient population is *less important* to your transition to practice as a nurse in your first year than with whom you practice and the support you receive from your team and administration. I would also argue that the question implies that medical-surgical nursing is not a specialty when, in fact, it is the single largest nursing specialty in the United States, with nurses caring for adults with a variety of medical or surgical issues (Academy of Medical-Surgical Nurses, 2024). But why are the people you work with and the support you receive from your team and administration more important than your practice setting when you graduate? A positive practice can decrease nurse burnout, improve nurse satisfaction, and positively affect nursing retention (Hargreaves & Pabico, 2020).

The characteristics of supportive work environments for new nurses have been studied, and two categories of these environments resonate as I reflect on the new-graduate transitions that I have directly observed and those that have been shared with me. Najafi and Nasiri (2023) describe an intimate, cooperative work environment with coworkers who show empathetic behaviors and have educational support as critical to new nurses' success. An intimate atmosphere is friendly, where coworkers cooperate during stressful situations, help one another's workload during challenging times, and feel safe sharing their feelings about difficulties with their colleagues (Najafi & Nasiri, 2023). Moira's story shows these glimmers of support among her nursing team as they come together to care for the patient in the trauma room. Later in this casebook, we will dive deeper into issues where newer nurses had different experiences and felt marginalized, unsupported, and not part of their team. Some challenges we faced in our position could not have been foreseen, like the transition to practice during the second wave of the COVID-19 pandemic that Grace had in Chapter 11 and the impact this had on her unit.

The New Nurse's Career Toolkit

Many emerging nurses find searching for their first nursing job very stressful. Keeping an open mind and using a systematic approach will make it more manageable. The American Medical Association (AMA, n.d.) published a toolkit to help structure career exploration for new physician job seekers. The physician toolkit was used as the foundation to develop the New Nurse's Career Toolkit; we have adapted and enhanced it with resources for emerging and new nurses as they look for their first or next career opportunity through seven steps.

Step 1: Identify Your Priorities—What Do You Want to Do? (AMA, n.d.)

Many things must be considered when deciding what positions to apply for. First, consider what motivated you to enter nursing and reflect on the clinical experiences you felt most aligned with as a student. Sometimes these are our favorite rotations because something "clicked" for us, or perhaps we thought we could make a difference for this patient population. Maybe you did not have the opportunity to work with a specific population during nursing school and would like to work in that area because you have always wanted to learn more about it. For example, in nursing school, you had clinical on an adult medicine floor where the nurses sometimes administered chemotherapy. However, you never had the opportunity to spend time in an outpatient infusion center.

Next, knowing what type of setting in which we feel most comfortable working is important. Many nursing programs traditionally have heavily emphasized acute care nursing, often in a hospital-based setting, and that may not be for you. Nursing education is evolving in many ways, one of which is to consider less the location where care is provided to patients and emphasize the spheres of care, which are our goals to address the healthcare needs of individuals, families, and populations and their care/services and to promote desired health outcomes (AACN, 2021). The spheres of care include disease prevention/promotion of health and well-being, chronic disease care, regenerative or restorative care, and hospice/palliative/supportive care, available across the lifespan (AACN, 2021).

Following are two questions to consider:

- In which sphere would you like to make an impact in nursing?
- With which population(s) would you like to work to see your impact through?

Step 2: Identify Your Priorities—How and Where Do You Want to Do It? (AMA, n.d.)

As you know, after you graduate from your nursing program, you must take the National Council Licensure Examination for Registered Nurses (NCLEX-RN; National Council of State Boards of Nursing [NCSBN], 2024). Your nursing program should advise you when to submit your electronic application to the nursing regulatory body (e.g., board of nursing) where you seek to be licensed and registered as a nurse. The NCSBN (2024) website (https://www. nclex.com/register.page) provides instructions on registering for this exam. You must consider the location or geographic setting where you would like to work. Some newer nurses want to work near their hometown or where they went to school or may decide to relocate to another area. This is an essential consideration as you begin to register for the NCLEX-RN, as you will have to decide in which state you wish to be licensed and registered to work as a nurse. For example, if you are from Connecticut, went to nursing school in Pennsylvania, and are applying to a nursing position in Texas, you can take the NCLEX-RN in any state because the NCLEX-RN is a national licensure exam; however, as you submit your application, you will have to select one state to apply for licensure and registry for your application (Nurse Licensure Compact [NLC], n.d.). Suppose that you decide to apply for licensure and registry in Texas but ultimately do not accept the position there and, instead, accept a role in Connecticut. In that case, you will have to follow Connecticut's processes for obtaining a license and registry as a nurse in the state after successfully passing the NCLEX-RN with the application for license and registry in Texas.

Nurse Licensure Compact

The NLC allows registered nurses (RNs) to possess multistate licenses, permitting them to work in their home and the other compact states (NLC, n.d.). The nurse's primary residence must be an NLC state to be eligible for a multistate license. At the time we are writing this casebook, 43 jurisdictions are part of NLC with some awaiting implementation and others with partial implementation in place (NLC, n.d.). An applicant for the NCLEX-RN or a nurse whose primary state of residence is not a compact state is not eligible for a multistate license; if they apply for licensure in a compact state, the nurse will be issued a single-state license (valid only in the state of issuance; NLC, n.d.).

Transition to Practice Programs

New nurses are expected to possess entry-level competencies at graduation, but research describes gaps in their role-related knowledge, skills, and clinical judgment (Rush et al., 2019). There is variability in the types of transition to practice programs (e.g., orientation, preceptorship, nurse residency) and their length (short: six to 12 weeks; intermediate: four to eight months; or long: 12 or more months; Charette et al., 2023, p. 1355). These programs aim to bridge the educational preparation-practice gap, yet the literature has yet to gain consensus on the structure of the most ideal and effective intervention to reach this goal (Aldosari et al., 2021; Rush et al., 2019; Ward-Smith et al., 2023). Some literature supports that new-graduate nurses participating in a comprehensive transition to practice program have higher commitments to their organization, increased satisfaction working with their colleagues, and lower intent to leave their positions (Grubaugh et al., 2023). Evidence supports that practice environments should pay particular attention to nurse well-being, support, and recognition of practicing nurses to support nurses as they transition to professional nursing practice and support remaining in their positions (Grubaugh et al., 2023). Regardless of what the transition to practice is called, supporting new-graduate nurses during their first year of practice is critical and helps mitigate transition shock, which can negatively affect their confidence as nurses and intention to stay in nursing practice (Koh et al., 2023). You should request information on what this program looks like with each potential employer.

Charette et al. (2023) studied the effectiveness of transition-to-practice programs on new-graduate nurses' clinical competence, job satisfaction, and perceptions of support. In studying the transition of a group of new-graduate nurses in Australia over 12 months, they identified the following themes within the milestones of their first year of practice that might be helpful for you to consider as you anticipate your transition to your new nursing role and first year of practice:

- Zero to three months: "You learn by getting out of student mode" (p. 1359).
- Three to six months: "I am more confident, calm, and in control" (p. 1361).
- Six to nine months: "I felt like I knew nothing, but I should have trusted myself more" (p. 1363).
- Nine to 12 months: "I am confident but still have a lot to learn" (p. 1363).

Source: Charette et al., 2023, pp. 1359–1363.

A preceptor is an experienced and competent registered nurse who serves as a role model and point person to newly hired nursing staff, filling the roles of educator, facilitator, mentor, and socializer (Joseph et al., 2022). Preceptors help new nurses develop their clinical reasoning skills, offer feedback, and provide opportunities for the new nurse to debrief, reflect, and ask questions (Powers et al., 2020). Sometimes the newly hired nurse follows a preceptor's schedule and has only one mentor, while at other times, the responsibility is shared among two or more nurses. While the added responsibility of orienting new staff may be very rewarding for the preceptor and credited toward career advancement, not all experienced nurses enjoy the role. In many settings, the experienced nurse might not be able to decline an offer to serve as a preceptor, and most often, preceptors are not compensated for this additional role. Those typically hold unit leadership positions such as preceptor and charge nurse with the experience and training to serve in these roles. If there are not enough people to serve in these capacities on a unit, experienced nurses hold these additional responsibilities frequently. We will explore the new nurse and preceptor relationships later in this casebook.

Why are we mentioning this when discussing what your orientation might look like? In reality, you are entering nursing during a time when burnout and job turnover are common. Your enthusiasm for starting your new position may not always be met with the enthusiasm, warmth, and support you deserve. Sometimes the preceptor does not make the best first impression, and the new nurse believes it is due to something they did, even if they just met. If this happens to you, *it likely has nothing to do with you.* Most preceptor-nurse relationships are positive and help the new nurse feel supported; improve their organizing, prioritizing, and communication/ leadership skills; and increase professional and job satisfaction for the new nurse (Joseph et al., 2022). Throughout your orientation, know that it takes considerable time for experienced nurses to share their knowledge and feedback. Express your gratitude lavishly and help others on the unit whenever possible. Despite your efforts, if you encounter nurses who are unprofessional, inappropriate, unsupportive, and uncivil, they should not be responsible for precepting you or other new nurses (Thompson, 2019). If you face challenges with your relationship with your preceptor, you should advocate for yourself and work with your nursing supervisor to improve your transition to the practice plan.

Step 3: Understand the Practice Settings Available (AMA, n.d.)

Traditionally, new-graduate nurses have been socialized to plan their first job to be in a hospital, working in acute care, typically in an inpatient hospital unit or in a critical care or ED setting. Working for a hospital or health system today can include primary and ambulatory settings, including specialty practices that offer specific services. Primary and specialty outpatient practices can also be privately owned, community-based, or a federally qualified health center, which is an outpatient clinic that qualifies for specific reimbursement systems under Medicare and Medicaid (Healthcare.gov, 2024). Nurses can care for patients in various settings, such as in their homes, schools, camps, prisons, health departments, hospices, and extended-care facilities. You do not have to limit your job search to one position, one hospital or health system, or one type of practice setting. Being open to exploring a variety of potential career settings may help you decide what is best for you. Keeping track of your contacts and deadlines will take organization.

Considering the "big picture" of whom you will interact with at each possible job, including those outside your interdisciplinary team, is essential. For example, as a pediatric nurse, I care for children from newborns to about 22 years of age and their families. When people ask me, *"How can you possibly work with sick children?"* I often respond that caring for children is fine for me and that the parents can sometimes present the real challenge. If a child comes to the ED after an injury and is critically ill, they require every ounce of my focus, clinical judgment, and experience. Once I meet their parents or guardians, I quickly try to gain their trust and partner to support their child.

When parents or guardians are in these types of situations where their child is critically ill or injured, they come as they are, meaning that they arrive with the communication skills and coping strategies that they have, and sometimes, due to a multitude of factors, they do not seem to be effective in either area. If parents are separated and have a contentious relationship, and the child is injured while under the other parent's supervision, things can become very tense. We practice family-centered care in pediatrics and promote family presence for most procedures outside of an operating room setting. With parental tensions and emotions running high, parents may try to target their frustration at me when I am preparing to start their child's IV by saying, *"You better get this on the first try."* For some nurses, even those who love children and are interested in the conditions that affect them, hearing comments such as this and being watched by parents as you perform procedures under pressure might be too much.

For those who do not mind this challenge, we learn to assess our and our patients' safety quickly, determine the best response to the parents' comments at the moment, and act on our next course of action. This type of expansion of the circle engagement with others in addition to your patient and typical interdisciplinary team is true in many nursing areas and should be considered. For example, in a surgical ICU, while caring for someone with a gunshot wound, your patient may also be in police custody with four-point forensic restraints and have a police officer at the bedside. On a burn unit, a fire marshal might contact the team with more information about the scene of a house fire. While working in a hospice facility, you may have many visitors with varying experiences with death and dying who visit your patients. Perhaps this sounds very obvious to some of you, and if that is the case, move on to Step 4. We want to make sure you think broadly about what might be involved in the holistic care of patients in your unit and your comfort with that possibility.

Step 4: Start Your Search (AMA, n.d.)

You can usually initiate your search several months before you want to start working; however, some new graduate programs have an earlier deadline. It is best to connect with each opportunity you apply to ensure you meet all deadlines. Most nursing programs offer career services and support, including resume reviews, interviewing strategies, and employer listings. Suppose you have graduated and are preparing to search for another position. In that case, most programs will continue extending these services to alums, so check in with your program to see if you have this continued resource.

Searching individual employers' electronic job postings on their websites is a good start for finding job postings. Setting up a profile on a business social media platform, such as LinkedIn, can help you with your job search in several ways. First, you can create your profile and connect with anyone whom you might know who works for your desired employer or whom you know professionally. You can also connect with your desired employer and receive news updates to keep you apprised of news affecting that organization that might be helpful to discuss if you are provided with the opportunity for an interview. If possible, search for recruiters at your desired employer, as they sometimes post available positions with deadlines on their business social media platform page. If you can connect with them, you might also be able to direct message them on the platform and query them about potential opportunities and if they have upcoming career fairs. Finally, you can search the connections of anyone else in your professional network (e.g., former colleagues, former faculty) to see if they have connections to anyone who might work at your desired employers. Perhaps they can connect with you, and you can inquire about the pathways by which they found their position.

To organize all of this information, you should maintain a spreadsheet or notes that include potential jobs with the name of the organization, location, contacts for the recruiter or manager with their email address and phone number, the status of your candidacy, and any important notes such as when you should plan to follow up. All written communications should start with a formal salutation (e.g., Dear Ms. Murphy). The absence of a formal greeting with an acknowledgment of the recipient's name is not considered professional (e.g., starting an email with "Hi" or jumping into the body of the message). Please do not assume that you can address the recipient by their first name unless they request that you do so. When on the telephone, the same holds; be sure to ask to speak to someone using their formal salutation. Thank those who support your receipt of the information. Following an interview in person, by phone, or over Zoom, send a thank-you email within 24 hours, written in a formal tone free of typos with a brief reference to any key points from the interview (Ortiz, 2023).

Step 5: Ask Questions (AMA, n.d.)

Before you think about the types of questions that you might want to ask during an interview, you should research the organization. Go to the employer's website and review the organization's mission and history to understand its culture and values better (AMA, n.d.). Their business social media site (e.g., LinkedIn page) is a great resource to follow as you prepare for the interview and receive news updates. It is also an excellent place to publish your professional achievements, which potential recruiters or employers may see. Many employers may also maintain a larger social media presence on platforms such as Facebook, Instagram, X, and TikTok. Use caution when following these accounts and giving them access to your personal information and activities outside work hours. In a recent poll, 70% of employers responded that every company should screen candidates' social media process during hiring (Cotriss, 2023). If you have a public account or follow the potential employer on social media, know that they can review the information you post anytime. Another great way to keep informed about an organization you are interested in is by setting up a Google alert. Visit google.com/alerts and enter the topic on which you want to set an alert (Google, 2025a), which might be the name of a medical center or healthcare organization. You can set how often you receive these updates to your Gmail account. You will receive links to stories about the word for which you set an alert. This might give you current information that will inform your answers during a job interview or even give you a bigger picture of what is happening at the organization. If you do not have a Gmail account, you can set one up for free by going to https:// accounts.google.com/ and selecting "create an account" (Google, 2025b).

Many resources are available to help you consider the questions you might be asked in an interview and what you should ask before accepting a nursing position. The career planning center at your school will often offer resources for preparing for an interview. Be prepared to dress professionally if you are interviewing on Zoom or in person. Most people wear at least business casual (pants, shirt/blouse), and some are more formal with suits/blazers. Always wear closed-toe conservative shoes. If you do not have these items, borrow them from a friend or invest in one professional outfit. Be mindful not to wear strong colognes or perfumes, as you will likely be in small spaces during the interview, and strong odors may be offensive to others. Cover tattoos and, when possible, remove facial jewelry for the interview. If this is not possible, choose subtle jewelry for the piercing, as you may not be aware of the employer's policies related to piercing in the workplace. If you are going to shadow immediately after the interview on the unit, it is OK to ask about what you should wear on interview day. Emerging nurses often wear their student scrubs to shadow days.

As part of the interview process, be prepared to answer questions that provide insight into your personality, attitude, communication style, and ability to work as part of a team. Remember to keep your answers focused on positive attributes desirable to the interviewer. I have often heard someone in an interview retelling a story to answer a question, and their response is pessimistic about the team, the type of work they were doing, or challenging workloads. Instead of using the opportunity to tell the story neutrally, they share negativity, and the response feels like they might bring this negative energy into their new work setting. Some questions for you to reflect on to help you prepare for your interview include the following:

- Can you tell us a little about yourself?
- Why did you choose nursing as a profession?
- What are your greatest strengths?
- What is a weakness you have, and how do you address it?
- What kind of work environment do you thrive in?
- Give an example of a time you were in a stressful situation. What happened, and how did you respond?
- What three words would your current employer/coworkers (clinical faculty) use to describe you and why?

Source: Adapted from Post University, 2023.

Emerging and new nurses are often very afraid of any type of clinical question that might be asked, but, while it is not impossible that this type of question will be posed, they are less common. Following are some examples for you to consider in preparing for your interview:

- If you had a patient with diabetes who was not communicative, what would you do?
- How would you respond if a provider approached you and yelled at you, referring to a patient who was not yours and whom you had not taken care of?
- If you were the nurse for a patient undergoing surgery, which preop and postop teachings would you discuss?
- If you are a nurse on a floor and one patient is experiencing a transfusion reaction, another patient is in pain, and a third patient has an angry family member demanding to speak to you, whom do you see first and why?

Source: Adapted from University of San Francisco, n.d.

I recently heard the following insightful questions from individuals interviewing for their first nursing position. These questions do not directly ask clinical questions; however, if they are answered thoughtfully, they can provide tremendous insight into a candidate's ability to receive feedback and advocate for patients.

- Can you provide an example of when you received feedback you disagreed with and how you handled the situation?
- What is an example of a mistake you made, and what happened?
- Describe a time when you had to stand up for something in the clinical setting.

Following are the American Nurses Credentialing Center's (ANCC) Pathway to Excellence® sample interview questions (n.d.) that you can ask during an interview:

- How would you describe the culture of your unit/organization?
- What is the onboarding process for a new hire? How does your organization support new employees?
- If a nurse needs additional help after orientation, what support is available?
- Which committees are direct care nurses invited to attend?
- What are the biggest challenges your nurses face daily?
- How has the leadership team helped them overcome these challenges?
- What is the current vacancy rate?
- What have been your most notable successes and failures during the past year?
- What programs does the organization have in place to support nurses' well-being?

Source: ANCC, n.d.

All the components of a job are important to consider, but the emotional and mental tolls are sometimes not asked about because we do not know what to ask. There are parts of the emotional response to caring for this patient that Moira does not mention. However, we will try to address the emotional response to caring for patients later in this casebook through other stories. Some things that may have taken a toll on Moria may have included caring for someone who intended to commit suicide yet was resuscitated potentially against their wishes. Her patient was unidentified, so the family could not be called to support the patient. She was caring for a patient who now needed a nurse with advanced critical care skills for a prolonged period beyond the regular scope of a new ED nurse, which can be overwhelming and scary.

Following are some questions you might want to reflect on and consider asking in your own words during an interview. You do not need to ask all of these questions, but instead, consider whether or not you have insight into the answers to these questions while you are in the interview process. If you do not have a sense for these answers, consider asking them in a way that makes you feel comfortable:

- How long does the typical nurse stay on the unit?
- What are the reasons the last three nurses left the unit?
- What types of situations take the most considerable toll on the nurses who work on the unit?
  - Can you describe a recent situation that challenged the staff emotionally and mentally?
  - How did organizational leadership support the staff?
  - Were any practice changes made after the situation?

- If nurses experience compassion fatigue from their work on the unit (i.e., negative responses to caring), what support is available to them?
- How do you advise new nurses working on the unit to address their experiences with the stress of working there?
- Can you describe the training nurses receive to communicate with patients and their families on the unit?
- What competencies must a staff nurse achieve before training as a charge nurse and preceptor?
- For the nurses you hired in the past year, are they currently serving as charge nurses and/or preceptors? When did they start those roles?
- Do nurses who work on this unit ever spend time together outside of work? If so, can you describe a recent event?
- Do members of the interdisciplinary team socialize outside of work? If so, can you describe a recent event?
- Can you describe your relationship with your physician leader counterpart? Can you describe a challenge that you recently faced together and the outcome?

You may have the opportunity to shadow a nurse on the unit as part of your interview process. Remember, that is still part of the interview process, and feedback from the nurse you are shadowing will be solicited. Be sure to inquire about appropriate attire for the shadow, and be mindful of your interactions with patients and staff. It is also an excellent opportunity for you to gain some insight into the position, but remember, it is only a tiny snapshot of the people, such as staff and patients, on the unit at that time. The following box provides additional questions you might want to ask the nurse you are shadowing and others you meet on the unit.

PRN (PLEASE READ NOW)

Additional Questions to Ask While You Are Shadowing

- How would you describe the culture of your unit in one word?
  - Can you please explain why you chose that word?
- How does the unit support new employees?
- What happens if a nurse needs additional support at the orientation's end?
- Can you describe a recent challenging day at work and how your colleagues responded?
- What are the biggest challenges you regularly face at work, and how does your supervisor address them?
- Are you aware of any colleagues who have been hurt on the unit? What was the communication from management around this, and what happened as a result?

Remember, it is essential to thank the staff who spoke with you about your interest in the position. Anyone you spend significant one-on-one time with should receive a personal thank-you. It is appropriate to send a group thank-you to those you only met briefly. Email thank-yous are received most quickly, but some hiring managers say that a handwritten thank-you makes a big statement as they are less common.

Step 6: Appraise Compensation (AMA, n.d.)

Compensation is an important consideration with any job, but remember that one number rarely tells the whole story (AMA, n.d.). Nurses in a registered nursing position in acute care are typically paid an hourly rate. When they work evenings, nights, and weekends, an additional payment of an off-shift differential is usually provided. The starting hourly rate for new-graduate nurses depends on the regional market, with the best-paying states for registered nurses currently the highest in California, Hawaii, Oregon, Massachusetts, and Alaska (U.S. News & World Report, 2024). Calculating what additional payments can be expected based on the proposed work schedule is an important consideration. Within working hours, ask whether the lunch break is unpaid (this is most common), meaning that you are at work an additional 30 minutes outside your paid hours. Required meal and break periods fall under state and not federal law; however, the U.S. Department of Labor (DOL) lists state standards (DOL, 2023). Finding out which provisions are in place so that you can always take a break during your shift and how you are compensated if you are unable to take your break due to patient care issues is important to find out in advance.

Under the Patient Protection and Affordable Care Act, employers with more than 50 full-time employees (or the equivalent of part-time employees) must provide health insurance to 95% of their employees or pay a penalty to the Internal Revenue Service (IRS, 2025). The type and tiers of coverage offered vary by employer, so take a careful look at your options. As you are evaluating which employer-offered insurance plan is best for you, be sure to check to see whether your current providers are in network, consider your health needs for the upcoming year (e.g., do you have major or minor care needs), and decide if you would like to manage your costs by having lower premiums or lower provider copays (UnitedHealthcare, 2024). Review prescription, dental, and vision plans. The Consolidated Omnibus Budget Reconciliation Act (COBRA) gives employees and their families the ability to extend health benefits for a short period during the transition between jobs, voluntary or involuntary job loss, death, or other life events (DOL, n.d.a.). You will likely see information about COBRA benefits in your package; you will not need them while you work in the position but may opt to use them if you leave the employer. Life and disability insurance are also common benefits, and it is often less expensive to purchase additional life insurance coverage from this employer-offered plan than seeking coverage privately.

Part and full-time employees receive paid time off (PTO), which varies by region and employer. Find out about sick leave and how much of your PTO must be used before using short- and long-term leaves. Be sure to find out the processes for selecting a vacation on your unit and how to request a single day of PTO during a scheduled period. Somewhat related to this, find out if the unit census drops and you do not need to work during your shift, if you floated to another unit, or if you must use your PTO to ensure consistent pay.

An employer is not required to offer a retirement savings plan; those who have established this benefit for their employees must adhere to minimum standards (DOL, n.d.b.). Many healthcare organizations plan such as a 403(b) plan (also called a *tax-sheltered annuity* or *TSA plan*), which is a retirement plan offered by specific 501(c)(3) tax-exempt organizations (IRS, 2024). While it may seem too soon to think about retirement when just starting your first nursing position, it is never too early. Automatic debits make savings easy and may help reduce your tax burden. A less common benefit offered to employees in the private and not-for-profit sectors but more common for those working for local, state, or federal governments is a pension. A pension is a retirement arrangement where the employer promises the employee who has worked for a specific period a regular payment from the day you retire for as long as you live (Pension Benefit Guaranty Corporation, 2021).

Other Benefits That an Employer May Offer You

Sign-on bonuses in exchange for a set work term are sometimes offered; however, make sure to explore the rationale for why these bonuses are being extended before you make your decision. While some employers offer sign-on bonuses to recruit nurses with specialized skills or experience, they are sometimes used to recruit during staffing shortages (Morris, 2023). Some larger employers are starting to offer assistance with student loans, usually for full-time nurses, with a monthly payment directly to the loan for a specified period (Weiss, 2024). A more common benefit is tuition reimbursement, an employer program that helps nurses receive additional education by providing financial assistance (Bright Horizons, 2024).

Employee wellness programs are also growing in popularity as an additional benefit. Most hospitals (83%) offer workplace wellness programs, including health screenings, health coaches, employee assistance programs, stress management and smoking-cessation programs, and even fitness benefits (Centers for Disease Control and Prevention, 2020). Details and associated costs are unique to the employer, so explore those resources and ask for clarification. Additional benefits such as pet insurance, adoption assistance, and credit unions are sometimes offered by larger employers.

Step 7: Negotiate Based on Your Priorities (AMA, n.d.)

When you successfully complete the interview process, you will have a job offer. This offer should include the work location, the shift/schedule requirements, and your hourly rate.

This may be offered to you verbally or by email, usually by human resources (HR), with written materials about the benefits program offered. HR or the manager provides a deadline to respond to this offer, which may be as quick as a few days. If this is your top position, then you may be ready to accept after reviewing the offer and considering any points you would like additional information about or if you would like to make any negotiations. If you are currently in the middle of interviewing or awaiting feedback from other potential employers, this may feel particularly stressful. You can ask for the grace of extending the deadline; however, they do not have to grant this to you. Depending on their response, you may have to decide on the offer before you have complete information from other potential employers.

As a new graduate, the starting salary offer may be set and not negotiable; however, you should always ask for consideration (Jean, 2023). Specialized skills and related experience may be a factor that can increase your salary; current recommendations are for a new college graduate to negotiate a range of no more than about 5% above the offer (Handshake, 2024). Other important quality-of-life factors that may not cost the employer are also good to consider in the negotiation process. Dates for an upcoming vacation or having a set day off each week to attend graduate school are two things for which I have heard new nurses successfully negotiate before accepting their first position. Larger organizations with PTO accrual policies will likely not be able to negotiate those offerings and offer you more vacation or sick time.

Most healthcare entities hire nurses as employees at will, meaning that work continues at the will of both the employee and employer, with each party able to end the relationship at any time (O'Neill et al., 2022). There might be a time, such as with an offer for a sign-on bonus or a new graduate residency agreement, when the employer may require that you commit to work for a set period. Before signing any contract or agreement, it is best to have a legal review. Even if specific requests are promised verbally to you by the employer, be sure to get all commitments in writing. An excellent way to have this documented if it is not offered to you is to follow up with an email requesting written confirmation of the request. For example, when you are offered the position, you tell the manager that you need a week off in March for your brother's out-of-state wedding. They assure you verbally that there should not be a problem; however, you could email the manager before you accept the position. An example might be as follows:

> Dear [name of manager],
>
> Thank you again for offering me the position [be specific regarding the name of unit, shifts, rotation]. When I [shadowed on the unit/interviewed], I was most impressed with [be specific about something you liked]. I am reviewing the offer

details and wanted to follow up on our conversation on [insert date] about my need to have [insert dates] off for an important, out-of-state family event. While I know that I am a new employee and there is a formal process for vacation requests on the unit going forward, ensuring that I have this time off is essential to my decision about the position. Can you please confirm this for me?

Sincerely,

[Your name]

Accepting your first nursing position requires information, significant thought, and reflection. That said, know that no job decision is permanent, and many opportunities are available for you in nursing now and in the future.

YOU MATTER: YOUR FIRST NURSING POSITION

Once you have passed the NCLEX-RN and are licensed to work, you have the opportunity to work in a variety of settings. Different jobs are right for different seasons and reasons in your life. Be proud of your decision to enter one of the most respected professions and all that is ahead.

Book Club Questions

1. Have you ever felt overwhelmed when in a new patient care scenario? What did you do to cope?
2. How can you be a support system to your coworkers?
3. How can you ask for help or advocate for yourself if you feel overwhelmed with your patient load? Who do you ask?
4. Reflect on your recent clinical experiences or your current role. Are the team members on your unit "your people?" If you are a new grad, what factors led you to select your position? For emerging nurses, what are some factors you are considering as you apply for new-graduate nurse positions?

About This Chapter's Authors

Moira Dougherty, BSN, RN

Moira was born and raised in the suburbs of Philadelphia. She graduated from Fairfield University's Marion Peckham Egan School of Nursing and Health Studies in 2022. Before graduating from nursing school, Moira was a resource float patient care technician at a community hospital during the COVID-19 pandemic and then transitioned to an ED tech position. Shortly after graduation, Moira moved to New York City to pursue her passion for emergency nursing. She is still in her original job and enjoys working in the ED's fast-paced environment. Outside work, Moira pursues her passion for competitive ballroom dancing, traveling, and spending time with family and friends.

Linda Roney, EdD, RN-BC, CPEN, CNE, FAAN

Linda is honored to provide the leader's reflection in this casebook chapter.

References

Academy of Medical-Surgical Nurses. (2024). *What is med-surg nursing?* https://amsn.org/About-AMSN/What-Is-Med-Surg-Nursing

Aldosari, N., Pryjmachuk, S., & Cooke, H. (2021). Newly qualified nurses' transition from learning to doing: A scoping review. *International Journal of Nursing Studies, 113,* 103792. https://doi.org/10.1016/j.ijnurstu.2020.103792

American Association of Colleges of Nursing. (2021). *The essentials: Core competencies for professional nursing education.* https://www.aacnnursing.org/Portals/0/PDFs/Publications/Essentials-2021.pdf

American Medical Association. (n.d.). *What to look for in your first or next practice evaluate the practice environment to match your priorities.* https://edhub.ama-assn.org/steps-forward/module/2767098

American Nurses Association. (2019). *Principles for nurse staffing* (3rd ed.). https://www.nursingworld.org/practice-policy/nurse-staffing/staffing-principles/

American Nurses Credentialing Center. (n.d.). *Pathway to Excellence® sample interview questions.* https://www.nursingworld.org/globalassets/organizational-programs/pathway-to-excellence/resources/2020-pathway-to-excellence-sample-interview-questions-4.3.20.pdf

Bright Horizons. (2024). *Learn about tuition reimbursement for nursing.* https://www.brighthorizons.com/benefits/tuition-reimbursement-for-nursing.

Centers for Disease Control and Prevention. (2020). *Hospital employees' health.* Workplace Health Promotion. https://www.cdc.gov/workplacehealthpromotion/features/hospital-employees-health.html

Charette, M., McKenna, L., McGillion, A., & Burke, S. (2023). Effectiveness of transition programs on new graduate nurses' clinical competence, job satisfaction and perceptions of support: A mixed-methods study. *Journal of Clinical Nursing, 32*(7–8), 1354–1369. https://doi.org/10.1111/jocn.16317

Church, C. D., Schalles, R., & Wise, T. (2023). The newly-licensed registered nurse workforce: Looking back to move forward. *Nursing Outlook, 71*(1), 101904–101904. https://doi.org/10.1016/j.outlook.2022.11.008

Cotriss, D. (2023). *Keep it clean: Social media screenings gain in popularity.* Business News Daily. https://www.businessnewsdaily.com/2377-social-media-hiring.html

Google (2025a). *Create a Google alert.* https://www.google.com/alerts

Google (2025b). *Create a Google account.* https://accounts.google.com/

Grubaugh, M., Africa, L., & Neisinger, K. (2023). Managing the Current Workforce: Status of New Graduate Nurse Well-being and Clinical Development 2018-2021. *Nursing Administration Quarterly, 47*(3), 257–268. https://doi.org/10.1097/NAQ.0000000000000585

Handshake. (2024). *Salary negotiation tips for the entry-level applicant.* https://joinhandshake.com/blog/students/salary-negotiations-for-the-entry-level-applicant/

Hargreaves, J., & Pabico, C. (2020). How to choose your first nursing job wisely. *American Nurse Journal, 15*(5), 30–31. https://www.nursingworld.org/globalassets/organizational-programs/pathway-to-excellence/resources/how-to-choose-your-first-job-wisely.pdf

Healthcare.gov. (2024). *Federally qualified health center (FQHC).* https://www.healthcare.gov/glossary/federally-qualified-health-center-fqhc/

Internal Revenue Service. (2025, January). Employer shared responsibility provisions. https://www.irs.gov/affordable-care-act/employers/employer-shared-responsibility-provisions

Internal Revenue Service. (2024). *Retirement plans FAQs regarding 403(b) tax-sheltered annuity plans.* https://www.irs.gov/retirement-plans/retirement-plans-faqs-regarding-403b-tax-sheltered-annuity-plans

Jean, J. (2023). Ask a nurse: How do I negotiate a higher salary? *Nurse Journal.* https://nursejournal.org/ask-a-nurse/how-to-negotiate-a-higher-salary/

Joseph, H. B., Issac, A., George, A. G., Gautam, G., Jiji, M., & Mondal, S. (2022). Transitional challenges and role of preceptor among new nursing graduates. *Journal of Caring Sciences, 11*(2), 56–63. https://doi.org/10.34172/jcs.2022.16

Koh, C. S. L., Ong, K. K., Tan, M. M. L., & Mordiffi, S. Z. (2023). Evaluation of a graduate nurse residency program: A retrospective longitudinal study. *Nurse education today, 126,* 105801. https://doi.org/10.1016/j.nedt.2023.105801

Morris, G. (2023). 7 different types of nursing bonuses explained. *Nurse Journal.* https://nursejournal.org/articles/different-types-of-nursing-bonuses-explained/

Najafi, B., & Nasiri, A. (2023). Support experiences for novice nurses in the workplace: A qualitative analysis. *SAGE Open Nursing, 9,* 23779608231169212. https://doi.org/10.1177/23779608231169212

National Council of State Boards of Nursing. (2024). *Registration process: How to register to take the NCLEX.* https://www.nclex.com/register.page

Nurse Licensure Compact. (n.d.). *Information for new nurse graduates.* https://www.nursecompact.com/files/2018NewGradsFactsheetFINAL.pdf

O'Neill, S. P., Woodruff, K., Sanchez, C., & Zappas, M. P. (2022, February 9). Nurses and contracts. *American Nurse.* https://www.myamericannurse.com/nurse-and-contracts

Oritz, J. (2023). *10 mistakes to avoid with a job interview thank-you email.* U.S. News Careers. https://money.usnews.com/money/blogs/outside-voices-careers/slideshows/mistakes-to-avoid-on-a-thank-you-email?slide=13

Pension Benefit Guaranty Corporation. (2021). *What is a pension?* https://www.pbgc.gov/about/who- we-are/retirement-matters/post/2013/04/17/What-is-a-Pension

Post University. (2023). *Popular professional interview questions.* https://post.edu/blog/popular-professional-interview-questions/

Powers, K., Pagel, J., & Herron, E. (2020, July 20). Nurse preceptors and new graduate success. *American Nurse.* https://www.myamericannurse.com/nurse-preceptors-and-new-graduate-success/

Rush, K. L., Janke, R., Duchscher, J. E., Phillips, R., & Kaur, S. (2019). Best practices of formal new graduate transition programs: An integrative review. *International Journal of Nursing Studies, 94,* 139–158. https://doi.org/10.1016/j.ijnurstu.2019.02.010

Thompson, A. (2019). An educational intervention to enhance nurse practitioner role transition in the first year of practice. *Journal of the American Association of Nurse Practitioners, 31*(1), 24–32. https://doi.org/10.1097/JXX.0000000000000095

Uchmanowicz, I., Lisiak, M., Wleklik, M., Pawlak, A. M., Zborowska, A., Stańczykiewicz, B., Ross, C., Czapla, M., & Juárez-Vela, R. (2024). The impact of rationing nursing care on patient safety: A systematic review. *Medical Science Monitor, 30,* e942031. https://doi.org/10.12659/MSM.942031

UnitedHealthcare. (2024). *3 tips for choosing your health insurance plan through work.* https://www.uhc.com/understanding-health-insurance/open-enrollment/understanding-coverage/tips-for-choosing-a-health-insurance-plan

University of San Francisco. (n.d.). *Sample nursing interview questions and tips.* Priscilla A. Scotlan Career Services Center. https://myusf.usfca.edu/sites/default/files/default/Career_Services/nursing-interview-ques.pdf

U.S. Department of Labor. (2023, January 1). *Minimum length of meal period required under state law for adult employees in private sector 1.* https://www.dol.gov/agencies/whd/state/meal-breaks

U.S. Department of Labor. (n.d.a.). *Continuation of health coverage (COBRA).* https://www.dol.gov/general/topic/health-plans/cobra

U.S. Department of Labor. (n.d.b.). *FAQs about retirement plans and ERISA.* https://www.dol.gov/sites/dolgov/files/EBSA/about-ebsa/our-activities/resource-center/faqs/retirement-plans-and-erisa-compliance.pdf

U.S. News & World Report. (2024). *Registered nurse salary.* Careers. https://money.usnews.com/careers/best-jobs/registered-nurse/salary

Ward-Smith, P., Peacock, A., Pilbeam, S., & Porter, V. (2023). Retention outcomes when a structured mentoring program is provided as part of new graduate orientation. *Journal for Nurses in Professional Development, 39*(4), E75–E80. https://doi.org/10.1097/NND.0000000000000849

Weiss, T. (2024). *Hospitals turn to shorter work days, signing bonuses and student loan forgiveness programs to try to retain nurses.* https://www.worklife.news/talent/hospitals-turn-to-shorter-work-days-signing-bonuses-and-student-loan-forgiveness-programs-to-try-to-retain-nurses/

CHAPTER 3

The Impact of Leadership and Support

Lauren Jamieson, BSN, RN, RNC-NIC; Michelle M. Kelly, PhD, CRNP, CNE, FAANP, FAAN; and Linda Roney, EdD, RN-BC, CPEN, CNE, FAAN

Learning Goals

1. Examine Katherine's strengths and challenges in caring for a critically ill neonate as a new-graduate nurse.
2. Value the role of nursing leadership in supporting new-graduate nurses in their transition to practice.
3. Describe the typical nursing chain of command structure in healthcare organizations and outline the key responsibilities associated with each role.
4. Discuss common leadership styles in nursing and provide one example of each.

'You Do Not Know What You Are Doing.'

By Lauren Jamieson, BSN, RN

Katherine began her nursing career right after graduating college with a Bachelor of Science in nursing following the COVID-19 pandemic. These years of nursing school and exposure to the field of nursing during such a transformative time surely painted nursing and health care in a different light than she knew previously. Katherine felt intimidated by the shoes she had to fill but was simultaneously inspired to see different realms of a hospital work together and support one another, like family, during such a discouraging time with limited resources. How could a future nurse not feel empowered when 2020 was the International Year of the Nurse? This lit a fire inside of her, and she wanted a nursing career, which was everything she hoped it would be. Katherine used this fire to fuel her desire to shoot for the stars after college. With this determination, she now found herself living her dream life. Katherine was now a registered nurse in a neonatal intensive care unit (NICU) working at her dream hospital on the West Coast in sunny California.

Throughout nursing school, Katherine was able to understand how diverse nurses are and the many hats they wear. What makes a nurse, and what makes a good nurse? From advocating for their patients, coordinating different hospital disciplines, being a shoulder to cry on, cleaning rooms, supporting families, and doing their nursing duties to assess and administer medications. Nurses are the ones who know patients best; their role is extremely versatile, and the amount of times a day nurses have to shift gears into an abundance of roles is endless. When Katherine thought of what it meant to be a good nurse, she thought about interactions she had in the hospital and of her professors' examples and her own ideas of what this meant. Katherine felt inspired to go above and beyond the nurses' basic tasks described in the textbooks, to embody the professors whom she looked up to and the nurses she worked alongside, and to wear many hats. But what about being the nurse who encounters a problem not addressed in basic textbooks? What about when a problem arises, and there are no hard-and-fast guidelines like those in a health assessment exam? Katherine felt there were parts of nursing that students could not learn through a textbook; they could learn only through experience. A textbook can give students guiding principles or a foundation to build on. Katherine wished someone could have tried to relay the true nuances of nursing and how they are so much more than what is written on the page.

When Katherine graduated and sought jobs, she pursued her goal of working in a NICU. It is a unit that provides detail-oriented, meticulous care to critically ill premature and newborn babies. Months of training go into the job, and learning is always ongoing. Her selling pitch as to why she would be a great candidate for this job as a new-graduate nurse was that the best way to stay at the cutting edge of any field is to educate the next generation of leaders. Instead of only hiring experienced nurses, Katherine knew she was worth investing in and that she, too, could be a leader in the future to help develop nursing and neonatal care. She offered fresh eyes, a fresh perspective, and any knowledge she was taught about that patient population would be at the forefront of her brain. Her drive and determination to learn would help her to succeed, and she certainly felt supported by peers, preceptors, nursing educators, and management upon arrival.

Katherine started her new job and was concurrently supported through a new-graduate residency program that met monthly. She met with people from leadership in her unit every few weeks to see what progress was being made on orientation and what changes could be made, if any. There was frequent outreach from leadership. Katherine felt as if she had found her place within nursing; she was doing important work, and she could see she was making a difference in patients' and families' lives. Katherine took the time to get to know families and understand why they chose the name they did for their baby and why it was important to them. She saw miracles, some heartbreak, some of the most critically ill patients and participated in baptisms, and, of course, the joys of a first bath. Katherine felt she was built with a strong foundation of knowledge to succeed at her job, but it was impossible for her to be prepared to handle every complex case and situation with grace and poise. Katherine wished there was some way to prepare beforehand for the difficult times in nursing that inevitably come with the job and when working in an intensive care unit (ICU) and how to maintain these resilient qualities that she knew made a good nurse and helped put the patient first.

In working in an ICU, nurses are tasked with handling critically ill patients. Specifically, in a NICU, nurses are tasked with caring for premature and newborn babies who mean the world to the parents and would do anything to save their lives. The walls of a NICU have seen every emotion one could imagine, and the high-stress environment can lead to an uncharacteristic display of emotions both from family members and hospital staff.

Parents want answers; they want nothing more than for their child/children to get healthy, grow, and get out of the hospital. These stressful circumstances often elicit an array of emotions, panic, and lashing out. Nurses often have an all-encompassing role, and they tend to be at the bedside the most, thus taking the brunt of the emotions from the family. Healthcare teams always encourage patients and their families to speak openly, participate in treatment choices, and promote their child's safety by being well-informed and involved in care. Yes, it is a nurse's duty to be willing to work with the family, find answers, and put the patient first, but in no occupation is it okay to relinquish respect and safety in return. As Katherine started to experience these moments of high stress with families while coming off orientation and completing her nurse residency program, she did not feel the same sense of support from nursing leadership as she had upon her arrival on the unit. Katherine was having a hard time deciphering if this was a normal sense of independence within the nursing field and on her unit or if she was right to question her experience.

Katherine worked on July 4 and was taking care of an infant who presented with some challenges. The baby was in need of intravenous (IV) access. Earlier in the day, IV access was attempted by the nurses, the nurse practitioners, the physician assistants, and even the pediatric surgical team, who came to the unit to try and place an ultrasound-guided peripheral IV with no luck. Time was running out, and the baby desperately needed some access to administer IV medications, fluids, and nutrition. The physicians attempted to call the father at home to ask for his consent for his child to get a surgically placed central line. The father was not willing to speak with the providers and hung up on them. They called him back, and he asked them to stop calling him. They tried to explain the importance of the central line and how time-sensitive it was, but again, he said he would not consent until he arrived at the unit. It was uncertain of exactly what time he would arrive as he did not have his own source of transportation to the hospital.

The healthcare team did have issues with this father in the past, so everyone was aware of the potential challenges that could lie ahead. Upon the father's arrival to the NICU, the surgical team was immediately available as they had been waiting to obtain consent for this procedure. One stipulation the father made was that he would give consent for the placement of the central line in the operating room only if the surgeon could promise the central line would not be placed in an arm. The father did not give any rationale as to the reasoning. The surgeon relayed that he would do his best to try to meet this request, but if it was medically necessary and became the only viable site of access, he may have to place the line in the arm. The father was not happy with this answer but signed the consent and allowed the healthcare team to take his child to the operating room for surgery.

The surgery went well, and the baby got his central line. The team did end up having to place it in the arm, and the father immediately expressed his frustration to the entire healthcare team. Everyone was trying to reassure the father that this was best for his child in order to help keep him medically stable and allow him to continue to grow and develop. As the team brought the baby back to the NICU, the father felt that Katherine and the team were too calm with regard to the situation. The father felt the team's emotions were lax and without care. Katherine moved the baby back into his bed when he suddenly began to have oral secretions that needed to be suctioned. Katherine asked the father if she could move around him to get to the wall suction, to which he responded that he was appalled that Katherine would ever ask him to move away from his child. The father told Katherine, *"You cannot speak to me that way, and I will not move."*

Katherine felt frustrated in the moment but knew that her patient came first. If she did not suction her patient, he would surely decompensate. As she watched the secretions pool in the infant's mouth, Katherine went around the father and grabbed the Yankauer suction. The father did not appreciate how Katherine approached the situation and immediately said, *"You cannot be taking care of my baby; I want a new nurse. None of this is OK! You do not know what you are doing."* For Katherine, this was hard to hear. How did something so innocent, such as going to suction a baby in distress, escalate to this level? Katherine felt confused and angry at what occurred. The charge nurse became involved and talked with the father. The father again relayed that he did not want Katherine taking care of his child that day or ever and that the way Katherine spoke to the dad was unacceptable. That warranted the charge nurse to reach out to the manager on call since it was a holiday (July 4) and no one from nursing leadership was there in person that day. Since the father was extremely unhappy with the situation, there was a discussion about whether the nurse should switch assignments with only two hours left of her shift. There were still assessments to be done and fluids to be hung, but the nurse quickly did her work and then steered clear from the bedside. The father claimed he would not return to the bedside until Katherine was out of the building and off the unit. Patient safety was compromised that day, and from that day forward, nursing leadership set the precedent that Katherine could not take care of that particular baby.

The following day, Katherine had a baby right next to that bedspace, and once again the father was enraged that Katherine was even in the vicinity of him and his child and demanded that she be moved. Per management, Katherine was not allowed to take care of that baby or any baby in the surrounding beds. Management relayed that this was for Katherine's safety. Katherine felt she was being punished for something that she did not do. Katherine was missing out on the opportunity to care for babies just because management had appeased this father and tolerated his disrespectful behavior. Instead of speaking with the father, setting boundaries for him, and attempting to support Katherine, management chose to phrase it as if it were for her safety. The question stood with Katherine: *If this man was a true threat, should he have visiting restrictions or precautions in place?* She felt the team should not bend and allow this father to dictate who could and could not take care of his baby when all nurses on the unit were trained competent professionals. From that day forward, there was a list of five-plus nurses on the unit who were not allowed to take care of this father's baby.

These decisions and actions by management made Katherine question whether she was truly supported by leadership and whether her voice mattered. By trying to care for her patient and reach the suction canister on the wall, her day-to-day care at work was being compromised. Katherine felt as if her supervisors were looking for a simple solution to the problem at hand. It would be easiest to remove the problem from the situation and not allow Katherine to care for that baby or anyone within the surrounding bed spaces to hopefully avoid further problems. Katherine felt that what was done was not right and that the father's actions and words should be held accountable. Katherine felt walked over yet limited in her ability to speak for more support. The problem had made it up through the chain of command in her unit, but she was unsure of what more she could do. As days went by, she still had encounters with this father. Katherine now went about her day in the NICU, seeking to avoid all interactions, if possible, with this father in the hope of bypassing any conflict.

Katherine reflected on the scenario and wondered if she should have stood up for herself more; she wondered if there was more she could have done in order to get a different outcome from management and the father.

Katherine knew that she was a good nurse, her intentions were good, and this altercation did not degrade her ability to provide pristine nursing care. She hoped to learn from this scenario and find ways to support herself and other nurses. Katherine thought back to her reasoning for wanting to work in the NICU and how she originally emphasized the importance of the best way to stay at the cutting edge of any field is to educate the next generation of leaders. How could she have been a leader? If she had the opportunity, how could she have rewritten her story and found her voice for herself and all the other nurses on the list who were no longer allowed to take care of that baby? Although Katherine would not wish this problem to occur to any nurse, it allowed her to brainstorm solutions to help facilitate respect, safety, and support for herself and her colleagues in the workplace.

'Bad Examples Are Good Teachers.'

By Michelle M. Kelly, PhD, CRNP, CNE, FAANP, FAAN

Katherine's story highlights several issues that stem from decisions made without considering the ramifications of those decisions. Too often in life and in health care, we are tempted to take the path of least resistance rather than explore the path strewn with hurdles. A NICU care team is typically comprised of the attending physician, nurse practitioner, fellows or residents, nurses, therapists, pharmacists, social workers or case managers, as well the unit leadership of nurse manager, educator, or clinical nurse specialists. Each member of the team has a role in providing safe and appropriate care for the infant.

If we were to pull Katherine's story apart further, we may find that the NICU care team made the first set of mistakes. It is likely this situation could have been avoided from the start. Katherine's story describes difficulties the NICU team experienced with the family related to unresponsiveness. Why was a case manager or social worker not already involved with the family? A NICU admission is stressful for the family. It is likely that the father's behaviors stemmed from psychosocial stressors that were exacerbated by having a critically ill child in the NICU. A solid relationship with a social worker or case manager may have helped the team to set up clear expectations for the family around communication and unit procedures. The child was put at risk when the parent refused to discuss the needed procedures. Hospitals that care for infants and children have policies for when parents are unreachable and life-sustaining treatments are required. An unreachable parent should have triggered those policies.

Another missed opportunity lay in failing to explore the father's concern regarding the placement of the central line in an arm. This was a very specific concern and one that needed to be explored. Why was the location a trigger for the parents? Was it due to a bad experience for themselves or another family member? Fear of loss of function in the arm? Were the risks and benefits not explained to the parents in a way they could understand? Katherine describes a fully assembled care team waiting to obtain consent from the father for the central line placement. When the father voiced his concern, did the surgeon or any member of the team ask him why that site concerned him specifically? It may not have changed the reality of the placement, but by taking time to explore the concern, it may have been alleviated. While it was not in Katherine's scope to explain the surgical risks, perhaps Katherine could have advocated for the family, asking the surgeon or the NICU care team to take that pause to explore the father's concern. It is likely that the central line placement, coupled with being asked to move to allow Katherine access to the patient in that immediate postprocedural period, became the "straw that broke the camel's back," sending the parent into a spiral. Again, communication faltered, and Katherine took the brunt of the family's frustration.

The situation came to a head over the holiday when the regular unit management team was unavailable. That means that the manager covering for the holiday was likely from a different unit, unfamiliar with the nature of NICU care and the stress families experience. The covering manager may not have been familiar with NICU policies. The covering manager's decision to appease that father and remove Katherine from the care team likely seemed like the path of least resistance, but it ultimately worsened the situation. Unfortunately, that decision was not corrected by the regular unit leadership, and the parent was allowed to dictate how care was provided not just to his child but to the whole unit.

There are times when family personalities and the nursing care team do not mesh and when the best outcome is to avoid those pairings. When requests of that nature are made by a family or by nurses, the unit leadership team and the NICU care team should explain that the request will be considered in assignments but that patient and unit needs will be the priority. Allowing a parent to dictate not only who can care for their child but also who can care for the infants in surrounding bed slots resulted in putting the entire unit at risk. Parents are unaware of nurse skill sets, acuity, or needs of infants on the unit. This behavior cannot be tolerated and needs to be addressed in meetings between the NICU care team, the unit leadership, and the family. In my career, these situations have, at times, resulted in the transfer of care to another hospital, which truly may have been in the best interest of all involved.

Katherine was left feeling unsupported and alone. That is not the feeling any new or seasoned nurse should experience and especially not in a NICU, where team care is essential to care for the smallest and most vulnerable infants. Once in the situation, Katherine felt little could be done to change course. When evaluating this situation from my vantage as a neonatal nurse practitioner, I wonder where the voices of the seasoned nurses were. Why did they not talk to Katherine and assure her that this situation was not about her but about the family's stress and psychosocial issues? Where was the nurse educator or the clinical nurse specialist who should have supported her and the rest of the nursing staff? Should an ethics committee meeting be convened to discuss the ramifications of the family's demands on the infant and the rest of the unit?

I would like to tell Katherine that, unfortunately, this would not be the last stressed, frustrated family in her NICU. This encounter taught her how a similar situation should not be handled. Unfortunately, bad examples are good teachers. The reality of NICU nursing is that we see families at their very worst when the anticipated event, the birth of a healthy child, is disrupted by an early or complicated delivery. However, one of the greatest joys of being a NICU nurse is teaching a family to care for that vulnerable child, guide them through the unexpected journey, and see them take that child home. To share that joy, we must accompany the family on the journey. We must walk the path that is sometimes arduous and fraught with obstacles. But we do not walk that path alone. We walk it as a team, the NICU care team and the family, always keeping in mind that we all want the same thing. The best possible outcome for the infant and the family.

Providing care in an ICU—whether it is a pediatric intensive care unit (PICU), NICU, or adult ICU setting—requires a special level of skill, compassion, and grace. When I was a new direct care nurse in a PICU, I would have a run of tachycardia in the elevator on my way to the fourth-floor unit. *Would my skills be enough? Would I have the compassion and grace to not only care for the child but to provide the support the family needed as well?* As a neonatal nurse practitioner, that anxiety continued, and I found myself saying the following words when covering the unit at night. Maybe these words can help you, too, or perhaps they will inspire you to find your own prayer or mantra that brings you peace when you need it most. They became my talisman to guide me and remind me that we all need skills, compassion, and grace.

PRAYER OF THE NEONATAL NURSE PRACTITIONER

By Dr. Michelle Kelly

Please watch over the infants in my care.

Let me be prepared for whatever challenge they face.

Let no harm come to them, at my hands or through my omission.

See them all safely through the night.

Safety Does Not Happen by Accident

By Linda Roney, EdD, RN-BC, CPEN, CNE, FAAN

Katherine's situation presented tremendous challenges for her in so many different ways. Taking pride in developing competency in the many dimensions of her work as a NICU nurse, the interactions with this parent and her team's lack of support left her empty. With nearly half of all NICU parents reporting depression, anxiety, and posttraumatic stress during hospitalization and up to half of NICU nurses and neonatologists reporting burnout, babies' complex medical needs and families' desire for answers that are yet to come place tremendous pressures on NICU staff (Grunberg et al., 2022). Katherine felt the weight of this pressure. While the story's focus was on the experience that challenged her, there were countless other moments in her nursing career that we did not get to hear about where she was the person that the families on her assignments wanted to care for their critically ill neonates. Even in adversity, Katherine demonstrates aptitude in the American Association of Colleges of Nursing essentials' (2021) domains 2 and 10 competencies and subcompetencies.

TABLE 3.1 **Examples of Domain 2: Person-Centered Care and Domain 10: Personal, Professional, and Leadership Development in This Exemplar**

Domain 2: Person-Centered Care	
2.1 Engage with the individual in establishing a caring relationship.	Katherine took the time to get to know the families in the NICU and honored traditions and rituals for her patients.
2.2 Communicate effectively with individuals.	Despite a very challenging dynamic with one parent, there were likely many patients and families who benefited from Katherine's care while she worked in the NICU.
Domain 10: Personal, Professional, and Leadership Development	
10.2 Demonstrate a spirit of inquiry that fosters flexibility and professional maturity.	Katherine identified mentors to support her professional growth in her preceptors, peers, management, and educators.
10.3 Develop capacity for leadership.	Katherine prioritized the safe care of her patients, putting her feelings aside. She thoughtfully reflected on situations that challenged her, considering opportunities for improvement in the future.

Critical partnerships with family involvement, known as *family-centered care,* born out of the relationships that neonatal and pediatric nurses and their interdisciplinary healthcare delivery teams have with the parents and families of their patients, is now a standard of care across the age and care continuum. In family-centered care, nurses collaborate with patients and their families (as they define their family) to determine how they will participate in care and decision-making (Institute for Patient and Family-Centered Care, n.d.). As Michelle highlights in her response, the father's behaviors in Katherine's story likely stemmed from psychosocial stressors that were exacerbated by having a critically ill child in the NICU. In ideal situations, as the team informs, engages, and empowers the parents, a collaborative relationship is nurtured based on mutual rapport and trust (Umberger et al., 2018). This relationship of mutual respect did not exist, leaving Katherine feeling vulnerable, unsupported, and powerless.

Know Your Chain of Command

Before this challenging situation, Katherine felt supported by the nurses, educators, peers, and management of her unit, but something changed during this challenge. As Michelle wondered in her reflection, where were the senior nurses in the NICU to support her? Senior nurses can help new-graduate nurses by creating a good working environment for all of the nurses and adjusting to their unit (Gregg et al., 2023). While experienced nurses tend to converse with novice nurses about tasks, they also spend time giving advice and exchanging positive talk (Chao et al., 2021). It is unclear if there was a missed opportunity for senior nurses to coach and advocate for Katherine in nursing leadership. Technically, senior nurses are in lateral positions compared with novice nurses if they work in the same capacity as Katherine. Still, their involvement in the unit had the opportunity to positively affect the situation in this example.

Charge Nurse

The charge nurse became involved when the patient returned from the operating room and the father was upset. The charge nurse is a registered nurse on a shift assigned, usually among other staff members meeting established organization criteria, to manage the flow of day-to-day patient care on a specific unit for a particular shift, including coordination to cover sick calls and arising issues and serve as a liaison to management (Rogers, 2019). While it is not currently the dominant practice model, permanent positions for charge nurses and role-specific development may lead to enhanced skill and expertise related to consistency of performance and charge nurse functions (Spiva et al., 2020). While no national data set reporting charge nurse financial compensation, they typically receive a nominal hourly differential as payment for their additional roles.

Healthcare organizations determine the job description, policies, and compensation for the charge nurse role. Jubinville et al. (2023) described the five essential skills of the charge nurse: leadership; interpersonal communication; clinical-administrative caring; problem-solving; and knowledge and understanding of the work environment. Charge nurses have extensive responsibilities and must use effective communication, influence, delegation, and interpersonal relationship-building to execute essential tasks, often in high-pressure situations (Medero et al., 2023). Charge nurses can have a substantial impact on quality outcomes. They should inspire healthcare organizations to support their development in a caring manner instead of throwing them into complex roles without providing them with training to be effectual frontline managers (Breedlove et al., 2022). Only some charge nurses receive a formal orientation to the role; if they do, it is usually by a peer who is also unprepared for the position (Dols et al., 2021).

In Katherine's story, the charge nurse talked with the father. The father again relayed that he did not want Katherine taking care of his child that day or ever. The charge nurse called the manager on call since it was a holiday and no one from nursing leadership was there in person that day. It is not in a charge nurse's purview to make decisions that affect outside of their shift without consultation from the next level of nursing leadership. Especially in a setting where the charge nurse assignment rotates daily, conversations that lead the charge nurse to make exceptions or decisions in favor of the family but are not mindful not to what is fair, appropriate, or in alignment with hospital policy can have significant implications. If the charge nurse decided that the path of least resistance with this father was to remove Katherine from her assignment for the rest of the shift, they would be setting the team up for a highly troublesome situation. The charge nurse needed to talk with the manager.

Nurse Manager

For simplicity's sake, we will refer to the next tier in the leadership structure as the manager. However, it can include people with the titles of nurse supervisor, patient service manager, assistant nurse manager, nurse manager, unit manager, or head nurse (Rogers, 2019). This title can also be unique to your organization. Some of the responsibilities of a manager include the following: handling staffing issues, such as creating staff schedules; supervising nursing personnel, including oversight of training and disciplining; managing financial and human resources for their unit; overseeing operations; serving as a liaison between nurses, providers, and upper-organization management; tracking unit performance metrics and creating performance improvement plans; and ensuring that the unit aligns with the strategic goals and legal and safety practices of the organization (American Nurses Association [ANA], 2023). Nurse managers typically report to a supervising nursing leader and ensure customer-focused service on their unit (Agency for Healthcare Quality and Research, 2018). The nurse manager translates the culture and strategy of the organization to the unit (González-García et al., 2021).

Despite statements by professional organizations for graduate education for nurse managers, some nurses are appointed to these positions without formal training. Some organizations provide leadership development programs that target either nurse managers already appointed to positions or emerging leaders who are likely to seek nurse leader positions ranging from three months to one year in duration (Warshawsky & Cramer, 2019). The American Organization for Nursing Leadership (2024), the American Association of Colleges of Nursing (2024), and Press Ganey (2024) provide excellent, evidence-based offerings for manager education, as do many healthcare organizations. Some staff nurses are promoted to the manager role while individuals come to a new unit to offer leadership.

Some larger units with extensive staff rosters have more than one manager. There might be one manager and several assistant nurse managers, sometimes offering coverage on off-shifts. It is important to ask who your primary leadership contact on the unit is (i.e., whom you should go to first if you have an issue) and if you should approach different unit leaders with different issues. It is okay to ask if this needs to be clarified for you. As Katherine describes, leadership may divide holiday coverage on larger units among the unit leadership team. More minor issues that can wait until nonholiday time (e.g., you would like to request a day off on the next time block) should wait, and calls to nursing leadership on holidays should be reserved for larger-scale issues that cannot be solved without leadership's input. While a nurse manager's responsibility is typically 24/7 accountability, prioritize outreach for advice only when an adverse outcome might occur without their input. A challenge in these high-emotion, urgent situations is that some involved in the subsequent days might not want to go against the precedent already established with the patient or family for fear of increased conflict.

You will likely meet your nurse manager as part of your interview process. You need to consider whether their leadership style aligns with how you work. Table 3.2 presents common leadership style for nurse leaders. Leaders tend to have a dominant style, but given the many facets of the role, other styles need to be called into action. For example, suppose a manager needs to step into a clinical role during a patient code with new staff. In that case, they may lean toward an autocratic leadership style, assigning roles and responsibilities to safely complete the emergency's work. However, in a different situation, if the same manager has to make a significant decision that affects the entire unit and makes the decision alone, the team will not be happy with their decision. Cummings et al. (2018) found that leadership focused solely on task completion is insufficient, and relational leadership practices need to be encouraged and supported by individuals and organizations to enhance nursing job satisfaction, retention, work environment factors, and individual productivity.

TABLE 3.2 Common Leadership Styles in Nursing

Leadership Style	Description
Autocratic	• Makes quick decisions with little input from employees and delegates tasks (ANA, 2023) • Great in an emergency • Increases follower perceptions of leader ability by drawing on functional leadership (Rosing et al., 2022)
Democratic	• Collaborative and focuses on team success (ANA, 2024) • Decision-making duties and power are shared with followers (Rosing et al., 2022) • Leadership is most appropriate for achieving follower trust and consensus-building (Rosing et al., 2022)
Laissez-faire	• Hands-off; puts faith in the experience of the team (ANA, 2024) • Enables nurses to make independent decisions (Alsadaan et al., 2023) • In negative contexts, has been associated with leaders who avoid responsibility
Servant	• Feels called to serve in leadership role (Demeke et al., 2024) • Focuses on employee development and individual needs (ANA, 2023)
Situational	• Analyzes the situation and determines the appropriate approach • Flexible enough to modify their approach based on the organization's or individual's needs (ANA, 2023)
Transactional	• Focuses on the tasks of the job (ANA, 2023; e.g., submitting staff hours to payroll)
Transformational	• Relational leadership style that helps employees develop their strengths (ANA, 2023) • Has a positive effect on employee satisfaction, engagement, and performance • Leaders work together in teams to identify what needs to be done and creates a vision to realize it with the group (Gebreheat et al., 2023) • Makes a great mentor; has been associated with adverse patient outcomes (Ystaas et al., 2023)

The nurse manager's job is important to the team and the unit's outcomes. Highly engaged and competent managers have nursing teams who deliver higher-quality care, miss fewer nursing care events, and are more likely to stay in their current positions (Warshawsky, 2023). Strong nursing leaders also significantly impact safety and patient satisfaction (Nurmeksela et al., 2021). As part of the research for preparing this casebook, I interviewed nurse managers about the challenges in their role. Katie, a new manager for just over a year after 35 years of bedside nursing practice at another organization, described the most challenging part of her new role. She stated that she was challenged to advocate for bedside nurses in meetings that her staff would never know about, related to changes others within the health system would like to implement that might negatively affect nurses' workload, practice, or satisfaction with their role. Katie described the sense of responsibility for tirelessly representing her nursing team in ways that they would likely never be aware of.

In Katherine's experience, she did not feel supported by her nurse managers, despite feeling supported in the past. The shock of the treatment by this father and the lack of support that Katherine felt from the management team closed communication. While all the details were not included in this story, we have to wonder how Katherine received this news about not being allowed to take care of that baby and any baby in the surrounding beds "for her safety." Katherine felt she was being punished by management. Because of the power differential between the new nurse (Katherine) and nursing management, she likely did not feel comfortable approaching the leaders for an open conversation. This situation was so different from any that she had been in before.

Director of Patient Services/Nursing Director

While the exact time might vary by organization, a nursing director/vice president role is mainly administrative. The director oversees the clinical services within a specific department and manages the department's budget (Rogers, 2019). Nurse managers in a related specialty, sometimes called a *service line*, will often report to the same director. In larger organizations, there might be directors for many different service lines (e.g., maternal-child health, cardiovascular health, musculoskeletal services), and the directors typically report to a chief nursing officer. This person would be Katherine's manager's boss.

House Supervisor

During off-shifts, such as nights, weekends, and holidays, a house supervisor (who might have other names that vary by organization, including off-shift nursing leader or off-shift executive) has administrative responsibility for the activities during that shift. They have many responsibilities that might differ from shift to shift but can include handling emergent staffing and scheduling needs and on-call systems, overseeing interfacility transfers, and ensuring administrative leadership during emergencies (Rogers, 2019). On a holiday, the hospital may have had a house supervisor whom the charge nurse could have called to offer administrative support for the issues with the father. Some hospitals do not use this role and, in its place, have unit managers share call responsibility. This may have been the case in this situation.

Chief Nursing Officer/Director of Nursing Services

The chief nursing officer and, in some smaller organizations, director of nursing services, are the senior nursing professionals within a health system, health-related organization, or governmental body who oversee their system's nursing professional practice and leadership and serve as part of the senior executive leadership team (ANA, 2024). They are accountable for overall professional nursing practice across a healthcare organization and typically report to its president and chief executive officer (ANA, 2024). Multiple service lines and related support services are usually linked to the oversight of a vice president. In some organizations, the title of vice president is used interchangeably with that of chief nursing officer/chief nursing executive. This person is the highest-ranking nurse in the organization.

Other Supports

The nurse educator Michelle mentioned, during the first encounter with the father, Katherine or any of the other nurses could have called social work to support the father through this most difficult time. Protective services should have been alerted by the charge nurse and manager at least about the concern that the father posed a risk to Katherine's safety. It sounded like the situation escalated with the father at the bedside. Katherine asked an appropriate question: *If this man was an actual threat, should he have visiting restrictions or precautions in place?* Implementation of visitor restrictions should carefully follow hospital policies.

Psychological Safety

A critical concept in this case is Katherine's psychological safety. *Psychological safety* is the climate where individuals feel free to express relevant thoughts and feelings without excessive self-censorship (Hughes-Reese, 2017). It is a critical antecedent for bringing up problems and challenging issues, especially in healthcare settings where nurses are attuned to hierarchical norms and may find it difficult to challenge members of the team if they have a lower professional rank and lower status on the team (Weiss et al., 2023). Katherine likely did not feel a sense of psychological safety as a new nurse on the team, and the events were so different from her other experiences on the unit so far that this reinforced this concept. In all her experiences up to this point, she had felt supported by her superiors, had had regular check-ins, and had had positive relationships with her patients' families. A decision was made "for her safety," but she was left feeling anything but safe. Psychological safety is a critical concept for all new nurses, and we will go into greater detail regarding it in Chapter 5.

Challenging Interactions With Patients and Families

Are challenging families unique to neonatal and pediatric nursing? Absolutely not. Research indicates that 15%–60% of patients are considered problematic by their providers, noting that patient and family behaviors can include rudeness, verbal abuse, and offensive language as well as threats of physically aggressive behavior and acts of violence (Fiester & Stites, 2023). Few training interventions are designed to support nurses when families' bad behavior escalates despite evidence that dealing with complex family dynamics is frequently cited (Zaider et al., 2016). There can be relational difficulties within the family that existed before a patient's current health state, such as poor communication, varying goals of care, or concern about the welfare of a family member, that can be unrecognized by staff but can be very problematic (Zaider et al., 2016).

PRN (PLEASE READ NOW)

- Do you think the father's comments to Katherine were rude, offensive, or abusive?
- What might be signs that his emotions were escalating and Katherine and the rest of the NICU team were unsafe?
  - If this had happened, what should Katherine and her coworkers have done?

In Chapter 4, we will explore concepts related to workplace violence more deeply and include steps to keep yourself safer at work.

YOU MATTER: TRUST YOUR INSTINCTS

Nursing demands are high, and it is well-documented that our profession is at high risk for burnout and abuse. Your physical, emotional, and psychological safety is of primary importance. If you are ever in doubt about whether a situation is appropriate or not, consider reframing the situation and ask yourself, *If I was in a public area (e.g., a bank) and someone acted this way toward an employee, what would happen?* If your answer is that the behavior would not be tolerated, then you have your answer. It is time to report this through your chain of command. If you feel that you are in immediate danger, activate your organization's public safety/police protocol for immediate safety support.

Book Club Questions

1. Have you ever felt treated unfairly by a patient's family member? What happened?
2. Who are some role model nurse leaders you have encountered? What qualities do you admire about them?
3. How can effective communication within the nursing chain of command improve teamwork and enhance patient care? What have you seen in practice?
4. Describe a time you felt marginalized while in your nursing role. What happened? What was your response? Did your supervisor support you? How or how not?

About This Chapter's Authors

Lauren Jamieson, BSN, RN

Lauren received her bachelor's degree from Fairfield University's Marion Peckham Egan School of Nursing and Health Studies in 2021. She is a graduate student working on her Master of Science in Nursing in nursing education from the University of Connecticut, with completion in 2026. She has received her RNC-NIC, Neonatal Intensive Care Nursing Core Certification, as her background includes working at the bedside in a level-four NICU. She is a part of her unit's education committee. She serves as a delivery room lab instructor to educate new NICU nurses about their role while attending newborn and premature infant deliveries. Outside of work, Lauren enjoys spending time with her golden retriever, taking trips to the beach, and finding new recipes to cook.

Michelle M. Kelly, PhD, CRNP, CNE, FAANP, FAAN

Dr. Michelle Kelly is an associate professor at Villanova University's M. Louise Fitzpatrick College of Nursing. She is a dual-certified pediatric and neonatal nurse practitioner with 30 years of experience providing care to children of all ages. She is an advocate for promoting the health of those born preterm across the lifespan, particularly related to neurodevelopmental and educational outcomes. She is a fellow in both the American Association of Nurse Practitioners and the American Academy of Nursing.

References

Agency for Healthcare Research and Quality. (2018, July). The role of the nurse manager | agency for Healthcare Research and Quality. The Role of the Nurse Manager. https://www.ahrq.gov/hai/cusp/modules/nursing/index.html

Alsadaan, N., Salameh, B., Reshia, F. A. A. E., Alruwaili, R. F., Alruwaili, M., Awad Ali, S. A., Alruwaili, A. N., Hefnawy, G. R., Alshammari, M. S. S., Alrumayh, A. G. R., Alruwaili, O., & Jones, L. K. (2023). Impact of nurse leaders behaviors on nursing staff performance: A systematic review of literature. *Inquiry, 60*, 469580231178528. https://doi.org/10.1177/00469580231178528

American Association of Colleges of Nursing. (2021). *The essentials: Core competencies for professional nursing education.* https://www.aacnnursing.org/Portals/0/PDFs/Publications/Essentials-2021.pdf

American Nurses Association. (2023). *Charge nurse vs. nurse manager: What's the difference?* ANA Nursing Resources Hub. https://www.nursingworld.org/content-hub/resources/nursing-resources/charge-nurse-vs-nurse-manager/

American Nurses Association. (2024). *What is a chief nursing officer/chief nurse executive?* ANA Nursing Resource Hub. https://www.nursingworld.org/content-hub/resources/nursing-leadership/chief-nursing-officer/

American Organization for Nursing Leadership. (2024). *AONL transition to nurse manager practice programs.* https://www.aonl.org/education/ttpcourses.com/siteassets/amn-insights/surveys/amn-healthcare-rnsurvey-2023.pdf

Breedlove, D. W., Amiri, A., & Arris, L. (2022). Evaluating the efficacy of an evidence-based charge nurse professional development activity at a highly complex Veterans Affairs medical center. *Journal for Nurses in Professional Development, 38*(2), E19–E24. https://doi.org/10.1097/NND.0000000000000824

Chao, L. F., Guo, S. E., Xiao, X., Luo, Y. Y., & Wang, J. (2021). A profile of novice and senior nurses' communication patterns during the transition to practice period: An application of the Roter Interaction Analysis System. *International Journal of Environmental Research and Public Health, 18*(20), 10688. https://doi.org/10.3390/ijerph182010688

Cummings, G. G., Tate, K., Lee, S., Wong, C. A., Paananen, T., Micaroni, S. P. M., & Chatterjee, G. E. (2018). Leadership styles and outcome patterns for the nursing workforce and work environment: A systematic review. *International Journal of Nursing Studies, 85*, 19–60. https://doi.org/10.1016/j.ijnurstu.2018.04.016

Demeke, G. W., van Engen, M. L., & Markos, S. (2024). Servant leadership in the healthcare literature: A systematic review. *Journal of Healthcare Leadership, 16*, 1–14. https://doi.org/10.2147/JHL.S440160

Dols, J., Ramirez, M., Hernandez, A., Allen, D., Kloewer, T., & Aguillon, V. (2021). Impact of evidence-based charge nurse education on charge nurse skills and nurse-specific metrics. *Journal of Nursing Administration, 51*(12), 630–637.

Fiester, A., & Stites, S. (2023). Using a mediator's toolbox: Reducing clinical conflict by learning to reconceive the "difficult" patient or family. *Journal of Teaching and Learning Resources, 19*, 11324. https://doi.org/10.15766/mep_2374-8265.11324

Gebreheat, G., Teame, H., & Costa, E. I. (2023). The impact of transformational leadership style on nurses' job satisfaction: An integrative review. *SAGE Open Nursing, 9*, 23779608231197428. https://doi.org/10.1177/23779608231197428

González-García, A., Pinto-Carral, A., Villorejo, J. S., & Marqués-Sánchez, P. (2021). Competency model for the middle nurse manager (MCGE-Logistic Level). *International Journal of Environmental Research and Public Health, 18*(8), 3898. https://doi.org/10.3390/ijerph18083898

Gregg, M., Wakisaka, T., & Hayashi, C. (2023). Senior nurses' expectations and support of new graduate nurses' adjustment in hospitals: A qualitative descriptive study. *Heliyon, 9*(8), e18681. https://doi.org/10.1016/j.heliyon.2023.e18681

Grunberg, V. A., Vranceanu, A. M., & Lerou, P. H. (2022). Caring for our caretakers: Building resiliency in NICU parents and staff. *European Journal of Pediatrics, 181*(9), 3545–3548. https://doi.org/10.1007/s00431-022-04553-1

Hughes-Reese, M. (2017). *Magnet tip: Cultivating psychological safety at the unit level*. American Nurses Association. https://www.nursingworld.org/organizational-programs/ana-consultation-services/tips-articles-and-videos/cultivating-psychological-safety-at-the-unit-level/

Institute for Patient and Family-Centered Care. (n.d.). *Patient- and family-centered care.* https://www.ipfcc.org/about/pfcc.html.

Jubinville, M., Tchouaket, E. N., & Longpré, C. (2023). Scoping review protocol examining charge nurse skills: requirement for the development of training. *BMJ Open, 13*(2), e067307. https://doi.org/10.1136/bmjopen-2022-067307

Medero, K., Goers, J. & Makic, M. (2023). Evaluation of a charge nurse leadership development program. *Nursing Management, 54*(7), 22–30.

Nurmeksela, A., Mikkonen, S., Kinnunen, J., & Kvist, T. (2021). Relationships between nurse managers' work activities, nurses' job satisfaction, patient satisfaction, and medication errors at the unit level: a correlational study. *BMC Health Services Research, 21*(1), 296. https://doi.org/10.1186/s12913-021-06288-5

Press Ganey. (2024). *Supporting the nurses at the heart of your facility.* https://www.press-ganey.com/consulting/nursing-consulting/

Rogers, S. (2019). *Who's who on the nurse's corporate ladder?* ProMed Certification. https://promedcert.com/blog/whos-who-on-the-nurses-corporate-ladder/

Rosing, F., Boer, D., & Buengeler, C. (2022). When timing is key: How autocratic and democratic leadership relate to follower trust in emergency contexts. *Frontiers in Psychology, 13*, 904605. https://doi.org/10.3389/fpsyg.2022.904605

Spiva, L., Davis, S., Case-Wirth, J., Hedenstrom, L., Hogue, V., Box, M., Berrier, E., Jones, C., Thurman, S., Knotts, K., & Ahlers, L. (2020). The effectiveness of charge nurse training on leadership style and resiliency. *Journal of Nursing Administration, 50*(2), 95–103. https://doi.org/10.1097/NNA.0000000000000848

Umberger, E., Canvasser, J., & Hall, S. L. (2018). Enhancing NICU parent engagement and empowerment. *Seminars in Pediatric Surgery, 27*(1), 19–24. https://doi.org/10.1053/j.sempedsurg.2017.11.004

Warshawsky, N. (2023). *The impact of high-performing nurse managers across clinical settings.* Press Ganey. https://info.pressganey.com/press-ganey-blog-healthcare-experience-insights/the-impact-of-high-performing-nurse-managers-across-clinical-settings

Warshawsky, N., & Cramer, E. (2019). Describing nurse manager role preparation and competency: Findings from a national study. *Journal of Nursing Administration, 49*(5), 249–255. https://doi.org/10.1097/NNA.0000000000000746

Weiss, M., Morrison, E. W., & Szyld, D. (2023). I like what you are saying, but only if I feel safe: Psychological safety moderates the relationship between voice and perceived contribution to healthcare team effectiveness. *Frontiers in Psychology, 14,* 1129359. https://doi.org/10.3389/fpsyg.2023.1129359

Ystaas, L. M. K., Nikitara, M., Ghobrial, S., Latzourakis, E., Polychronis, G., & Constantinou, C. S. (2023). The impact of transformational leadership in the nursing work environment and patients' outcomes: A systematic review. *Nursing Reports, 13*(3), 1271–1290. https://doi.org/10.3390/nursrep13030108

Zaider, T. I., Banerjee, S. C., Manna, R., Coyle, N., Pehrson, C., Hammonds, S., Krueger, C. A., & Bylund, C. L. (2016). Responding to challenging interactions with families: A training module for inpatient oncology nurses. *Families, Systems & Health, 34*(3), 204–212. https://doi.org/10.1037/fsh0000159

CHAPTER 4

Incivility, Bullying, and Other Types of Workplace Violence

Anabelle Murphy, BSN, RN, CCRN; Maria Bautista Durand, MSN, APRN, FNP-C, CPNP-PC; and Linda Roney, EdD, RN-BC, CPEN, CNE, FAAN

Learning Goals

1. Describe Anabelle's strengths and challenges in her first nursing position.
2. Analyze descriptions of nursing interactions to identify potential signs of incivility or bullying.
3. Reflect on the four types of workplace violence (WPV) and identify ways to identify each.
4. Select characteristics that place a patient or visitor at greater risk for bringing violence against a nurse.

'I Felt That What Little Confidence I Had Built Up Was Wiped Clean.'

By Anabelle Murphy, BSN, RN, CCRN

I have been in intensive care for the entirety of my almost two-year nursing career. This is a statement with a lot of weight and typically a lot of judgment. For a long time, it was difficult and even frowned upon for new nurses to start in intensive care. This is a narrative that I am passionate about changing. Intensive care nursing is not for everyone, but those passionate about critical care nursing should be able to find and pursue a career that fulfills those passions. My passion for critical care came after a shadowing opportunity in high school, in a neuro intensive care unit (ICU) in which I would later work as a critical care tech. This allowed me to see how short life can be as well as the importance of appreciating the small things and taking advantage of our short time on Earth. I wanted to be a bright spot in our patients' hardest days while also receiving the opportunity to think critically and provide care to the whole person, including the family. One of my favorite things about being a critical care nurse is critically thinking about each patient individually and focusing on the "why" of each intervention being added to benefit the specific patient. There is so much variety in critical care; even when you think you've seen it all, there are opportunities to learn something new every shift.

As a new grad, I had a great opportunity to relocate to another region of the country to take a critical care nursing position at a world-renowned medical center. Many nurses before me had to fight tooth and nail to get into the ICU, and now some newer nurses don't have to "do their time" in other specialties before coming to the ICU. You have probably heard or even asked other nurses, *"Do I have to start in med-surg after graduation?"* I did not, and I want future nurses to know that you don't have to if that is not the type of nursing you want to practice. While I was a student nurse, I worked in the intensive care setting as a tech and later transitioned to a different hospital to work in intensive care when I became a nurse. I mention this change in hospitals because although it was my first nursing job, I had some awareness of what an ICU setting was like and was able to compare the energy and interactions between staff on both units. These observations grounded me in the fact that not all units are the same. A little bit more about me: I was a student-athlete in college, an excellent student, and I consider myself to be strong-willed and not afraid of conflict or not being liked.

The first unit I worked on as a nurse immediately following graduation was a transplant-surgical ICU. Surgical ICUs often have the reputation of being extremely task-oriented, attracting intense employee personalities, and frequently having to work with surgeons with extremely high expectations. Knowing these things did not drive me away from this unit; I had the chance to work with many high-acuity patients and see a variety of procedures that are once-in-a-lifetime opportunities. The nurses on this unit had various experiences, ranging from new-grad nurses to those with more than 20 years of experience. From the learning perspective of a new nurse, being surrounded by this level of experience was comforting. However, I quickly learned that some of the more experienced nurses weren't as supportive of the next generation of nurses and believed that you should suffer to learn how to "really" be a nurse. By no means was I expecting to be babied and hand-held through my new-grad days; however, I did not expect to be thrown to the wolves. For example, something unique to my unit was that each shift chose its assignments during the pre-shift huddle. This meant that the night-shift charge nurse (for me, it was when I had about one year of experience when I started rotating into this role) read through each patient with a brief summary of what was ahead during the upcoming shift. This included important drips, travel plans for procedures, and any other pertinent information such as code status and sometimes psychosocial and family information. It is beneficial for the unit staff to know a bit about all the patients if something happens while the primary nurse is at lunch or has stepped away. Anyway, after all the patients are read through and the night-shift charge nurse offers input on any complex assignment pairings or identification of patients with a high volume of tasks, it is up to the next shift of nurses to choose which patients they want. Sounds great, right? Great if you have seniority, that is. The registered nurse (RN) with the highest seniority picks their assignment first, usually leaving the new grad with the least experience to have the last pick, which is often a sick patient in precautions, a patient with many needs and complex family dynamics, or a patient with any number of reasons that a senior nurse might not pick them. This system has pros and cons; if you are a senior nurse, you will likely get the "best assignment" in the unit. However, on many occasions, I felt that this practice created hostility within the unit in several ways. For one, travel nurses always pick last after new grads, and preceptors with new nurses could override everyone else's choices and bump a nurse who was back from the previous day and wanted the same assignment. I have seen all of these scenarios and the vibe they can create in a unit for the day. I have been the new grad getting the worst assignment, and I have also been the slightly more experienced nurse getting bumped by an orientation assignment. It can lead to very unsafe scenarios, such as nurses fresh off of orientation getting a very sick patient whom they are not yet ready to care for independently. The argument can go either way: Sick patients are a great experience for growing new nurses, but sometimes these nurses are not yet equipped to handle an acute change by themselves, and a resource is not always available to help them.

This happened to me. There was a patient who was very sick, with a very contagious and stigmatized illness, on top of his significant ICU needs. Due to the infectious nature of the patient's underlying disease, many older nurses avoided this assignment. They claimed that certain nurses should not take it because of children or families at home. This led to the assignment falling on new grads consistently instead of establishing a fair rotation of the patient and fairer exposure. After taking this assignment for two days out of four, I went to my assistant manager and expressed my concerns about the assignment and my sincere care for the patient. The only solution the unit management offered me was to switch to one of the other units for the next shift rather than develop a fairer system for rotating this patient assignment. While this created a lot of stress for me at the time, I am grateful for some of the difficult patients and situations I encountered due to this assignment practice, as I believe they made me a better and more experienced nurse. On another shift, I was assigned a critically ill, long-term care patient and an open bed, meaning that I would likely be getting the next admission. I got an admission from the operating room who had desaturated to 14% during admission. We had the patient on our monitor but were switching from the transport ventilator to the room ventilator. Despite being surrounded by experienced nurses, I felt panicked over not knowing what to do. One of my coworkers started to ventilate the patient with the Ambu bag, and we recovered the oxygen saturation to 100% with adequate sedation and ventilation. Being new, it took me longer than it now does to complete all the admission tasks and ensure that I provided adequate care to my other patients.

I was behind in my work for most of the night, could not take a lunch break, and had to stay after my shift to finish my charting. I gave report to a more senior nurse at shift change. There were things that I had missed, such as giving 2 grams (g) of magnesium instead of 4 g for a magnesium level of 1.6. Our unit protocol was to replace electrolytes overnight based on lab values drawn with midnight labs. This wouldn't be considered a med error, but per the order protocol, the patient needed 2 g more than I had already given. I offered to hang the additional bag of magnesium before I left at the end of my shift, but the oncoming nurse declined my offer. She educated me on the importance of electrolyte replacement at the bedside, and I assumed that that was all she could do. When I returned the following night, she advised me on a few additional things I had missed from the previous shift. What I did not know until a few nights later was that she had written an *anecdotal* on all of the things that I had missed about which she had already educated me at the bedside. An anecdotal in our unit would be the equivalent of getting written up. It is not necessarily a safety or event report but a note from RN to RN that is discussed with management and goes into your employee file. One of those things was that my turns had been charted incorrectly, and she assumed that I did not turn the patient during my shift. She did not consider that I could have made a mistake in the charting during the chaos of my shift. This frustrated me because I thought she was supporting my learning as a new nurse and was not transparent about writing the incident up without my knowledge.

I took what she said, and it made me into a very hyperaware, anxious, and almost neurotic nurse for every shift after that. I felt that what little confidence I had built up was wiped clean. I felt like every nurse on my unit was out to get me (except that they weren't). When I reflect on this event, it still frustrates me. Yes, I learned from it and became even more detail-oriented and careful in the care of my patients, but it also felt like a personal attack to show that she had more power over me because she was an experienced nurse. The assistant nurse manager was the one to review this anecdotal with me. He even told me, off the record, that it was done to prove that she was senior to me. While I had heard about nurse bullying in nursing school classes, this felt like my first introduction to this negative practice. I was led to go about the rest of my shifts in fear of my coworkers. Nurses share many similar qualities, such as being perfectionists, high-achieving, goal- and detail-oriented, kind, and caring and having the desire to be liked and be part of a group. The desire to be liked is not specific to nursing, and the range of stress and emotions we encounter can create a toxic work environment. Humans as a whole want so much to be liked by other people; whether they are "cooler" or more experienced, they will do almost anything to gain the approval of others. This can be seen in lateral bullying, which is mean to younger coworkers because they haven't found their place yet or won't fight back out of fear of your experience. I have also seen this in break rooms during lunch: Coworkers gossip about their coworkers, some of who may even be out on the floor that day. It lowers the morale of the entire unit when people speak so negatively about others. Although these experiences I have described are not ones I would wish on anyone else, it has allowed me to take extra time in my workday to offer help to my coworkers, especially newer nurses, and avoid speaking poorly of my colleagues or participating in that type of gossip to make friends.

With all that being said, you might feel hopeless or fearful about your future nursing job. Please do not worry. I share this because I wish I had known about this when I was looking for my first nursing position. While I wish horizontal and lateral violence never happened in nursing, it is important to note that this is not the case on every unit. After so many negative work experiences had altered my outside life, I leaped to find a new job, hoping that changing hospitals would lead me to positive, non-cliquey units just like all of my friends claimed to be working in for their first positions. *And I was successful.* I love my current job in critical care nursing. My one piece of advice here is to feel the vibes of the unit culture rather than choosing a job for the title or prestige of the hospital. It can feel risky and nerve-wracking, but growth happens outside of your comfort zone, and sometimes taking the leap to a job or a place you are unsure about is the thing you need the most. I know it did for me.

'How Does It Feel to Be Stupid Again?'

By Maria Bautista Durand, MSN, APRN, FNP-C, CPNP-PC

Anabelle is a *warrior* who has overcome many challenging situations early in her nursing career. I commend her strength and perseverance in not giving up on our profession. Anabelle's experiences demonstrate her attempt to make the best of the situation and learn from it.

You may have heard the unfortunately familiar saying that *nurses eat their young.* I have been a nurse for way too long, and I can't recall when I first heard this statement, whether it was in nursing school in the 1990s or when I started my first nursing job. The saying reminds me of belonging to a *sorority* or *fraternity* of nursing in your unit or hospital. There is a time when hazing occurs for the new nurse, whether they are a new-graduate nurse or just a new nurse to the unit. Like a rite of passage to the nursing culture of the unit. This concept of hazing in nursing brings a hostile, stress-inducing, nonproductive, and dangerous environment to the nursing unit. This is not an environment where a new-graduate nurse can learn and thrive. According to Tradewell (1996), the rite of passage begins when the new-graduate nurse enters the organization and transitioning from being a nursing student to adapting as a new nurse to the hospital setting begins. This rite of passage is crucial in forming the new nurse's identity in their nursing unit and organization. It can only be a positive experience for the new-graduate nurse if there is support built in by the organization's leadership to foster an easy transition.

The organization's top leadership must know this potential "hazing" phenomenon for these vulnerable new-graduate nurses and the importance of establishing resources to support them and their supervisors/managers. Exposure to a work environment that is highly stressful and does not provide support from leadership or colleagues can create a negative foundation for workplace bullying among nurses. This unpleasant environment can lead to emotional distress, amongst many other psychological symptoms, which can cause adverse effects that could possibly lead to burnout or leaving the work environment (Galanis et al., 2024). Galanis mentions the concept of compassion satisfaction, which is a positive idea for the nurse's mental health. Strengthening cooperation and good working relationships enhances compassion satisfaction (Galanis et al., 2024). The organization should be aware of this concept and create programs that foster this idea to prevent burnout and nurses leaving the work environment.

When I compare my first new-graduate job with Anabelle's, there are differences between our experiences. Her first job was in a transplant-surgical ICU. ICUs are typically viewed as high-stress units due to the nature of the patient population admitted to these units. These patients are the *sickest of the sick*. In most of the cases, *time is of the essence* for these patients. The nurse needs to be knowledgeable about everything related to their patient, whether that is changes in lab values, vital signs, or physiological. Prompt identification of these changes with their ICU patient is crucial to the patient outcome, adding additional stress to their workday. Studies have shown that nurse bullying is more likely to occur in high-stress settings (Edmonson & Zelonka, 2019).

In comparison, my first nursing job was on a medical-surgical ward with mainly surgical patients. The patient population for the unit was primarily stable surgical patients. The unit was relaxed and nonstressful and had a sense of community. There was a mix of seasoned nurses who had been there for 20-plus years and nurses with fewer than 10 years of experience. When I started, I was one of two new-graduate nurses. We were the *newbies,* but we both felt welcomed. I felt a sense of belonging to the unit. We were included in conversations, potlucks, and unit outings. New-graduate transition programs did not exist when I started nursing. I was fortunate to have a supportive preceptor available to me to reach out to with any questions or concerns. My preceptor later became a mentor after I finished orientation. There was a sense of community in the unit. Everyone helped each other out regardless of who you were. I would feel comfortable asking another nurse about a patient's situation, medication, or treatment. It did not matter if the nurse was not my assigned preceptor. I looked forward to coming to work, meeting new patients, and learning new things. It was not a stressful environment. Do not get me wrong—I also had my share of challenging patients, but I had my community of nurses to contact for help and advice. My transition from nursing student to new nurse was a positive experience.

In contrast, Anabelle did not have as positive of a transition experience as I did. The older nurse's mentality that you should suffer to learn how to be a nurse suggests that they believe new nurses need to do their time and learn from their negative experiences or mistakes. This practice is the rite of passage for their unit. These nurses support the theme of nurses eating their young. I am sure these veteran nurses had the same negative experience when they were new nurses. They experienced a lack of support and had to figure things out the hard way. The idea of passing on suffering is never a good theme for the unit. It is already stressful enough to start working in a new position, plus adding the responsibility of caring for a sick patient can push someone over the edge. This stressful environment does not allow the new nurse to transition into the profession smoothly but places barriers for them to grow. Ultimately, it can contribute to patient safety issues, nurse burnout, and stress.

Fast-forward 25 years. I have my advanced practice RN degree. My first nurse practitioner (NP) job was in a pediatric orthopedic practice. I experienced another great transition from bedside nurse to advanced practice nurse. Again, there was a sense of community, a feeling of being welcomed, and support where I could reach out to any provider for help. Eventually, I left this practice to return to the hospital where I started my nursing career. This same hospital was where I'd felt welcomed and a sense of belonging. This next NP job was in the trauma program, part of the pediatric surgery division. I looked forward to coming back and seeing my old friends and colleagues. The patients I would care for and manage would be on the unit where I used to work as a bedside nurse. Seeing my old friends and colleagues in my old nursing unit was like a reunion. They were welcoming and incredibly supportive toward me. I imagined my transition would be seamless because I was already an experienced NP and knew most of the people I would interact with. I would only need to learn the idiosyncrasies of the pediatric trauma population.

Well … my first day with my new pediatric surgery NP group was not what I had imagined. At the time, there were four NPs in the department, and their experience ranged from five to 20-plus years. The NP with 20-plus years of experience approached me while I was reading a pediatric surgery textbook and asked me, *"How does it feel to be stupid again?"* and then laughed and walked back to her desk. I was dumbfounded and could not reply to her. One of the other NP colleagues heard this, wanted to remove me from the situation, and asked me to take a lunch break with her. Not knowing her purpose, I told her that I had already eaten. She asked me to go to lunch with her again and lightly grabbed my arm, and we walked out together. This colleague of mine was my support person in this new job and has become my confidant. She told me not to mind that coworker and that she was like that to her and every new NP who starts in the department. You must prove yourself to her. Prove your knowledge and competence. Learn things on your own, like she did 20-plus years ago. Here is the mentality of nurses: *They eat their young.* I could not believe that this was happening to me after all these years. I was a seasoned RN and an experienced NP but a "new" pediatric surgery NP. I survived the *hazing* with the support of the other three NPs in the department. After some time, this seasoned NP engaged with me and shared some of her knowledge and tips, and I can now call her a friend and colleague. Going through this hazing process made me learn that I would never want another individual to go through that process. My other NP colleagues and I have changed the culture in our department. We offer a nurturing and welcoming environment where anyone can ask a question and no question is a dumb one.

As a student nurse, you may have come from experiencing a nurturing environment where you felt supported while you were in school. During your nursing program, you may have had fellow students, friends, colleagues, and professors to lean on and assist you. During your clinical rotations, you may have felt supported by your clinical instructors and the staff nurses on the unit. When you were caring for your assigned patients, you could rely on these people for help and guidance. Negative experiences, as Anabelle describes, are a culture shock for them during their transition from student nurse to novice new-graduate nurse. Maybe some of you were unable to build these positive relationships while in nursing school. If this is your situation, I encourage you to be open to finding a confidant at your workplace. This person could be your "preceptor" or fellow nurse colleague with whom you feel comfortable sharing experiences. If you do not have a person at work, share your experiences with family or friends outside of work. It is always better to share your experiences with someone to gain an outsider's perspective who can offer support and advice.

Receiving positive feedback, getting life lessons, and having the opportunity to teach give individuals a sense that they are valued and that someone is investing in them, which can bring a sense of worth. Anabelle's situation of not correcting her patient's electrolyte imbalance per the protocol and the nurse coworker teaching her at the bedside about the importance of replacing electrolyte imbalance and other pertinent clinical information made her feel valued until she heard from management. Anabelle thought this coworker was investing in her as a nurse colleague and that she could be someone to confide in and turn to for support. Unfortunately, this was not the case.

Power and politics can take many forms in the workplace. Leaders should be exemplary and model positive behavior so that their staff can thrive. The unit's culture can be reflective of the leaders who are managing. The behaviors that occur can be a trickle-down effect from the top. Anabelle mentions an example when she had to discuss her write-up with a unit leader, and the conversation was far from offering support to her but rather offering excuses that accepted the negative behavior. This leadership style is not ideal and can damage the person and unit; therefore, in my opinion, it should be eliminated.

Anabelle's new-graduate experiences were negative situations that did not support her transition from student to new-graduate nurse. Her challenges did not help build her self-esteem or promote her sense of importance and competence. These qualities are vital in transitioning from student to new nurse and foundational in building workplace self-confidence. Anabelle rose above these challenges and found a place to thrive and grow professionally. Like Anabelle, do not be discouraged if you are in a similar negative situation. I believe that you can turn a negative situation into a positive learning experience. Knowing the circumstances that occurred to you, be the change agent if the opportunity arises. Be the nurse leader you would want to have. Know that there is always light at the end of the tunnel, yet it may not be where you are. Take notes, reach out to a mentor or friend to talk with, and know that you are a valued person and are worthy!

That's Not Just the Way They Are; They Are a Bully.

By Linda Roney, EdD, RN-BC, CPEN, CNE, FAAN

The desire to be accepted and included implies that a person wants to belong to one's environmental or social group (Patel et al., 2024). This is true for nurses when they select a place of employment and want to feel part of the team. Key concepts to create a sense of belonging in nurses have been studied and described to include the perception of being part of the team, having a connection to the community, and feeling trusted, valued, and accepted (Patel et al., 2024). As we consider the theory of marginalization as it applies to the experience that Anabelle describes, it was clear that she felt marginalized, meaning "casting aside of groups that are considered 'other' within society" (Pratt & Fowler, 2022, para. 2). How can this be? Nurses aim to protect, promote, and optimize the health of their patients, preventing illness, facilitating healing, alleviating suffering, and advocating for the care of individuals and families (American Nurses Association [ANA], n.d.). How could nurses treat their coworkers this way?

Even in adversity, Anabelle demonstrates strength and aptitude in the American Association of Colleges of Nursing essentials' (2021) domains 2 and 10 competencies and subcompetencies.

TABLE 4.1 **Examples of Domain 2: Person-Centered Care and Domain 10: Personal, Professional, and Leadership Development in This Exemplar**

Domain 2: Person-Centered Care	
2.3 Integrate assessment skills in practice.	Anabelle developed a robust assessment skill set to care for a complex, critically ill patient load.
2.6 Demonstrate accountability for care delivery.	Anabelle stated, "One of my favorite things about being a critical care nurse is critically thinking about each patient individually and focusing on the 'why' of each intervention being added to benefit the specific patient."
Domain 10: Personal, Professional, and Leadership Development	
10.2 Demonstrate a spirit of inquiry that fosters flexibility and professional maturity.	Anabelle reflected on her experiences and stayed committed to her professional growth. She explored and pursued new opportunities that were a better fit for her.

The discussion of WVP may make it seem like it is about "us" (the team) versus "them" (the patient, the visitors, or an authorized individual), and, as we will discuss later in this chapter, that is sometimes the case. Another harsh reality is that nurses can encounter WVP from other healthcare team members. *Incivility* is "one or more rude, discourteous or disrespectful actions that may or may not have negative intent behind them" (ANA, 2024a, p. 2). These can range from subtle belittling to overt hostility (Alsadaan et al., 2024) and include rudeness, excessive competitiveness, social exclusion, inaction, and other forms of disrespect (Pattani et al., 2018). Incivility can be rude and discourteous actions, gossiping and spreading rumors, and refusing to assist a coworker (ANA, 2015). It can be from another nurse or any other healthcare team member.

Bullying entails repeated, unwanted, harmful actions intended to humiliate, offend, and cause distress in the recipient and often involves a misuse of power, creates feelings of defenselessness and injustice in the target, and undermines an individual's rights (Edmonson & Zelonka, 2019). It may be directed from the top down (employers against employees), from the bottom up (employees against employers), or horizontally (employees against employees; ANA, 2015). In the situations that both Anabelle and Maria describe, they encountered workplace incivility and, for Anabelle, possibly bullying. Organizational factors related to incivility among healthcare providers include departmental silos, poor leadership, a culture of silence, and the existence of power cliques (Pattani et al., 2024). Bullying is more likely to occur in high-stress settings with high-stakes outcomes, heavy workloads, and low job autonomy (Edmonson & Zelonka, 2019).

The *culture of silence* refers to the inability of leaders to recognize, acknowledge, and confront incivility (Pattani et al., 2024) and bullying (Edmonson & Zelonka, 2019). Where were the leaders in the situation Anabelle describes?

Where were the informal leaders on the unit, other staff nurses with more experience, who could have stepped up to support her? We do not hear about them, but it is clear that Anabelle channeled the leader within to advocate for herself. She reports that when she needed a break from the highly contagious, high-stakes patient assignment, her manager offered only to float her to a different unit for relief. When she discussed the "anecdotal" with management, he told her off the record that the nurse did this to prove she was "senior" to Anabelle.

Edmonson and Zelonka (2019) state that workplace bullying requires the right environment to thrive. Supervisors and managers who lead by intimidation and fear tend to foster the same in their staff. Nurse managers have some of the highest-pressure positions in health care and lack authority in all situations, yet have a high level of accountability. Bad managers often adopt a leadership style modeled by toxic supervisors in the past, which tends to intensify under pressure. When bullying becomes part of an organization's culture, these behaviors persist, even as individual nurses come and go (Edmonson & Zelonka, 2019). I have even seen it persist when there is a change in leadership, but nothing had been previously documented, and now, on top of being a leader in a new area, they are creating a case to support staff against the toxic behaviors of a bully.

Root causes of incivility can stem from issues outside of personality. They may be signs of burnout, depression, or other stresses (Pattani et al., 2024). Bullying is more likely to occur in high-stress settings with high-stakes outcomes, heavy workloads, and low job autonomy (Edmonson & Zelonka, 2019). The workload Anabelle describes was heavy, and patients were gravely ill, but that is no excuse. The culture Anabelle worked in for her first position did not do enough to stop staff from feeling marginalized.

On an employer level, there are many things that the manager, senior leadership, and organization need to focus on preventing and intervening in relation to workplace incivility and bullying, which we will touch on later in this chapter. However, the focus of this casebook is to help you develop the tools to address this situation if you are in it as an RN. In its position statement on incivility, bullying, and WPV, the ANA (2015) identifies the Workplace Bullying Institute (WBI)'s (ANA, 2024b) three-step action plan as a resource for nurses to address bullying. First, you must recognize the behavioral signs of workplace bullying, including verbal abuse, exclusion, intimidation, undermining of work, and unfair treatment. It must be consistent to be considered bullying. If you believe this is happening to you, you need to keep a detailed record of the bullying behavior, including the dates and times it occurred and any witnesses during the interaction. You want to assess for patterns in your notes to ensure that the behavior is a repeated pattern and not an isolated incident (WBI, 2024).

Next, if you feel safe in doing so, address the bully and ask them to stop their behavior using "I" statements, such as "*I feel uncomfortable when you make comments about my work.*" Tell the bully that their behavior is not OK with you and must stop immediately. If you feel uncomfortable addressing the bully, speak with a colleague or human resources (HR) to help you develop a plan to address the person. Speak up early and follow your organization's internal policies that address workplace incivility and bullying (WBI, 2024). After you have reported it, be sure to ask your supervisor to provide feedback on how the situation was handled (WBI, 2024).

What do you do if you feel you are not being listened to by your supervisor when you share that you have experienced workplace incivility or bullying? They may respond as the assistant manager did to Anabelle, acknowledging that the person was using their experience on the unit to marginalize her. However, regardless, Anabelle felt that she must have done something to deserve to be treated this way (and although those may have been her feelings, she did nothing to deserve this).

Following are potential responses to give your supervisor if they minimize or tell you things like *"that is just the way they are"*:

- Do you think that it is OK for the person to treat me this way?
- The Joint Commission (TJC) and the ANA state that employers must address workplace incivility and bullying concerns to ensure safe working environments.
- I am asking you to address the behaviors of [insert person's name] and not ignore them. Do you need more from me to help you address their behaviors?

Document the summary of your conversation as an email to your supervisor following your meeting. If they do not commit to taking action immediately, it is time to go to HR or—in the cases where you might have a relationship—your manager's supervisor.

Workplace incivility costs are high, directly affecting nurse well-being while indirectly affecting patient outcomes through reduced care involvement and worsening care quality (Alsadaan et al., 2024). Anabelle shared with us that she left that unit and found happiness and a positive work environment in another ICU at a different medical center. Her decision to leave her first position was a costly loss to the employer. Orienting a new-graduate nurse can cost up to $96,000 (Perron et al., 2019). Finding nurses to replace those who leave takes a lot of time; in 2023, the average time to fill an open critical care nurse position with an experienced nurse in the United States was 99 days. With a 19.4% annual turnover rate in critical care, the financial and staffing impacts are tremendous (NSI Nursing Solutions, 2024). If you face a similar situation and are not finding a resolution that improves your working conditions, leaving and finding a new position as Anabelle did might help you work in a setting where you are better appreciated and valued.

Violence Is Not Part of the Job

So much of your time in nursing school is focused on learning to provide nursing care to your patients without significant preparation focused on keeping you physically and emotionally safe at work. It is sometimes beyond our comprehension that we could be injured while caring for others. Many join the nursing profession because of deep compassion for others and then find it heartbreaking to learn that WPV is a common occurrence that nurses must face (ANA, 2024a). The stories that Anabelle and Maria share are examples of lateral violence, one of the four types of WPV that nurses can encounter in the healthcare setting.

Healthcare workers are five times more likely than employees in other fields to experience WPV (U.S. Bureau of Labor Statistics [BLS], 2024). Violence can occur in any healthcare setting, but it occurs most often in emergency department (EDs), psychiatric units, geriatric/long-term care units, and waiting areas (Centers for Disease Control and Prevention, 2024). One in four nurses report having been physically assaulted (ANA, 2022). For something so common in the workplace, we do not start talking about it soon enough in nursing programs. As nurses, we need to adopt a zero-tolerance policy for WPV directed toward ourselves and our coworkers and to normalize reporting all incidents of WPV that occur in clinical settings to eliminate the current phenomenon of underreporting WPV events. Song et al. (2021) reported that nurses may not report WPV if they perceive the aggressive behavior to be unintentional—that is, related to patient illness—or if it was nonphysical violence, often believing that dealing with WPV is part of being a nurse and that if they reported it, nothing would change. These findings align with the continued narrative of marginalization in nursing—that nurses do not matter. This change needs to happen now and with all of us.

TJC revised the standards of employer responsibility related to preventing WPV effective in 2022 (TJC, 2021). As part of these standards, hospitals must conduct an annual analysis of their WPV prevention program; establish processes for continually monitoring, internally reporting, and investigating WPV; and provide training, education, and resources to address prevention, recognition, response, and reporting of WPV (TJC, 2021). Verbal abuse is the most common type of WPV that nurses encounter. Jeong and Kim (2018) found that 17.3% of nurses had been verbally abused once a day by their patients and 15.9% by patients' families, with 61% reporting that WPV had a direct impact on their intention to leave their job and 97.2% of participants having endured WPV but not reporting it. WPV directly affects nurses' intention to leave their current position as well as their job satisfaction (Stafford et al., 2022).

According to the National Institute for Occupational Safety and Health (NIOSH; 2024), there are four types of WPV: type 1: criminal intent violence; type 2: client violence; type 3: worker-on-worker violence; and type 4: personal relationship violence. In type 1 WPV, known as *criminal intent violence*, the offender has no legitimate relationship with the business or its employees, and it is usually a crime of violence (NIOSH, 2024). An example of this would be the devastating case of visiting nurse Joyce Grayson, who was murdered in the home of a patient where she was providing nursing care (Collins, 2024). Regarding type 2 WPV, *client violence*, the client is the most common type of violence in healthcare settings where patients, their family members, and visitors commit an act of violence on a healthcare worker (NIOSH, 2024). An example of this was when a gunman entered a medical building with an AR-15–style semiautomatic rifle, targeting a specific surgeon who treated him and killing two physicians, a patient, and a hospital employee (Hanna & Watts, 2022).

Type 3 WPV, *worker-on-worker violence*, also known as *lateral or horizontal violence*, can range from verbal and emotional abuse to homicide (NIOSH, 2024). The cases that Anabelle and Maria describe are examples of type 3 WPV. In type 4 WPV, *personal relationship violence*, the attacker has a violent relationship outside of the workplace that affects the work environment (NIOSH, 2024). While we will focus on types 1 through 3, some of the strategies might help address personal relationship violence in the workplace. If you or someone you care about is a survivor of domestic violence and needs support, please contact the National Domestic Violence Hotline at 1-800-799-SAFE (7233), text "START" to 88788, or access the hotline's live chat and additional resources on its website (https://www.thehotline.org/get-help/).

The BLS (2024) reports that nearly three-quarters of violence-related workplace injuries in the United States are to healthcare workers. The incidence of WPV is very high in units caring for older adults and children or laboring and postpartum women, psychiatric units, and emergency rooms (Cheung et al., 2017). Verbal abuse, sexual harassment, and physical abuse are common (Liu et al., 2019). More than 80% of nurses report that they have experienced at least one type of WPV act in the past year (National Nurses United, 2024). This number should not be tolerated in any profession, especially in nursing, where the goal of our profession is to help others. WPV has serious implications for both the nurse and the organization as it is directly related to increased job stress, absenteeism, burnout, sleep disorders, post-traumatic stress disorder, fear, and suicide (Kafle et al., 2022). Healthcare organizations have deployed strategies to protect staff and prevent nurses from violence by offering training sessions focused on de-escalating violence to build a culture of safety (Crisis Prevention Institute [CPI], 2024); installing panic buttons, locks, and metal detectors; screening visitors by hospital security; adding flags to the electronic medical record alerting staff to past violent events; implementing one-on-one monitoring; and promoting the use of tools for assessing violence risk level (McCollum et al., 2024).

Security Personnel

Healthcare organizations offer security personnel to protect patients, staff, visitors, and assets (Shongwe et al., 2023). This can be seen in a recent national survey, where 21% of hospitals employed police officers and 72% employed nonsworn security personnel (Saadi & Ray, 2023). Also, law enforcement officers may interact with patients and clinicians in the hospital, such as in the ED, when someone under arrest seeks medical care, investigates crimes, and provides security, which averages about one-third of the time, and interacts with about 2% of the patients, as noted in a study at one urban trauma center (Alur et al., 2022).

What Can You Do?

Your employer will offer you annual training, usually in the form of online modules, to ensure compliance with TJC standards related to WPV. Some employers also offer additional training to nurses and other healthcare workers in high-risk areas such as the ED and psychiatric units. If training is available to you, take it. As nurses, we are trained to provide holistic, patient-centered care, and many of the skills to keep ourselves and our healthcare environments are not intuitive.

De-Escalation

The CPI (2022) created 10 de-escalation tips, which are as follows. Nurses can use these to respond to defensive behavior to avoid a physical confrontation with someone who has lost control of their behavior:

1. Be empathetic and nonjudgmental. Take the time to listen, and wait to come up with a response.
2. Stand at least 1.5 to 3 feet away from a person who is escalating to give personal space; this tends to decrease a person's anxiety.
3. The more a person loses control, the less they hear your words and the more they react to your nonverbal communication. Be mindful of your gestures, facial expressions, movements, and tone of voice.
4. Remain calm, rational, and professional.
5. Watch and listen carefully for the person's real message about their feelings and offer supportive words in response.
6. Ignore challenging questions and redirect focus on how to work together to solve the problem.
7. Set limits with short, clear, and enforceable limits.
8. If you can offer a person options and flexibility, you may be able to avoid unnecessary altercations.
9. Give the person a chance to reflect on what is happening in silence so that they can determine what they will do next.
10. When a person is upset, they may be unable to think clearly. Allow time for decisions.

Source: CPI, 2022.

Know Safety Procedures in Your Work Area

Most clinical settings have a process for alerting coworkers, and you may need help with an escalating patient. While some units have discretely placed panic alarms that directly call protective services, other areas might have workplace modifications that offer the same resource. For example, in some healthcare settings, computer workstation keyboards are labeled with the exact combination of keys to press if a staff member feels unsafe and needs protective services immediately. After the combination of keys is set, an immediate alert is sent to protective services with the location of the call for help.

In all clinical situations, whether or not you sense they can escalate to WPV, patients and their visitors should never block your access to the door or exit. When you walk into a patient's room and feel that you do not have complete and unencumbered access to the door, politely make the modifications so that you have clear and immediate access to the door at all times with no one and nothing in your way. Nurses often work in tight spaces, and Katherine's story describes her difficulty navigating to access the suction to clear the secretions from her patient's airway. Also, keep your pathways to emergency equipment clear as much as possible. Heavy equipment and excessive supplies not in use should not be kept in patient care areas as they can be thrown at or used to hurt you. Healthcare settings usually have specific guidelines around patient visitors, but there are times when those limits are waived—for example, with the death of a patient. As nurses, we know the importance of having loved ones around in difficult times, but in many settings in which we work, we may witness strong emotional reactions to bad news. Any time you make an exception as the nurse to allow more visitors than usual, especially during a tragic time, alert protective services to be on standby, and if you feel the situation may warrant it, ask them to be physically present on the unit outside of the room. They are trained to keep our environments safe. In these interactions that might be high-stress and emotional, be sure to speak briefly and clearly, with clear limits (e.g., "You may have five people in the room. If someone else comes and wants to visit you, someone will have to swap out with them."). Manage expectations with all patients and families up front, and always lean toward decisions that will keep you and your coworkers safe if things escalate.

#EndNurseAbuse (ANA, 2024)

While there are times when a security officer is present to protect staff, there are many times when, because of the care they provide, nurses are alone with patients and visitors who can hurt them. #EndNurseAbuse is the ANA's campaign to prevent WPV (ANA, 2024b). Approximately two nurses per hour are assaulted in the acute care setting, resulting in an average of 57 assaults per day in the United States (Press Ganey, 2022). These data are based on what is reported; it is estimated that only 20%–60% of incidents are reported (ANA, 2024b).

More still needs to be done. In 2022, TJC's new revised WPV prevention standards were enacted. WPV is now defined as:

> an act or threat occurring at the workplace that can include any of the following: verbal, nonverbal, written, or physical aggression; threatening, intimidating, harassing, or humiliating words or actions; bullying; sabotage; sexual harassment; physical assaults; or other behaviors of concern involving staff, licensed practitioners, patients, or visitors. (TJC, 2021, p. 1)

TJC's Workplace Violence Prevention Standards apply to hospitals, including critical access hospitals, behavioral health care, and human service organizations (TJC, 2021). Table 4.2 summarizes these new standards and how they affect you if you work as a new nurse. The new requirements underscore WPV as an organizational issue that necessitates a systems approach (Arnetz, 2022). This is a tremendous paradigm shift that new nurses should understand. If something happens and a new nurse encounters WPV, it is not their fault and reflects a system failure. Abuse is never your fault (ANA, 2024b).

TABLE 4.2 Workplace Violence Prevention Standards and the New Nurse

The Joint Commission Standard	Why the New Nurse Should Care About This
Standard EC.02.01.01: The hospital manages safety and security risks. EP 17: The hospital conducts an annual worksite analysis related to its WPV prevention program. The hospital takes actions to mitigate or resolve the WPV safety and security risks based upon findings from the analysis.	The hospital should share information with the new nurse and the entire staff about what steps they take annually to address and mitigate WPV and security risks at the enterprise level.
Standard EC.04.01.01: The hospital collects information to monitor conditions in the environment. EP 1: The hospital establishes a process(es) for continually monitoring, internally reporting, and investigating the following (that relate to WPV): • Injuries to patients or others within the hospital's facilities • Occupational illnesses and staff injuries • Incidents of damage to its property or the property of others • Safety and security incidents involving patients, staff, or others within its facilities, including those related to WPV	The new nurse should be generally aware of the steps that the hospital takes to monitor for WPV, how to report WPV and issues of property damage due to violence, and who is part of the investigation team if something is reported. Transparency in this process supports a culture of safety.

(Continued)

TABLE 4.2 **(Continued)**

The Joint Commission Standard	Why the New Nurse Should Care About This
Standard HR.01.05.03: Staff participate in ongoing education and training. EP 29: As part of its WPV prevention program, the hospital provides training, education, and resources (at time of hire, annually, and whenever changes occur regarding the WPV prevention program) to leadership, staff, and licensed practitioners. The hospital determines what aspects of training are appropriate for individuals based on their roles and responsibilities. The training, education, and resources address prevention, recognition, response, and reporting of WPV as follows: • What constitutes WPV • Education on the roles and responsibilities of leadership, clinical staff, security personnel, and external law enforcement • Training in de-escalation, nonphysical intervention skills, and physical intervention techniques, and response to emergency incidents • The reporting process for WPV incidents	New nurses and other staff should be aware of what their ongoing training regarding WPV prevention. When possible and if appropriate to the client population, new nurses should have the opportunity to practice nonphysical intervention skills, physical intervention techniques, and response to emergency incidents in simulation. This regular training should also include what are the types of events that should be reported and how to do so. WPV is underreported, and only through accurate reporting can healthcare environments become safer.
Standard LD.03.01.01: Leaders create and maintain a culture of safety and quality throughout the hospital. EP 9: The hospital has a WPV prevention program led by a designated individual and developed by a multidisciplinary team that includes the following: • Policies and procedures to prevent and respond to WPV • A process to report incidents in order to analyze incidents and trends • A process for follow-up and support of victims and witnesses affected by WPV, including trauma and psychological counseling, if necessary • Reporting of WPV incidents to the governing body	New nurses and other staff should be aware of and have access to the information included in the policies and procedures at their organization to prevent and respond to WPV. This regular training should also detail the types of events that should be reported and how to do so. All staff should be aware of how to access trauma and psychological counseling, if necessary, following a WPV event. Following a WPV event, if counseling services are not offered, the new nurse should know that they are entitled to this support and how to advocate for this.

Nonetheless, nurses should be prepared to address this in the work setting. In some settings, nurses may have to deal with aggressive patients daily, whereas in others, it is a less common occurrence. Your work setting should provide you with training that includes strategies and tools to recognize aggressive patients in your practice setting, de-escalation models, and interventions for defusing aggression (TJC, 2019).

New nurses need to use situational awareness, assess the presence and purpose of individuals, survey the environment, and recognize clues for escalating behaviors (ANA, 2024b). Table 4.3 presents patient- and visitor-related risk factors for WPV. Even though it could potentially take more time, work with a buddy in situations where a patient has the potential to be aggressive (ANA, 2024b), and always have a position close to the door of the room. Do not ever let the patient or visitor come between you and the room's exit. Be aware of objects that can potentially be used to hurt you in the room, and have them removed before you enter. I consider this with each new patient encounter, whether it is at the beginning of my shift and I have just received report or at each transition of care where I receive a new patient.

If the objects cannot be removed due to their role in your patient's treatment, put distance between the patient and their access to the item.

If you sense a patient is escalating as you start a procedure or other activity requiring concentration, stop what you are doing and ensure your safety. Threatening comments by a family member as you are about to start an intravenous line on your patient, such as *"You'd better get this on the first shot, or else,"* do not contribute to your success or focus. Even when I have heard these comments from a parent, I remove the tourniquet, ensure my position of safety, and use my tools to de-escalate the situation. If the comments worsen and I sense that I am potentially in an unsafe setting, I

TABLE 4.3 **Patients', Visitors', and Unauthorized Individuals' Risk Factors for Workplace Violence**

Demographics	• Male • Lower education • Higher social status
Low impulse control	• Mental disorders • Influence of drugs and/or alcohol • Poor treatment adherence
Personality	• Style of control and dominance
Experience	• Poor previous experience • Patient dissatisfaction • Unexpected/high cost of services • Legal cases • Patient death
Additional considerations	• Complex family • Too many or no visitors • Siblings and spouses

Source: Based on Kumari et al., 2020.

remove myself from the room. If the patient's condition does not permit me to leave and the visitor—perhaps even a parent—threatens my or my team's safety, I ask security to speak with and remove them so that I can continue my important work. Please refer to your employer's policies and education about what to do if you encounter an escalating or violent patient or family member.

One final comment about encountering violence in the workplace: Your priority is to remain safe. I mention this as there have been times when I have seen violent acts at work, and I felt an intense need to keep my patient safe. As caregivers, we naturally want to help, but that does not mean we put ourselves in harm's way. We do not have the advanced training that security and police officers have regarding rescuing someone from a violent situation. Let me give you an example. A few years ago, I was walking onto the unit at the beginning of my shift and saw a man forcing a woman against the wall with a knife to her throat as their newborn lay supine on the bedside cot. While the baby was not safe, at that exact moment, the man was threatening the woman was turned away from the infant, and my hospital's safety protocol was to push the panic button so that the security team could intervene in the situation. They came to the floor in less than 60 seconds, restrained the aggressor, and removed him from the unit. We were then able to attend to the infant and her mother. I do not want to imagine what could have happened if we did not follow protocol.

PRN (PLEASE READ NOW)

Policy Matters

In April 2021, H.R. 1195, the Workplace Violence Prevention for Health Care and Social Service Workers Act, was passed by the U.S. House of Representatives and then went to the Senate as S. 1176, where it was sent to the Senate's Committee on Health, Education, Labor, and Pensions and introduced to the Senate in 2023 (S. 1176—Committee on Health, Education, Labor, and Pensions 118th Congress, 2023–2024). This bill would require the U.S. Department of Labor to address WPV issues by setting standards that employers would have to protect workers from WPV. Nurses should care about this act because it calls for enhanced safety measures, prioritizes violence prevention, and offers a nationwide federal standard for WPV prevention. As of March 2025, the bill remains in the Senate Committee on Health, Education, Labor, and Pensions, where it was referred after introduction. No further legislative action has been reported since its referral to the committee. In June 2022 during the 117th Congress, the Safety From Violence for Healthcare Employees Act (SAVE) Act was introduced in Congress to protect hospital personnel from violence. The SAVE Act would make assault on healthcare workers a federal crime. In the 118th Congress, the SAVE Act was reintroduced into both chambers (House, H.R. 2584, and Senate, S. 2768). Also as of March 2025, the SAVE Act remains under consideration in both the House and Senate. The American Hospital Association continues to urge Congress to pass this legislation to ensure healthcare workers' safety at protection levels currently offered to flight crews, flight attendants, and airport workers (American Hospital Association, 2024).

YOU MATTER: STAYING SAFE AT WORK

When you go to work each day with a passion for caring for others, incidents of WPV can catch you completely off guard. You have learned to identify the signs that need action in this casebook and throughout your nursing education. Trust your instincts when you sense something is wrong, and consult outside resources for support. All nurses have the fundamental right to feel safe at work. This includes psychological safety. Nursing demands are high, and it is well documented that our profession is at high risk for burnout and abuse. Your physical, emotional, and psychological safety is of primary importance. If you are ever in doubt about whether a situation is not appropriate, consider reframing the situation and ask yourself, "*If I was in a public area (e.g., a bank) and someone acted this way toward an employee, what would happen?*" If your answer is that it would not be tolerated, then you are experiencing WPV. It is not part of your job description to tolerate any forms of WPV. Be proactive about keeping yourself, your coworkers, and others in your practice area safe, because you matter.

Book Club Questions

1. After reading this chapter, what is your definition of feeling safe at work? What would you do if you did not feel safe?
2. Have you ever witnessed or experienced incivility or bullying in the workplace? Is there anything you would change in your response to the bully today?
3. Are there ever circumstances in which it is OK for patients or visitors to direct violence toward you and other members of the healthcare team? How would you keep safe?
4. You report feeling bullied by your preceptor to your nurse manager, bringing documentation of the dates, events, and names of witnesses. They tell you to "grow up" and not be so sensitive. What are your next steps?

About This Chapter's Authors

Anabelle Murphy, BSN, RN, CCRN

Anabelle is originally from the East Coast, south of Boston. She graduated from Fairfield University's Marion Peckham Egan School of Nursing and Health Studies in 2022. Her nursing career started as a critical care tech in a neuro ICU in Boston, where she fell in love with the critical thinking and complexity of the intensive care patient population. After finishing nursing school, she moved to Cleveland to work in a transplant-surgical ICU. After a year-and-a-half there, she obtained an Adult Critical Care Registered Nurse (CCRN) certification and transitioned to a level one trauma-surgical ICU. Outside work, Anabelle enjoys lifting weights at the gym, reading, and discovering new coffee shops.

Maria Bautista Durand, MSN, APRN, FNP-C, CPNP-PC

Maria's nursing career began more than 20 years ago when she worked as a Children's Hospital Los Angeles (CHLA) staff nurse on a surgical unit. After she received her NP degree in 2011 from Azusa Pacific University, she worked in a pediatric orthopedic practice, specifically in orthopedic trauma. Her current position is at CHLA as the hospital's trauma NP, a position in which she started working in 2015. She is an active member of several pediatric trauma professional organizations, such as the Society of Trauma Nurses, and is currently serving as the clinical director at large. She is also an active member at the Pediatric Trauma Society. She has presented at national conferences and has multiple publications in pediatric trauma. Her passion for teaching led her to join Azusa Pacific University and the University of California, Los Angeles, School of Nursing as a faculty member in the school's Advanced Practice RN programs. Maria has been married for 22 years. She has a son, a daughter, and two dogs. She enjoys the outdoors, traveling, and trying new food places.

References

Alsadaan, N., Ramadan, O. M. E., & Alqahtani, M. (2024). From incivility to outcomes: Tracing the effects of nursing incivility on nurse well-being, patient engagement, and health outcomes. *BMC Nursing, 23*(1), 325. https://doi.org/10.1186/s12912-024-01996-9

Alur, R., Hall, E., Khatri, U., Jacoby, S., South, E., & Kaufman, E. J. (2022). Law enforcement in the emergency department. *JAMA Surgery, 157*(9), 852–854.

American Association of Colleges of Nursing. (2021). *The essentials: Core competencies for professional nursing education.* https://www.aacnnursing.org/Portals/0/PDFs/Publications/Essentials-2021.pdf

American Hospital Association. (2024, October 31). Advocacy issue: Save act: AHA. Advocacy Issue: SAVE Act. https://www.aha.org/advocacy/advocacy-issues/2024-10-31-advocacy-issue-save-act

American Nurses Association. (2015). *American Nurses Association position state-ment on incivility, bullying, and workplace violence.* https://www.nursingworld.org/globalassets/practiceandpolicy/nursing-excellence/incivility-bullying-and-work-place-violence--ana-position-statement.pdf

American Nurses Association. (2022, April 21). Workplace violence in nursing. Workplace Violence in Nursing: Dangerous & Underreported. https://www.nursingworld.org/practice-policy/work-environment/end-nurse-abuse/workplace-violence/

American Nurses Association. (2024a). *Unreported workplace violence. Why is this so common?* https://www.nursingworld.org/content-hub/resources/workplace/unreported-workplace-violence---why-is-this-so-common/

American Nurses Association. (2024b). *Workplace violence/#EndNurseAbuse.* https://www.nursingworld.org/practice-policy/work-environment/end-nurse-abuse/

American Nurses Association. (n.d.). *Nursing: Scope and standards of practice* (4th ed.). https://www.nursingworld.org/practice-policy/scope-of-practice/

Arnetz, J. E. (2022). The Joint Commission's new and revised workplace violence pre-vention standards for hospitals: A major step forward toward improved quality and safety. *Joint Commission Journal on Quality and Patient Safety, 48*(4), 241–245. https://doi.org/10.1016/j.jcjq.2022.02.001

Centers for Disease Control and Prevention. (2024, May 16). *Common reasons for workplace violence.* Common Reasons for Workplace Violence. https://wwwn.cdc.gov/WPVHC/Nurses/Course/Slide/Unit3_6

Cheung, T., Lee, P. H., & Yip, P. S. F. (2017). Workplace violence toward physicians and nurses: Prevalence and correlates in Macau. *International Journal of Environmental Research and Public Health, 14*(8), 879. https://doi.org/10.3390/ijerph14080879

Collins, D. (2024). *Employer of visiting nurse who was killed didn't protect her and should be fined, safety agency says.* Associated Press. https://apnews.com/article/connecticut-visiting-nurse-killed-5cc5b9ebf6a68df638fe00ff2243cbb2

Crisis Prevention Institute. (2024). *CPI training for health care facilities.* https://www.crisisprevention.com/industries/health-care/

Crisis Prevention Institute. (2022, June 8). CPI's top 10 de-escalation tips revisited. CPI's Top 10 de-escalation tips revisited. https://www.crisisprevention.com/blog/general/cpi-s-top-10-de-escalation-tips-revisited/

Edmonson, C., & Zelonka, C. (2019). Our own worst enemies. The nurse bullying epi-demic. *Nursing Administration Quarterly, 43*(3), 274–279. https://doi.org/10.1097/naq.0000000000000353

Galanis, P., Moisoglou, I., Katsiroumpa, A., & Mastrogianni, M. (2024). Association between workplace bullying, job stress, and professional quality of life in nurses: A systematic review and meta-analysis. *Healthcare* (Basel, Switzerland), *12*(6), 623. https://doi.org/10.3390/healthcare12060623

Hanna, J., & Watts, A. (2022, June 2). *Gunman who killed 4 at Oklahoma medical building had been a patient of a victim, police chief says.* CNN. https://www.cnn.com/2022/06/02/us/tulsa-hospital-shooting-thursday/index.html

Jeong, I. Y., & Kim, J. S. (2018). The relationship between intention to leave the hospital and coping methods of emergency nurses after workplace violence. *Journal of Clinical Nursing, 27*(7-8), 1692–1701. https://doi.org/10.1111/jocn.14228

Kafle, S., Paudel, S., Thapaliya, A., & Acharya, R. (2022). Workplace violence against nurses: a narrative review. *Journal of Clinical and Translational Research, 8*(5), 421–424.

Kumari, A., Kaur, T., Ranjan, P., Chopra, S., Sarkar, S., & Baitha, U. (2020). Workplace violence against doctors: Characteristics, risk factors, and mitigation strategies. *Journal of Postgraduate Medicine, 66*(3), 149–154. https://doi.org/10.4103/jpgm.JPGM_96_20

Liu, J., Gan, Y., Jiang, H., Li, L., Dwyer, R., Lu, K., Yan, S., Sampson, O., Xu, H., Wang, C., Zhu, Y., Chang, Y., Yang, Y., Yang, T., Chen, Y., Song, F., & Lu, Z. (2019). Prevalence of workplace violence against healthcare workers: A systematic review and meta-analysis. *Occupational and Environmental Medicine, 76*(12), 927–937. https://doi.org/10.1136/oemed-2019-105849

McCollum, M., Garcia, J., & Lesandrini, J. (2024). Empowering nurses in an era of workplace violence. *Nurse Leader, 22*(3), 251–257. https://www.nurseleader.com/action/showPdf?pii=S1541-4612%2823%2900360-9

National Domestic Violence Hotline. (2024). *Need help now? We are here for you.* https://www.thehotline.org/get-help/

National Institute for Occupational Safety and Health. (2024). *Types of workplace violence.* https://wwwn.cdc.gov/WPVHC/Nurses/Course/Slide/Unit1_5

National Nurses United. (2024, February 5). *NNU report shows increased rates of workplace violence experienced by nurses* [press release]. https://www.nationalnursesunited.org/press/nnu-report-shows-increased-rates-of-workplace-violence-experienced-by-nurses

NSI Nursing Solutions. (2024). *2024 NSI national healthcare retention and RN staffing report.* https://www.nsinursingsolutions.com/documents/library/nsi_national_health_care_retention_report.pdf

Patel, S. E., Varghese, J., & Hamm, K. (2024). Defining a sense of belonging in nursing—An evolutionary concept analysis. *Journal of Professional Nursing, 54*, 151–163. https://doi.org/10.1016/j.profnurs.2024.07.003

Pattani, R., Ginsburg, S., Mascarenhas Johnson, A., Moore, J. E., Jassemi, S., & Straus, S. E. (2018). Organizational factors contributing to incivility at an academic medical center and systems-based solutions: A qualitative study. *Academic Medicine, 93*(10), 1569–1575. https://doi.org/10.1097/ACM.0000000000002310

Perron, T., Gascoyne, M., Kallakavumkal, T., Kelly, M., & Demagistris, N. (2019). Effectiveness of nurse residency programs. *Journal of Nursing Practice Applications & Reviews of Research, 9*(2), 48–52.

Pratt, A., & Fowler, T. "Deconstructing bias: Marginalization." The NICHD Connection. *Eunice Kennedy Shriver National Institute of Child Health and Human Development*, National Institutes of Health. 13(145):6. June 2022.

Press Ganey. (2022, September 8). *On average, two nurses are assaulted every hour, new Press Ganey analysis finds.* https://www.pressganey.com/news/on-average-two-nurses-are-assaulted-every-hour-new-press-ganey-analysis-finds/

S. 1176—118th Congress (2023–2024): Workplace Violence Prevention for Health Care and Social Service Workers Act. (2023, April 18). https://www.congress.gov/bill/118th-congress/senate-bill/1176

Saadi, A., & Ray, V. E. (2023). Police violence in health care settings in US media coverage. *JAMA Network Open*, 6(11), e2342998. https://doi.org/10.1001/jamanet workopen.2023.42998

Shongwe, L., Hanft-Robert, S., Cossie, Q., Sithole, P., Roos, T., & Swartz, L. (2023). Role of security guards in healthcare settings: A protocol for a systematic review. *BMJ Open*, 13(5), e069546. https://doi.org/10.1136/bmjopen-2022-069546

Song, C., Wang, G., & Wu, H. (2020). Frequency and barriers of reporting workplace violence in nurses: An online survey in China. *International Journal of Nursing Sciences*, 8(1), 65–70. https://doi.org/10.1016/j.ijnss.2020.11.006

Stafford, S., Avsar, P., Nugent, L., O'Connor, T., Moore, Z., Patton, D., & Watson, C. (2022). What is the impact of patient violence in the emergency department on emergency nurses' intention to leave? *Journal of Nursing Management*, 30(6), 1852–1860. https:// doi.org/10.1111/jonm.13728

The Joint Commission. (2019, January 28). *Quick safety issue 47: De-escalation in health care.* https://www.jointcommission.org/resources/news-and-multimedia/newsletters/ newsletters/quick-safety/quick-safety-47-deescalation-in-health-care/

The Joint Commission. (2021). *R3 report issue 30: Workplace violence prevention standards.* https://www.jointcommission.org/standards/r3-report/r3-report-issue-30-workplace-violence-prevention-standards/

Tradewell, G. (1996). Rites of passage: Adaptation of nursing graduates to a hospital setting. *Journal of Nursing Staff Development*, 12(4), 183–189.

U.S. Bureau of Labor Statistics. (2024). *Injuries, illness and fatalities.* https://www.bls.gov/ iif/factsheets/workplace-violence-2021-2022.htm

Workplace Bullying Institute. (2024, May 18). *Action plan.* https://workplacebullying. org/action/

CHAPTER 5

Together We Thrive

Building Stronger Teams for Greater Impact

Bridget Morrissey, BSN, RN; Sean Elwell, DNP, RN, NE-BC, TCRN, EMT; and Linda Roney, EdD, RN-BC, CPEN, CNE, FAAN

Learning Goals

1. Define *psychological safety* and explain how it applies to the situation described by Bridget.
2. Compare traditional communication models with the *CUS Tool* in addressing concerns within healthcare settings.
3. Appraise the benefits to the team when using the model "How to Get Straight A's as a Coworker."
4. Distinguish the hierarchy and roles of the medical team in a healthcare setting.

'He Said WHAT?'

By Bridget Morrissey, BSN, RN

When I was 22, I was hired as a new-grad nurse at a local community hospital. I interned on the Medicine floor during college, facilitating a smoother transition during the dreaded "new-grad" year that many young nurses dread. A large part of my identity at this job was found in being a team player. I modeled the behaviors that I would want to see in another nurse. Whether it was picking up an extra shift, assisting other nurses with their rounds, making small talk with my older patients, or staying an extra hour after work, I craved feeling useful. I loved hearing a 93-year-old woman say that I had *"a lovely disposition"* and when my coworkers called me a *"lifesaver."* My coworker Megan said, *"Bridget's sparkly. She always comes to work with this much enthusiasm."* She reaffirmed that I was achieving what I set out to do—I wanted to be a positive light in a challenging unit. Even though I was fresh off orientation and was responsible for caring for six patients, I was eager to take on the challenge. One night, I had a heavy assignment of five total-care patients, each requiring time-consuming care. I was ready to make it another great night. Little did I know that my one ambulatory patient would cause me to call into question the team I wanted desperately to join.

This particular patient was a 31-year-old woman. I was initially wary because the senior nurses had passed her around like a hot potato. No one could handle her for more than one shift. With only three months of nursing experience, I was cautiously optimistic. I enjoy being challenged, and I am not a quitter.

When I received a report from a dayshift nurse, he highlighted a milelong list of as-needed (PRN) medications on his computer screen. He also gave me a piece of paper with his personal phone number: *"If something happens during the night, call me. I will tell the manager that I'm the one culpable."* When I asked him to explain further, he simply wished me luck with my assignment.

As I was overloaded with information, my strategy was to breach this patient head on. I wanted some sense of agency in this situation. My technique was to overcome preconceived notions about this patient that I had acquired from the other nurses over the past few weeks. I attempted to dazzle her with a silly sense of humor. I complimented her nails, cracked jokes about a basketball game she was watching (a sport I know nothing about), and made small talk in hopes of easing both of us. *"If you don't have any questions, I'm going to introduce myself to my other patients, and I will return shortly to check up on you,"* I said with a smile.

The patient's mother and I had conflicting agendas. She rang the call bell incessantly. Before I could introduce myself to my next patient, she was reporting that her daughter was in excruciating pain and nausea. When I asked the patient about these symptoms, she remained silent. I promised to reassess shortly and repeated that I needed to see my other patients for the time being.

While I was next door with another patient, the mother from the other room followed me inside and demanded that I see her daughter. I guided her to the exit, saying that I would see her within the hour. The mom began screaming profanities at me. I apologized to my older patient and followed the mother out the door.

The daughter was lying in bed watching television, in the same position she had been in a few minutes ago. The more senior nurses encouraged me to call security and have the mom removed because of her language. My pride prevented me from making the call. I wanted to be liked. If I were to ask for a security escort, the mom would shoot to hell any chance of us developing a friendly rapport. I genuinely believed there was a way that I could salvage this relationship and that we could collaborate to care for the patient. I wanted to turn the tide and be the person on the floor who could foster a connection with this family.

Looking back, I should have asked security to usher the mom out of the room. I could have had a more honest conversation with the patient about her pain levels without a helicopter parent stifling us. Instead, I asked the patient if she was comfortable having the mom in the room, and she replied, *"Yes, of course."* When I asked about her pain level, she repeated verbatim the mom's statement about increasing pain.

I assessed the chart and saw that she did not have any scheduled pain medications. The doctor had placed several PRN orders that could be administered as needed. The chart showed that Amy had administered all of the medications at the same time last night. Amy had been a senior nurse on the unit for more than 25 years. She was one of my mentors. I questioned her indication for administering a concoction of dangerous medications at the same time rapidly through an intravenous—including 2 milligrams (mg) of Ativan, 4 mg of Dilaudid, and 10 mg each of morphine, Benadryl, and Zofran, to top it off. I pulled Amy aside and asked, *"Is it safe for her to receive all of these?"*

I explained my hesitations to her and was stunned by her response. Amy shrugged and said, *"She is so difficult. I can't keep fighting her. Nothing bad happened last night when I gave them. You will be fine if you give them all."* A pit sat in my stomach when I thought of giving all of these medications to an 80-pound girl who was parroting her mother's words. Potential risks ran through my mind: respiratory distress, risk for falls, dizziness, and headaches. I admired Amy and wished that I could trust her judgment, but my instincts compelled me to seek another opinion.

I escalated the question by paging the resident responsible for her during the night. I explained the mother's reaction and my apprehension in administering the medications. *"Can you please come to the bedside and do an assessment?"* He refused, saying, *"I have been inundated with complaints about this lady every night for weeks. I'm not going to talk to her again."*

"I understand—it's difficult to deal with her for one shift, so two weeks is definitely difficult. But I don't feel comfortable administering these doses of medication all at once in her current state. I don't want the effects to stack or cause respiratory distress."

He sighed and said, *"Listen. Hypothetically, no, it isn't safe to give this kind of cocktail to a 38-kilogram woman. But if you don't, the mom will make the rest of your shift a living hell. Just give the medications so she'll be off your back, and you can focus on your other patients. I'll be in the emergency department. If she passes out, call me."*

Nothing could have prepared me for this apathetic response. This physician had completely dismissed all of my concerns without regard for patient safety. My blood was boiling as I explained the situation to my charge nurse, Mary.

Meanwhile, the patient's mom interrupted repeatedly. *"Why are you incapable of bringing the doctor here? Does he think you're incompetent, too? My daughter deserves better than a teenage nurse."*

I was getting nowhere. The entire staff on my floor dismissed this patient as too difficult and refused to examine the indications for why these medications were ordered and strategize more effective timing.

I should be able to figure this out on my own, I remember thinking. I wanted to communicate effectively with challenging patients through my merit without calling for help. Throughout my nursing residency, I had strived to be the ideal coworker, but no one was willing to reciprocate my efforts when I needed guidance. I needed to find someone with similar values who would collaborate on my team, not the pessimistic side that Amy and the physician had joined. With this in mind, a lot must be said about using your critical thinking and establishing a rapport with your patients. However, these efforts are more often fruitless with abusive patients and families. When someone makes it their mission to target you, forcing a friendly relationship is not going to reach a therapeutic place. I needed to focus on boundaries to get this train back on its tracks, and I needed to outsource help.

In a last-ditch effort, I decided to arc this up one more time. It was my first time calling the nursing supervisor. Nora was 4 feet 10 inches of pure might. I have seen nurses duck into corners when they catch wind of her Danskos clicking on the hospital tile floors. With a shaky voice, I felt like the biggest tattletale in the hospital as I relayed my woeful shift to her.

"He said WHAT?" Nora yelled into the receiver.

The other women at the nurses' station looked at me and mouthed, *"Nora?"* You never had to ask when someone was on the phone with Nora; everyone could hear her even when she wasn't on speakerphone.

"Promise me that you will ignore everything that stupid doctor said. Meet me outside the Med Room; I'll be there in three minutes."

Nora ripped a piece of paper and drew a table for me. *"Here are the medications ordered. You're going to administer Dilaudid now. This is the strongest and will relieve the worst of the pain. You will reassess her in 15 minutes—focus on breathing. If she looks worse, call me. If she seems OK, you will reassess in another 30 minutes and administer the Ativan slowly over two minutes. Wait another 15 minutes. OK, this will get you to 1, so you'll check on her after 15 minutes and wait another hour. If she keeps asking for medications, you can offer Benadryl. With any luck, they'll sleep, but if not, then you can give the Zofran at 2:15. Do you feel better about this? Is there anything that you want to change?"*

In typical fashion for that night, the patient's mom heard us in the hallway and stormed out, slamming the door. *"I demand to speak with the doctor this instant and refuse to talk to anyone who isn't an MD!"*

Nora shrugged and, with a cheeky smile, said, *"Sorry. We aren't MDs."* She turned toward me and asked, *"Can I help you with anything else?"*

Relief coursed through my veins. It meant everything to have someone take the time to listen to me, ask for my opinion, and honor the words that I was saying. Her intentionality and generosity shone a light into the reality of being a team player when your colleagues are at their lowest. She was my hero during a frustrating and isolating shift. Every time new grads ask me questions, I prioritize approaching my answers with the same intensity and collaborative spirit Nora showed me.

I wish I could end this rigamarole by saying that the rest of the shift was easy-peasy and that Nora's method worked like a charm: The patient was grateful for my efforts to keep her alive and breathing, nominated me for a Daisy Award, and even bought me a latte in the morning. However, none of that would be true. I followed Nora's timeline and completed thorough respiratory assessments of my patient, all while facing bipolar responses from the patient and mother. Sometimes they would completely ice me out and refuse to answer any assessment questions. At other times, they would pelt me with insults, hoping that I would crack. One moment, the mother would yell, *"You're withholding care from my daughter!"* Fifteen minutes later, she would be tearful, crying about an abusive healthcare system.

These women drained every ounce of sparkle that I possessed. I left feeling conflicting emotions. I had been holding in tears for the past 12 hours, refusing to give this mother any satisfaction in seeing me cry or using it as another piece of leverage to deem me an unfit caretaker. To my surprise, I also felt a sense of satisfaction. That morning, I clocked out, knowing that I had turned every stone and done everything in my arsenal as a new grad to protect this vulnerable patient. Regardless of her perception or the perception held by her family, I was her advocate—even if they could not see the bigger picture yet.

After this highly emotional shift, I struggled to decompress and sleep during the day because I was scheduled to work that same night at 7 p.m. It was customary in my unit to have the same patients when you worked multiple shifts in a row. This allowed for a more consistent caregiver who was aware of the patient's baseline and had a deeper understanding of their medical history. As I was leaving, I spoke with the daytime charge nurse and requested not to have this patient for a second shift in a row. To this day, this is the only time I have ever made such a request. It had become a point of pride that I never requested to change my assignment. It marked me as resilient, cooperative—and a good teammate. I was happy to face patients with more demanding personalities. However, this shift made me realize that I could not handle being verbally assaulted for two nights in a row for my own mental health, but especially for the sake of my other patients. My five total-care patients were unnecessarily placed at risk because my attention was divided.

Being a dedicated nurse does not mean sacrificing your values or placing yourself in an uncomfortable position. You can advocate for your patient and your needs while supporting the rest of the unit; these things are not mutually exclusive. The best coworkers are not the people who pick up the most shifts or show up for work 15 minutes early or even the people who offer to help turn your *C. difficile* patients—team players are conscientious collaborators.

None of my patients have ever made me feel as inept as these women did on that fateful April night. While I was in the eye of the storm, it meant everything to have Nora validate my concerns, offer suggestions, and encourage my opinions. For me, experience brings confidence. I am strengthened by my previous experiences, even the ones that were unpleasant in the moment. I aim to use this knowledge daily as a nurse who cultivates an encouraging work setting.

Effective Teams Are Only as Strong as the Players

By Sean Elwell, DNP, RN, NE-BC, TCRN, EMT

Every one of us has a story about why they got into the nursing profession. Without getting into boring details, my "why" was to be part of a team who provided care to others when they needed it most. I quickly realized that I could not do that alone. I am dependent on the entire multidisciplinary team. The nursing profession is deeply rooted in team dynamics. Effective teams are only as strong as the players within that team and their commitment to their shared mission.

New Nurses

New-graduate nurses are often excited to begin their careers. While each may have taken a different approach to beginning their careers, each new nurse has completed a rigorous educational program. While this can sometimes seem daunting, new nurses must remember that this is just the foundation for their practice. New-graduate nurses must adjust to their new roles and new environments. This can often be challenging, as they must learn new skills, processes, and procedures. The environment, or culture, can affect the success of the new nurse and the care they provide to patients.

The development of credibility has been listed as an important component of new-graduate nurses' orientation into their new roles. This process is defined as developing trust in one's nursing practice and gaining the trust of others (Lyman et al., 2020). While this may sound simple, it may be one of the most important foundational pieces to ensure that new nurses are successful. Why is credibility important? As nurses attempt to build credibility within their team, it can be difficult to speak up. In the shift that Bridget described, she struggled with her ability to speak up when she felt that the previous nurse had administered too many medications. She was attempting to build credibility with not only the care team but also the patient and family. Establishing a relationship with a patient or family who is challenging can be difficult. There is no singular piece of advice that builds credibility within the team. Sometimes credibility is built through time, experience, and observation. Establishing a relationship with patients and family members starts with honest communication, mutual respect, and trust.

While there are many keys to success, effective communication and professional behaviors are two of the most important aspects (Aydogdu, 2023). Nurses beginning their careers are seeking mentorship within their respective environments. These nurses need support and guidance to be successful in their new role (Ephraim, 2020). Nurses often model the behaviors that preceptors display. These nurses value the role of their mentor and seek their acceptance. Nora, in her role as the nursing supervisor, highlighted the importance of mentorship in this scenario. She collaborated with Bridget and was intentional with her direction. Nora's presence brought a sense of relief to the bedside nurse and provided validity to her concerns, which had previously been overlooked.

As Michelle discussed in Chapter 3, psychological safety is a relatively new concept in the nursing profession but is especially important to newer nurses. This concept is rooted in being a shared belief among team members, which allows individuals to feel comfortable sharing ideas, providing feedback, and, ultimately, speaking up for safety without fear of consequences (Lyman et al., 2020). As nurses enter the profession, they face many difficult challenges to navigate. In many cases, they are learning a new organization, role, and culture.

Difficult Experiences

Managing difficult families is something each of us will have to encounter. There are varying levels of difficult patients and family members, and there is no single recipe to manage these challenges. In this specific case, the parent appeared to be the individual driving the negative interaction. While the patient exhibited negative behavior, this appeared to be in response to the parent's displayed behavior. Parents or caregivers can negatively affect the team dynamics crucial to optimal patient care. The behaviors of this specific family were incredibly challenging—so much so that the thought of more than one shift spent managing this family was unbearable.

One of the ways that we can manage our response is by understanding why we are frustrated with the interaction with our patient, family, or caregiver. The think-feel-act cycle is one strategy that can be used to understand our patients or families during difficult experiences (Naidorf, 2023). The cycle has four phases, which include the patient arriving or assuming care, the clinician having thought about the patient, the clinician's thought causing a feeling, and those feelings driving the clinician's actions

(Naidorf, 2023). In this case, the patient had been on a unit for a period of time prior to the nurse assuming responsibility. The opinion of the nurse was actually formed prior to her even meeting the patient. The thoughts and opinions of the care team and their previous experiences caused the nurse to have feelings and opinions before the first patient interaction. Imagine the impact those experiences would have on your feelings before entering the patient's room. It is clear in the scenario that Bridget was experiencing a level of anxiety and was overwhelmed with the amount of information she had received.

Bridget should have been applauded for not allowing her feelings to drive her decisions. She could have easily given a "cocktail" to the patient and looked the other way. Instead, she chose to do what was best for the patient. There are many strategies for de-escalating difficult patients and families. Through research, we have discovered the 10 domains of de-escalation, which are as follows (Naidorf, 2023):

1. Respect personal space.
2. Do not be provocative.
3. Establish verbal contact.
4. Be concise.
5. Identify wants and feelings.
6. Listen closely to what the patient is saying.
7. Agree or agree to disagree.
8. Lay down the law and set clear limits.
9. Offer choices and optimism.
10. Debrief the patient and staff.

Changing the behavior of this patient and their parent was not likely. Understanding our thoughts and opinions while using the 10 domains of de-escalation can make these types of interactions less painful.

Bridget used her past experiences and knowledge to respond to this scenario. While de-escalation may not have been on her mind, she did meet several of the domains of de-escalation. In this case, Bridget could have benefited from agreeing to disagree, laying down the law, setting limits, and offering choices. While the mother was incessant that the patient immediately needed pain medications, the two could have concluded with both parties agreeing to disagree. Perhaps the most important domain would have been to set limits. Bridget self-identified that involving security or removing the mom would have been beneficial. It is also acceptable to share with families what behaviors will and won't be tolerated. We are human, too. Just because Bridget is a healthcare provider does not mean that she is a human punching bag.

Harm Prevention

The reporting of errors has recently come more into the spotlight. Historically, error reporting was avoided, as this practice was perceived as punitive. Lyman et al. (2020) share that new-graduate nurses can preserve their credibility when team members embrace errors as opportunities for improvement. This allows new nurses to normalize error reporting while maintaining their clinical competence (Lyman et al., 2020). While the nurses in this scenario may not have made an error, their actions could have caused harm to the patient. Nurses should be encouraged to speak up any time they have a concern. One way to empower team members is by using the CUS Tool (American Hospital Association [AHA], 2024a). This tool uses keywords to communicate to the care team that you have concerns. Upon hearing these words, the care team pauses to discuss the concern and agree on a solution. The *C* begins the conversation by stating, "*I am concerned.*" Should the concern not be addressed, the *U* follows with "*I am uncomfortable.*" Finally, the *S* stands for stating, "*This is a safety issue.*" The *S* in the *CUS* should stop the line and allow the team to refocus on the task at hand (AHA, 2024b).

The CUS Tool is part of the TeamSTEPPS® suite of evidence-based tools that can be used by anyone who wants to improve communication and teamwork in health care (AHA, 2024b). You will see some chapters will have a "TeamSTEPPS Tip" (the first one is below) that will help you consider the real-life application and a point to consider about using the tool.

TeamSTEPPS TIP

The CUS Tool is an outstanding way to communicate when you have concerns; however, be prepared that after you receive information, you may find out that your concerns are not justified and that you just needed more information.

Remember, just because you raise a concern with CUS doesn't necessarily mean that you're in the right. Consider that there could be a rational explanation for something you've perceived as a problem or mistake—and if there is, be prepared to move on.

It might be helpful to say something like, "OK, thanks for clarifying. I'm glad we cleared that up."

Source: AHA, 2024a.

If the healthcare industry intends to improve the care provided and encourage error reporting, a culture of inclusiveness is needed. This means being available for team members to report errors, seeking input, and recognizing team members for speaking up for safety (Munn et al., 2023). Error reporting is encouraged but can be successful only if team members feel safe to speak up about the problem they are encountering. Fear is frequently cited as a main barrier to error reporting (Munn et al., 2023). Prioritizing high-functioning teams who communicate effectively will help change team dynamics and maximize psychological safety (Munn et al., 2023).

Mentorship

If we were to informally poll our colleagues about what they deemed most important to their initial success, many would say that they had a strong, supportive preceptor. The bond that frequently develops between a preceptor and a new nurse can have lasting impacts. Research suggests that a successful transition to practice depends on the role of the preceptor (Lyman et al., 2020). Preceptors often build trust with new-graduate nurses. This is strengthened by portraying a willingness to teach and answer questions provided by new nurses (Lyman et al., 2020). Lyman and colleagues report that nurses feel less safe around colleagues when they hear them gossiping and do not feel that they support the team (Lyman et al., 2020). While preceptors often make great mentors, they are not the only option. In fact, there are times in which the preceptor is not a good choice for being a mentor. Nora stepped into the mentorship role in this case. She instantly gained Bridget's trust and portrayed confidence in managing the patient. Should a nurse find themselves with a preceptor or mentor who is not a good fit, it is OK to raise that with the leadership team. A nurse is not expected to continue in a partnership that is not conducive to their success.

Team Dynamics

Nurses play an integral role in the care team. Unfortunately, there are often hierarchal issues within the team. Whether perceived or actual, providers often assume a hierarchal role by giving orders to nurses (Aydogdu, 2023). These team dynamics can often affect interpersonal relationships. Interactions between team members can sometimes be challenging. We have all experienced a time when communication did not go as planned. The perception of our teams often begins before individuals ever interact. Aydogdu completed a study of nursing students and found that interactions during clinical rotations affect future relationships within the interprofessional team (Aydogdu, 2023). Regardless of the role one is in, being supported by the entire team is important. There are a number of ways that teams can be supportive of each other. New-graduate nurses have reported that feeling supported by their team and organization is important to their psychological safety (Lyman et al., 2020). One of the ways this occurs is by team members providing a respectful response when team members ask questions or raise concerns (Lyman et al., 2020). Unfortunately, in this scenario, the team members did not support the new nurse or provide respectful responses when concerns were raised. These responses can lead to intimidation within the care team.

Successful teams are rooted in the professionalism of those team members. Interpersonal relationships are necessary to provide high-quality care to patients (Aydogdu, 2023). Nurses represent the largest profession within healthcare organizations. Interactions with the nursing team must be effective to ensure the treatment plan is appropriate and patient outcomes are optimal (Aydogdu, 2023).

Throughout the chapter, we discussed psychological safety. While this concept alone does not ensure a supportive team, research demonstrates that promoting psychological safety among nurses and interdisciplinary teams positively affects error reporting (Munn et al., 2023). In this case study, the nurse's mentor and the interdisciplinary team did not create a welcoming environment. Fortunately, the nurse did not settle for the responses she was receiving. She took it upon herself to advocate for her patient and advocate for appropriate nursing practice. As a relatively new nurse, this can be difficult. This nurse prioritized the safety of the patient above all else.

There are times when team members should feel empowered to escalate their concerns. Each organization may have a different method for elevating challenges. In this case, Bridget escalated this issue to the nursing supervisor. Each team member should know the appropriate escalation pathway for their organization. This may include using nursing leaders, physician leaders, or an on-call structure. Escalating challenges can be stressful, but given the correct environment, these conversations can empower and ultimately improve patient care.

The scenario presented in this section was full of challenges. Since the care team was not aligned in managing this patient, debriefing the events would have been valuable. *Debriefing* is the dialogue between two or more people to discuss the actions and thought processes involved in a particular patient care situation (Gabriel et al., 2021). The care team debriefing this challenging episode would allow the care team to manage the associated stress, reach a resolution on the care plan, and proactively plan for future scenarios.

Self-Care

Beginning a new chapter in your professional journey can be full of challenges. New nurses often put hours of thought into choosing the right organization and environment to begin their practice. Once they have started in their new role, they should take every opportunity to engage in their team by building relationships, sharing ideas, and reporting errors (Lyman et al., 2020).

A healthy work environment is crucial within the healthcare profession. To ensure the healthiest work environment, team members must value the nursing profession, understand role boundaries, and train in effective communication and conflict management (Aydogdu, 2023). Before graduation, students must complete training to advance leadership, teamwork, and communication skills (Aydogdu, 2023). This training and education will provide a foundation for navigating the changing landscape within the healthcare world. Chapter 12 will help you identify self-care strategies that effectively decrease stress and promote your sense of well-being.

Playing on the Team

By Linda Roney, EdD, RN-BC, CPEN, CNE, FAAN

If you are reading this book, your life and academic experiences were likely dramatically affected by the COVID-19 pandemic. Perhaps you did not have the opportunity to use a microscope complete your anatomy and physiology labs, so you were assigned videos to watch at home. Or perhaps you spent countless hours meeting with your teacher and class by Zoom while you and half of your class alternated with who could be in person with the teacher to de-densify the classroom. Each individual has their own story about how the learning that brought them to this point differed from what had been for those nurses before them. You are not afraid of hard work and have displayed significant determination. Your ability to face challenging and ambiguous situations shines through all you do.

Maybe you are at the point in this casebook when you read Bridget's story where you are wondering a few things about yourself such as the following after working so hard to get into nursing school and complete your program:

- Will my coworkers, patients and their families, and my supervisors even like me?
    - What will I do if they do not?
- What would I have done if I had been in Bridget's situation that night? Would I have given all of the meds as ordered?
- Will I find my "Nora" where I work? What happens if I do not?
- What if my new team rejects me?
- I have worked hard to become a nurse. Will I even like it?

Bridget felt so many emotions that night at work. She wanted to be liked by her patient and mother, and she could do nothing to win them over. Her colleagues were giving her what she knew was terrible advice, and she needed clarification on why they would take this risk. She felt uncertain and did not know what to do next in this situation, in which the patient's mother did not display mutual respect and violated multiple boundaries with Bridget and the other patients on the unit. Bridget felt abandoned when her physician colleague would not come and evaluate the patient when she asked. She felt the sting of the words *"teenage nurse"* when the patient's mother said her daughter deserved better than Bridget. Bridget knew she deserved better than to be treated disrespectfully by her patient's mother but did not let it get in the way of her being her patient's advocate, stating, *"Regardless of her perception or the perception held by her family, I was her advocate—even if they could not see the bigger picture yet."*

With all of the shift events, Bridget took the initiative to demonstrate competency in some of the American Association of Colleges of Nursing essentials' (2021) domains 2 and 10 competencies and subcompetencies.

Let's look at Table 5.1 to see how Bridget provided person-centered care and demonstrated personal, professional, and leadership development.

Bridget shared feelings about wanting to be liked on her unit by her coworkers, and she took pride in her reputation as a hard worker. She brought her enthusiasm and "sparkle" and took pride in how her coworkers perceived her. Bridget worked hard to contribute to her team; the following box provides some quick tips on being a great coworker. While they may sound obvious, you will be surprised how implementing these practices can help you feel like part of the team.

TABLE 5.1 Examples of Domain 2: Person-Centered Care and Domain 10: Personal, Professional, and Leadership Development in This Exemplar

Domain 2: Person-Centered Care	
2.1 Engage with the individual in establishing a caring relationship.	Bridget showed empathic and compassionate care despite not feeling respected by the family.
2.2 Communicate effectively with individuals.	Bridget strived to meet her patient and her mother where they were to try to deliver person-centered care and apply emotional intelligence to the situation. She sought feedback from others when she faced communication challenges and applied new learned info to the situation.
Domain 10: Personal, Professional, and Leadership Development	
10.2 Demonstrate a spirit of inquiry that fosters flexibility and professional maturity.	Bridget reflected on the patient orders and trusted her judgment when others told her to go against her gut. When she needed additional resources to inform her care, she sought the guidance of the nursing supervisor and used that feedback to provide care. She identified a mentor that was outside of her immediate team to support her in making safe decisions.
10.3 Develop capacity for leadership.	By not giving into the status quo, Bridget demonstrated tremendous leadership skills. She called outside resources when she was dealing with a difficult situation where there seemed to be no good answer. She acknowledged her own implicit bias (wanting to be liked) and acknowledged this challenge with this family. Bridget knew that it was time to challenge what safe practices the other team members had been doing just to appease the family and gathered the information she needed to make the decision that was safest for her patient. Her authentic leadership shone when she stated, "Regardless of her perception or the perception held by her family, I was her advocate—even if they could not see the bigger picture yet."

Belonging in Your New Home as a New Nurse

> Fitting in and belonging are not the same thing. In fact, fitting in is one of the greatest barriers to belonging. Fitting in is about assessing a situation and becoming who you need to be to be accepted. Belonging, on the other hand, does not require us to change who we are; it requires us to be who we are. (Brown, 2012, p. 231)

Think about your childhood. Who is the first friend you can remember? What are some of the things that you remember about them? Did they ask you to sit next to them on the school bus? Did they share their snack with you? Did they ask you to play with them on the playground? You probably went home from school that day and told your family you made a friend. That friend made you feel like you *mattered*.

Working as a nurse is not always as fun as an afternoon at the playground, nor must you be best friends with your coworkers. However, you do need to feel like you belong.

A sense of belonging is crucial to whether new graduate nurses are willing to continue working in nursing (Ching et al., 2022). New nurses yearn for acceptance, care, attention, encouragement, and support from their colleagues but often feel like outsiders or intruders. They possess certain expectations about their nursing role before they enter the workforce. However, once there, they usually discover discrepancies between the actual nursing environment and the one they imagined, leading to loneliness, anxiety, and restlessness (Ching et al., 2022).

Li et al. (2023) studied new nurses' clinical sense of belonging and turnover intention. A clinical sense of belonging is the nurse's perception of the healthcare team's requirement for acceptance, respect, and support from coworkers or patients. The risk of the turnover intention of new nurses with a "poor clinical sense of belonging" was 0.62 times that of new nurses with a "rich clinical sense of belonging," which was statically significant (odds ratio = 0.62, $p < 0.01$; Li et al., 2023). Of a sample of 123,000 registered nurses across the United States who answered their organization's Press Ganey employee engagement survey in 2022 and 2023, nearly one in four nurses who were in their organization for two years or less left their organization between those two years, with disengaged nurses 2.2 times more likely to leave than those who were highly engaged (Doucette, 2023).

Who Gave You That Order?

Many new nurses need clarification on the titles of coworkers they encounter when they start working in the clinical setting. Knowing their training and educational background helps them navigate their new work environment and interact with providers.

Medical Students

To apply to medical school, an individual must complete prerequisite coursework that varies by program and typically includes behavioral science, biology, biochemistry, inorganic and organic chemistry, and physics (American Association of Medical Colleges [AAMC], 2024). They must earn a bachelor's degree, but the major does not have to be a science degree; the candidate needs to meet the academic requirements of the medical school. All medical schools in the United States require the Medical College Admission Test, a standardized, multiple-choice, computer-based test that tests knowledge in areas of biology, chemistry, physics, behavioral health, and critical reasoning skills (AAMC, 2024).

Medical school is a four-year graduate curriculum. The first two preclinical years are focused on learning about basic medical concepts, the structure and functions of the body, diseases, diagnoses, and treatment concepts (AAMC, 2024). Clinical rotations, sometimes called *clerkships*, occur during medical school's third and fourth years. Like nursing school, the total hours required by program and state vary (AAMC, 2024). During the fourth year, most people apply for a residency program. Licensure as a physician involves taking three tests for the United States Medical Licensing Examination (USMLE): step 1 (usually after the second year of medical school), step 2 (usually in the fourth year of medical school), and step 3 (usually taken after the first year of residency; USMLE, 2024). Patient orders that medical students might request must be reviewed and co-signed by a resident or attending physician.

Residents

Usually, during their third year of school, medical students typically decide on the clinical specialty they would like to pursue for their career path. Medical students apply for residency programs, usually across the country, in the specialty that they hope will be their career. The process is competitive, stressful, and involves what you may have heard referred to as "matching." Candidates apply using an online application hosted by the National Resident Matching Program (NRMP; https://www.nrmp.org/). The NRMP uses a computerized mathematical algorithm to place applicants into their most preferred residency and fellowship positions. The agreement is binding, meaning that they are told where they must go to complete residency, and the decision is final. This immersive clinical residency, essentially the individual's first job in medicine, lasts three to seven years, with surgical residencies lasting at least five years (American College of Surgeons, 2024). The residency is paid, and the average salary in the United States is currently $67,400 and usually increases slightly each year, but half of residents have at least $200,000 in debt from medical school (Robbins, 2023). First-year residents are sometimes called *interns*, and those in the other years of their clerkship are called *residents*.

Fellows

Following residency, many physicians are ready to work in their chosen professional setting and must find a job. For some specialties, orthopedic and pediatric surgery are examples; additional specialty training in the form of what is called a fellowship is over one to three years (Mayo College of Medicine and Science, 2024). Some physicians complete a fellowship at an institution where they were residents.

Attending

Those who have completed their residency and a fellowship are not required for their jobs, or those who have completed their fellowship will then look for a position as an attending physician or surgeon. An attending physician is responsible for a patient's overall care in a hospital or clinic setting and may also supervise and teach medical students, interns, and residents involved in the patient's care (National Cancer Institute, 2024).

Advanced Practice Providers

Advanced practice providers are physician assistants and advanced practice nurses. The term *mid-level provider* or *practitioner* is derogatory because it implies their care is not as good as physicians'.

Physician Assistant

Also called *physician associates*, physician assistants (PA) must complete a program of study that leads to a bachelor's degree. Some people choose a science-related major while they complete the required coursework to apply to PA programs. Applicants must complete at least 1,000 hours of health-care experience or patient care experience to apply to PA school. While there are some programs that a student can apply to as a high school senior, complete their bachelor's degree, and be granted a position in the graduate PA program after meeting specific admissions criteria, most PA programs are postgraduate. PA school is typically 23 to 27 months, with at least 2,000 hours of structured clinical education. Following program completion, the PA student takes the Physician Assistant National Certifying Exam and can apply for state licensure and start working as a PA.

Advanced Practice Nurses

Advanced practice registered nurses (APRNs) include nurse practitioners, clinical nurse specialists, nurse anesthetists, and nurse midwives who meet the licensure, accreditation, certification, and education requirements for advanced nursing practice in their role. Currently, APRNs are educated at the graduate level in a master's or doctoral program (usually a Doctorate of Nursing Practice). Nurse practitioners can practice independently in 27 states after meeting the state licensing board's requirements (American Association of Nurse Practitioners, 2024).

What Is a Hospitalist?

Hospitalists are primary care providers, like family physicians or practitioners, but they are trained to treat hospitalized patients (Cinteza, 2023). Before adopting a hospitalist model, primary care providers would have to visit and place orders for their patients for their routine care, and the specialists would prescribe the therapies specifically associated with why the patient was admitted to the hospital. Let us consider the example of an infant who falls out of their parent's arms onto uncarpeted steps. The child is admitted to the hospital for observation as he has a skull fracture. The neurosurgical team would place all of the orders related to monitoring and caring for the infant for their injury, but if the child also had a diaper rash, something that an infant would typically see their pediatric primary care provider for, the hospitalist, the child's acting pediatric primary care provider at the hospital, would be the provider the nurse contacted for the order for a diaper rash ointment.

This is an area that can be quite time-consuming and, frankly, frustrating for nurses. There are gray areas, of course, when you are working with multiple provider teams caring for one patient, which can be confusing for a new nurse to know who to ask. Sometimes, a neurosurgical resident from a specialty service will do the team a favor and order the diaper ointment when the nurse requests it, but then the next time a different resident is on, they refuse, which leaves the new nurse confused. When admitted to the hospital, each patient is admitted to a specific service (e.g., orthopedics, oncology, plastic surgery), and the attending physician is ultimately responsible for their care. Take notice of who your preceptors reach out to in different situations to gain a sense of the pathways at your new job.

Teamwork Makes the Dreams Work

Throughout your nursing school experience, you have heard about collaborating with the interdisciplinary team. We spent much time reviewing the various types of providers you may work with, as this often needs to be clarified for new nurses. You may have had some interaction with providers, but sometimes not as much as you will in your new position. You may have observed roles such as watching a physical therapist empower patients with the skills they need to get out of bed for the first time after surgery or an occupational therapist reteach someone how to button their clothes after a stroke. Instead of providing an exhaustive list of all the possible incredible interdisciplinary collaborators that you might work with—because, at this point in your nursing career, you likely know many of them—let us briefly talk about how you work with collaborate as a member of an interdisciplinary team.

No one would argue that nurses are busy; however, let me gently remind you that so are the other interdisciplinary team members. We get so consumed by the tasks on our electronic health record that we sometimes greet our interdisciplinary colleagues as if we are stunned when we see them, like uninvited house guests inside our messy house. If you work regularly with some collaborators, then you will quickly develop a relationship, rhythm, and flow with them. For those with whom we work less often, be the first to reach out to coordinate goals of the day. This can ensure the comfort of our patients (premedicate), give us time to let our patients know the plan for the day (anticipatory guidance), and help with all of our workflows.

YOU MATTER: WE CAN DO THIS TOGETHER!

In this case, Bridget reached out to old and new friends for help with a difficult situation. She went outside her comfort zone to find a supervisor, who helped her exactly how she needed. If you are not satisfied with your current situation related to anything in your nursing practice, do not settle. Find your Nora. They are out there, and when you have the chance, be Nora for someone else.

There is a lot going on in your first nursing position, but one of the greatest investments you can make is getting to know the people with whom you work from all disciplines. Taking the time to be the first to introduce yourself, ask others questions about how their weekend was, and get to know more about them personally will cultivate and strengthen your professional relationship. It will also increase your sense of belonging at work, which is crucial to how you feel about your career in nursing.

Book Club Questions

1. Have you ever been asked to do something you were uncomfortable doing in your nursing role? What did you do?
2. What makes a good coworker?
3. Have you ever felt like you did not fit in at work? How did you resolve the situation?
4. Who would you call first if you had a problem with your patient? What information do you need to gather and consider before you make a call?

About This Chapter's Authors

Bridget Morrissey, BSN, RN

Bridget was born and raised in suburban Connecticut. In 2022, she graduated from Fairfield University's Marion Peckham Egan School of Nursing and Health Studies. Following graduation, her nursing career started in adult medicine at a community hospital. She now works in a neonatal ICU, where she participates in little miracles every day. In her free time, she spends time with her family and friends as well as reading, journaling, hanging out on the beach, and listening to hours of Taylor Swift.

Sean Elwell, DNP, RN, NE-BC, TCRN, EMT

Dr. Sean Elwell is the senior director of Emergency Services, Critical Care Transport, and the Pediatric Trauma Center at Nemours Children's Hospital in Wilmington, Delaware. He has been employed with the organization for more than 21 years, starting as an emergency medical technician (EMT) before becoming a registered nurse. Sean completed his Doctor of Nursing Practice through Wilmington University and is a graduate of Drexel University, where he graduated summa cum laude with a master's degree in nursing leadership and health systems management. Sean has written numerous articles for publication and presented at regional and national conferences. He is actively involved in several professional organizations nationally, including the Society of Trauma Nurses, where he is a past president. He also serves on the board of directors for the Board of Certification for Emergency Nursing, currently serving as secretary/treasurer.

Sean is also active in the community and sits on various boards and committees. He has volunteered with the Elsinboro Fire Company for the past 25 years and served in various leadership roles, including emergency medical services/rescue captain and vice president. He is an active EMT and firefighter and is the company's chief.

Sean is also the mayor of Elsinboro Township in Salem County, New Jersey. He is in his 18th year serving as an elected official. Sean served as deputy mayor for four years and has been mayor for the past 14 years. In addition, he served as president of the Salem County Association of Local Government and on the New Jersey Conference of Mayors board of directors. He currently serves on the executive board of the New Jersey League of Municipalities (NJLM). In November 2024, Sean became the first vice president of the league, and in November 2025, he will assume the role of president for the NJLM.

References

American Association of Colleges of Nursing. (2021). *The essentials: Core competencies for professional nursing education.* https://www.aacnnursing.org/Portals/0/PDFs/Publications/Essentials-2021.pdf

American Association of Medical Colleges. (2024). *Your journey from premed through residency.* American Association of Medical Colleges. https://students-residents.aamc.org

American Association of Nurse Practitioners. (2024). *State practice environment.* https://www.aanp.org/advocacy/state/state-practice-environment

American College of Surgeons. (2024). *How many years of postgraduate training do surgical residents undergo?* https://www.facs.org/for-medical-professionals/education/online-guide-to-choosing-a-surgical-residency/guide-to-choosing-a-surgical-residency-for-medical-students/faqs/training/

American Hospital Association. (2024a). *CUS: AHA TeamSTEPPS video toolkit.* https://www.aha.org/center/project-firstline/teamstepps-video-toolkit/cus

American Hospital Association. (2024b). *TeamSTEPPS® video toolkit.* AHA Center for Health Innovation. https://www.aha.org/center/project-firstline/teamstepps-video-toolkit

Aydogdu, A. L. F. (2023). Interpersonal relationships of the nursing team in the work environment according to nursing students: A qualitative study. *Nurse Education in Practice,* 103861. https://doi.org/10.1016/j.nepr.2023.103861

Brown, B. (2012). *Daring greatly: How the courage to be vulnerable transforms the way we live, love, parent and lead.* Hay House.

Ching, H. Y., Fang, Y. T., & Yun, W. K. (2022). How new nurses experience workplace belonging: A qualitative study. *Sage Open, 12*(3). https://doi.org/10.1177/21582440221119471

Cinteza, M. (2023). Hospitalist? Internist? Who else? *Maedica, 18*(4), 545–546. https://doi.org/10.26574/maedica.2023.18.4.545

Doucette, J. (2023, November 29). *The state of nursing turnover and key nurse retention strategies.* Press Ganey. https://info.pressganey.com/press-ganey-blog-healthcare-experience-insights/the-state-of-nursing-turnover-and-key-nurse-retention-strategies

Ephraim, N. (2020). Mentoring in nursing education: An essential element in the retention of new nurse faculty. *Journal of Professional Nursing, 37*(2). https://doi.org/10.1016/j.profnurs.2020.12.001

Gabriel, P. M., Smith, K., Mullen-Fortino, M., Ballinghoff, J., Holland, S., & Cacchione, P. Z. (2021). Systematic debriefing for critical events facilitates team dynamics, education, and process improvement. *Journal of Nursing Care Quality, 37*(2), 142–148. https://doi.org/10.1097/ncq.0000000000000581

Li, G., Wu, Y. T., Asghar, A., & Zhong, Y. (2023). New nurses' turnover intention and clinical belonging, based on latent class analysis (LCA). *Nursing Open, 11*(1), e2077. https://doi.org/10.1002/nop2.2077

Lyman, B., Gunn, M. M., & Mendon, C. R. (2020). New graduate registered nurses' experiences with psychological safety. *Journal of Nursing Management, 28*(4), 831–839. https://doi.org/10.1111/jonm.13006

Mayo College of Medicine and Science. (2024). *Residencies and fellowships.* https://college.mayo.edu/academics/residencies-and-fellowships/surgery-specialties/

Munn, L. T., Lynn, M. R., Knafl, G. J., Willis, T. S., & Jones, C. B. (2023). A study of error reporting by nurses: The significant impact of nursing team dynamics. *Journal of Research in Nursing, 28*(5), 354–364. https://doi.org/10.1177/17449871231194180

Naidorf, J. (2023). Dealing with difficult patients and their families. In *An emergency physician's path* (pp. 443–449). Springer. https://doi.org/10.1007/978-3-031-47873-4_64

National Cancer Institute. (2024). *Attending physician.* https://www.cancer.gov/publications/dictionaries/cancer-terms/def/attending-physician

Robbins, R. (2023). *Annual income rises: Medscape resident salary & debt report 2023.* Medscape. https://www.medscape.com/slideshow/2023-residents-salary-debt-report-6016676#1

United States Medical Licensing Exam. (2024). *Eligibility.* https://www.usmle.org/bulletin-information/eligibility

CHAPTER 6

Beyond Blame

A Dose of Understanding in Medication Errors

Anna Mulac, FNP-BC; Laurie Nolan-Kelley, DNP, RN, CNL, CEN, TCRN, EMT-P; and Linda Roney, EdD, RN-BC, CPEN, CNE, FAAN

Learning Goals

1. Describe a just culture and relate it to Anna's story.
2. Appraise essential components of nursing documentation.
3. Describe the value of the role of the electronic health record (EHR) and, specifically, the nurse's documentation in regulatory/verification processes, legal matters, reimbursement, research, and quality improvement.

'I Felt So Betrayed and Hurt.'

By Anna Mulac, BSN, RN, FNP-BC

The Situation

A few weeks after my three-month orientation, training mainly on the day shift as a new-grad nurse on a medical surgical floor, I was swiftly moved to the night shift. My mind was still groggy from the process of becoming nocturnal since this was a couple weeks into my transition, as I took the typical walk up the 32 stairs to my floor. Anxiety shot through my chest as I read my assignment for the day. It included a full patient load with multiple patients marked as a 5. A 5 on my floor meant that the patient was a heavy workload for the nurse either medically, physically, or combatively. I located the exhausted day-shift nurse and received report on all my patients.

When the nurse left, I received a call that emergency medical services (EMS) transport was ready to take one of my patients to another facility, and I needed to report ASAP. To my dismay, neither paperwork, belongings, nor the patient were ready for transport. While I was scurrying to accomplish those tasks, a coworker told me my other patient was screaming into the hall for pain medications, and another patient was ringing their call bell. I thought back to what I learned from nursing school and the National Council Licensure Examination and remembered to prioritize. I asked a certified nursing assistant to assist with the call bell while I attended to the screaming patient first. However, I had to rush since the transport team told me they could only stay for another five minutes until they had to leave, with or without the patient.

I briskly walked to the other side of the unit toward the sounds of moaning. My patient reported 10/10 pain and showed major signs of discomfort. I looked at the electronic medical record on the phone and saw that no one had administered the oral pain med in more than eight hours. I pulled it out of the Pyxis; scanned it into Epic, the EHR; and then gave it to the patient. Now breaking a sweat, I rushed back over to finish with the transport team just in time. Only then could I finally sit at a computer to plan the rest of my med pass. At that moment, I noticed something that I had not seen before. My patient's oral pain medication was prescribed as needed for every 10 hours. My heart dropped into my stomach as I realized I had just given a controlled pain medication two hours early.

I immediately checked on the patient, and they were alert and oriented, wide awake, and still writhing in pain. Then I followed the protocol without hesitation by immediately calling the physician and telling them what happened. Their response was to give the patient another dose of the exact same pain medication immediately because their pain was still a 10/10. This comment somewhat soothed my nerves because it meant the physician was not concerned about the dose being too high. While still keeping an eye on the patient, I finished the protocol and wrote an incident report. I continued to work nonstop for the next 10 hours. During this time, I anxiously waited to hear from my manager. However, the shift ended, and I did not even see my manager. Instead, I had to go home with a deep anxiety settling in my gut. Leaving the hospital for the night, which was actually sunrise, I slipped into my car and immediately called each member of my family and cried to them about what happened.

Aftermath

Two weeks went by without any further talk of the incident. My anxiety about it still existed, but I pushed it to the back of my mind in order to continue caring for other patients. That quickly changed when, in the middle of my shift, I finally got called into the manager's office. It felt like my heart was racing but also in the pit of my stomach at the same time. I was never a troublemaker and was always at the top of my class, so I was entering into the unknown. I looked around the tiny office that both the day- and night-shift managers shared, and I saw all the statistics on the floor surrounding me, such as central line–associated bloodstream infections, falls, and catheter-associated urinary tract infections. The night-shift manager told me to sit down in one of the two chairs in the small office and shut the door behind me. This not only scared me because that meant she didn't want anyone to hear our conversation but also surprised me because she knew my name since this was our first conversation that had lasted longer than "Hello."

The nurse supervisor brought out the incident report and another sheet and went over the situation. After any clarifications for the report were addressed, she asked me what I had learned. I acknowledged that I need to slow down and be more cautious with PRN, or as-needed, medications, because the Pyxis and Epic will allow you to give those early. Also, I explained that I needed to ask for help when necessary. I promised that this mistake would never happen again. At that moment, I was proud that I finished speaking without tearing up. She then handed me a pen to sign a paper about our discussion, which she called "the write-up." Leaving the room, I actually felt better about the situation. No one was hurt, and I had learned some valuable lessons as a new nurse.

Immediately after I left the room, my coworkers asked me how it went, and I explained everything. My coworkers appeared shocked that I did not seem upset. They went on to explain that a write-up stays on record with the hospital and keeps a nurse from moving specialties for over a year. At that time, my dream was to apply to the intensive care unit (ICU) residency program. Pulling up the email for the application confirmed what my coworkers were saying. I felt betrayed and hurt that my manager had neglected to explain the significance of signing the paper. It also felt like I was being crucified for my first mistake, which had not harmed anyone. As I fought back tears, my coworkers attempted to cheer me up and guide me. They said that this was the reason they often did not come forward with innocuous mistakes, and they recommended that I not tattle on myself next time. In shock by what I just heard, I looked around at all of these compassionate and intelligent nurses and wondered how the profession had reached this point. Without people's willingness to admit their mistakes, problems within systems will remain. We will not be able to learn from each other, and the same mistake can repeat itself over and over again.

Reflection

We know that to err is human, and nurses are no different. In this experience, the current system severely punished me and others who own up to their mistakes, which naturally encourages people to be less open when errors are made. Additionally, the experience left me with feelings of insignificance. I felt like I was just another cog in the machine. My manager did not care about my career aspirations and, frankly, never asked. The average turnover on this floor was eight months, and I stayed for a year. I was unable to apply to that ICU program and ultimately realized I wanted to work in the outpatient setting, where I now love my job and my manager.

'Every Nurse Has Worked This Shift.'

By Laurie Nolan-Kelley, DNP, RN, CNL, CEN, TCRN, EMT-P

Every nurse has worked this shift: the one where you arrive talking to yourself to gear up for 12 hours of multitasking. You walk briskly and push aside all thoughts outside of your unit and your work responsibilities. You have an assignment, and you will do important work. You remind yourself to listen carefully as you take report. You will need to prioritize based on your patients' acuity. You must delegate what you can. You will likely be interrupted, so you need to focus. You mustn't rush to the patient making the most noise. First, you must learn who is the most fragile and needs you immediately.

As Anna describes, every nurse also knows the effect of inadequate or incomplete handoff. When EMS arrived unexpectedly, she was unprepared for a patient's discharge and had to regroup. I share here what I believe is a less-known truism: There are two kinds of nurses: those who have made a med error and those who will. How the nurse responds says a lot about him or her. And how the nurse leader responds speaks volumes.

As a nurse practicing in a leadership role it is my responsibility to balance the demands of patient care with the needs of my team; however, I must also understand the hospital's needs. I have made the choice to practice in the space between these two worlds that may, at times, seem diametrically opposed. In my earliest experience as a new nurse, I alternated between *"Hey, look at me—hanging meds, charting assessments, teaching patients and families ..."* and *"I am so over my head. I don't think I was paying attention in school that day."* As a leader, I take ownership of my actions, but I am also accountable for the behaviors of my employees, individually and collectively and the consequences of those behaviors. Team successes belong to the team. Team failures, errors, and shortfalls belong to me as the nurse leader. (Side note: Intentional abuse, risk-taking behavior, and disregard for safety are very rare, and those are the exceptions to the thoughts I am sharing now.)

As leaders, we must question when we lose sight of our novice nurse selves, and remind ourselves to stay in touch with that part of our professional history. Now, when things go wrong, when an error occurs, it is my failure. I say that because, as a leader, I must accept that I failed to put in place, or demand that the hospital put systems and processes in place, that make it nearly impossible for that event to happen. In this case, the medication order was verified. The Pyxis released the dose. Epic allowed the medication to be given without a warning. The charge nurse was either unaware that a novice nurse was overwhelmed or failed to intervene. Systems and leaders failed Anna. Any of these failures might create a setting where the error is possible; the combination allowed it to happen. Accidents result from multiple system failures, brilliantly illustrated by James Reason (2016) in the Swiss cheese model of how accidents and errors occur. The cheese is the barrier, and the holes in the cheese are flaws in the system. When the holes align, the failure gets through the holes in the barrier and reaches the patient (Reason, 2017).

Consider, too, the supervisor's intent in taking disciplinary action. What did she hope to achieve in her meeting with Anna, and what was the goal of penalizing her? Disciplinary action taken against a novice nurse does not protect future patients or the hospital. It undermines one nurse and contributes to a culture that covers up inherent flaws. It exposes patients to greater risk. Since the Institute of Medicine (IOM) published *To Err Is Human: Building a Safer Health System* (2000), which exposed and explored medical errors, hospitals, professional organizations, and colleges of nursing have embraced the concepts of just culture as a way to encourage self-reporting and systems engineering in healthcare to prevent errors.

Anna made an error. In a just culture, she should be consoled. She should also be encouraged to speak openly about her experience, alert her colleagues to a near-miss or precursor safety event, and take action to correct the system flaws that allowed this error to reach the patient.

Anna was not given the support she needed. She was forced to delay in pursuing her chosen nursing specialty and perceived herself as a failure. She might have asked the supervisor what could be done differently, although, considering this supervisor's leadership style, the answer would likely have been extremely unhelpful, such as *"Be more careful next time."* She might also have explained that she reported her own error, hoping that others might learn from it. While interviewing, a novice nurse should investigate the hospital's nurse residency program. How much orientation and preceptor support are provided, and for how long? Ask the interviewer about the old adage that nurses eat their young. Consider inquiring about errors: *"Can you tell me about a time a nurse made an error and how you (or the hospital) responded?"* Listen for keywords when questioning how the hospital responds to errors and safety events. If the response includes the words *just culture, console, coach,* or *second victim,* the hospital is embracing best practices and high-reliability principles (Boysen, 2013; Ozeke et al., 2019).

In his research into management styles, Andrew Schmidt (2008) developed an instrument to measure "dysfunctional and destructive behaviors" by leaders. Employing this tool, studies exposed a positive correlation between toxic leadership in nursing and patient harm (Labrague, 2021). In the scenario Anna shared, she was balancing demands, so she took a moment to stop, think, and prioritize. This is a recognized high-reliability skill. When she identified an error, she took immediate action to protect her patient. She demonstrated that she incorporates high-reliability processes into her practice. These actions should be applauded, not penalized. Most importantly, shame has no place in a mentoring relationship.

When nurse leaders speak of their responsibilities, we generally address administrative expectations first. We are responsible for staffing, unit or department operations, schedules, equipment, and supplies, or ensuring competencies, for example. Rarely do we put mentoring novice nurses at the top of the list. Yet, the manner in which nurse leaders guide the development of the nurses they supervise reflects on leaders' own self-awareness and commitment to lifelong learning. The American Association of Colleges of Nursing (n.d.) identifies an essential part of nursing leadership as the intentional development of nurses and nurse leaders of the future. The tenth domain, Personal, Professional, and Leadership Development, calls for self-reflection and a commitment to personal growth but also for leaders to advocate for the nursing profession and to mentor others' in their growth and accountability. The supervisor in this scenario failed, both as a mentor and as a nurse leader.

The hospital in this story lost a conscientious, self-aware nurse. The nursing profession suffered a setback when Anna abandoned her pursuit of critical care training. Countless critically ill patients were deprived of the attentive, professional care she would have provided them had she been welcomed into the profession by an authentic, supportive nurse leader, mentored in the development of her practice, and inspired to do the same for the next generation of nurses.

To Err Is Human

By Linda Roney, EdD, RN-BC, CPEN, CNE, FAAN

If you have not had the chance to read *To Err Is Human* (IOM, 2000) while in nursing school, I highly recommend it. While the book is more than 25 years old, it is central to how we practice health care today. It helps us look at Anna's situation with an understanding that while she was punished for her role in the situation, the problem was systemic and needs that lens to fix it; otherwise it will continue to happen. The typical initial reaction when there is an error is to find and blame someone (IOM, 2000); in that case, it was Anna. Even when an error appears to be caused by one person, it is most often due to multiple contributing factors. Blaming an individual does not change these factors, and the same error will likely happen again (IOM, 2000). Lancaster et al. (2022) describe *just culture* as one in which medical errors often result from problems in error-proofing organizational systems and structures rather than a mistake made by a well-intentioned person directly involved in an incident. This ensures a fair approach, and it is important to note that some errors warrant disciplinary action.

Even in adversity, Anna demonstrates strength and aptitude in the American Association of Colleges of Nursing essentials' (2021) domains 2 and 10 competencies and subcompetencies.

TABLE 6.1 Examples of Domain 2: Person-Centered Care and Domain 10: Personal, Professional, and Leadership Development in This Exemplar

Domain 2: Person-Centered Care	
2.1 Engage with the individual in establishing a caring relationship.	Despite feeling overwhelmed by the many simultaneous needs of her patients at the beginning of her shift, Anna prioritized empathetic and compassionate care of her patients.
2.3 Integrate assessment skills in practice.	Anna was able to distinguish between normal and abnormal health findings as she recognized that her patient was in severe pain.
2.4 Diagnose actual or potential health problems and needs.	With multiple demands, Anna was able to prioritize her patients and when she recognized her error, she called the provider about the current situation, what had happened, and her assessment.
2.5 Develop a plan of care.	After recognizing her error, Anna was aware and anticipating any potentially adverse outcomes of the medication administration.
2.6 Demonstrate accountability for care delivery.	Anna appropriately delegated to the certified nursing assistant.
Domain 10: Personal, Professional, and Leadership Development	
10.1 Demonstrate a commitment to personal health and well-being.	Anna engaged in guided and spontaneous reflection on her experience with the medication error and the aftermath of the situation to promote her wellness and resiliency. While the incident impacted her plan for applying for the critical care residency, she showed commitment to her professional development and created a new path.

Documentation

There are many reasons why we document care in a healthcare record. De Groot et al. (2022) describe the clinical documentation process as a way for nurses to continuously reflect on their entire process (assessment, diagnosis, care planning, implementation, and evaluation) of providing direct nursing care to patients. This process can take up to 41% of their shift (De Groot et al., 2022). Each entry in the medical record, from routine assessments to complex interventions, has financial implications. Missing, incomplete, or unclear documentation can lead to revenue loss for the organization, as services that are not documented accurately may not be billed (American Health Information Management Association, 2022). While it is well known that adequate nursing staffing positively affects patient and nurse satisfaction, it can also provide an advantage to hospitals and result in better financial performance. Hospitals facing financial uncertainty have reduced nursing staffing to increase profitability, which worsens the problem (Everhart et al., 2013). Adequate staffing results in nurses having more time for better documentation of the excellent care they provide, which, in turn, helps organizations receive better payment for services.

I have been asked by many emerging nurses what they are supposed to document. The question is rooted in wanting to do what is best for their patients and often prioritizing the actual patient care over writing what was done when pressed for time (American Nurses Association [ANA}, 2010). Although the ANA's *Principles for Nursing Documentation: Guidance for Registered Nurses* (ANA, 2010) was published before more sophisticated EHR were commonplace in health care, their principles remain at the core of excellent documentation.

The Uses of Nursing Documentation

Our nursing documentation is essential for communicating within the healthcare team (ANA, 2010). We provide our assessment of the patient and their status at the snapshot of time that we record. Technology gives us other tools to help support this (such as when your abnormal vital signs are automatically documented into the patient's flowsheet or when you get a fingerstick and when you return the device to the docking station, the information is transmitted to the EHR. You must know and comply with your clinical unit's and healthcare organization's documentation standards. They may include the following: assessments, clinical problems; communication with other healthcare providers regarding the patient, communication, and education of the patient, family, and third parties (e.g., home care agencies); medication administration; order acknowledgment, implementation, and management; patient clinical parameters; patient responses and outcomes, including status changes; and plans of care for the patient's social and cultural needs (ANA, 2010, p. 5).

Documentation Tips

Before charting, ensure that you have the correct chart open (Nurses Service Organization [NSO], 2024). As nurses, we are toggling throughout our day through the multiple pages of the multiple patients on our assignment's medical record. In addition to the areas listed in the section above (The Uses of Nursing Documentation), chart precautions or preventive measures are used to ensure the safety of your patients and others (NSO, 2024). An example of this might be that you maintained seizure precautions on your patient, complying with hospital guidelines that include the bed in a low position, suction and oxygen at the head of the bed, and padded side rails. Some EHRs have a drop-down menu of items to click, while in others, especially if the type of precaution is not typical for your patient population, you may have to write it in as part of your narrative note. Record any outreach, including phone calls and secure mobile messaging on hospital-approved devices, to a provider or another team member about a patient, including the exact time, message, and response (NSO, 2024). If they did not respond, document when you tried contacting them again. Follow your unit policies for escalating unreturned communication based on the service's organizational chart. Reviewing Chapter 5 about provider hierarchy may be helpful in providing background information as you prepare for these interactions.

If a patient or caregiver refuses a treatment or medication, document it and report it to the covering provider. If appropriate to your unit policies, report it to your nursing supervisor (NSO, 2024). While we all get busy, chart as much as possible in real time. Bringing a mobile computer into your patient's room might not be possible with every patient encounter throughout your shift, but make a point to chart as soon as you leave the room. It is too easy to forget details later (NSO, 2024). Do not chart a patient's symptoms without documenting how you responded to them (NSO, 2024). For example, if your patient reports leg pain, you must also chart how you responded to their concern, such as their pain assessment scale and rating and that you provided PRN acetaminophen as ordered. When someone tells you something that needs to be documented, use quotation marks and properly attribute the remarks to the correct person (NSO, 2024).

Try to document as objectively as possible. The patient was wearing a yellow jewelry band on their left fourth digit that was removed and given to the security officer is better than "The patient was wearing a gold wedding ring on their finger." Do you know that it was gold? You are not a gemologist, so document your patient's belongings as plainly as you do their assessments. Just the facts, without emotion and with few, if any, details that you did not directly observe yourself.

Who Reads What You Wrote?

In addition to the team (now and in the future) who is caring for the patient, you need to be aware that other individuals and representatives of organizations can view your documentation to promote high-quality care.

Regulation and Legislative Mandates (ANA, 2010)

As a nursing student, you may have heard the terms *The Joint Commission* and *the State* or *DPH* (*Department of Public Health*). The Joint Commission

(TJC) is a nonprofit organization that accredits and certifies healthcare organizations and programs in the United States. Its primary role is to ensure that healthcare facilities meet standards of care (TJC, n.d.). While the exact term and nuances vary by state, each state's department of public health ensures compliance with state licensing laws and federal certification regulations in its role as the state survey agency for the Centers for Medicare & Medicaid Services, for which it certifies facilities to receive Medicare and Medicaid reimbursements (California Department of Public Health, n.d.). Chart audits from these and other accrediting and certifying agencies, such as trauma center verification, may be reviewed to gather information about compliance with an issue or protocol or in response to a reported adverse event. Organizations have very strict guidelines about the timeline and what needs to be reported, and your employer can share these with you.

Legal Personnel (ANA, 2010)

Patient documentation is essential evidence in legal matters, and incomplete, inaccurate, untimely, or false documentation can put healthcare organizations and providers at risk of liability (ANA, 2010). There are specific processes that those in the legal system must pursue in order to obtain copies of the medical record for review.

Reimbursement (ANA, 2010)

Nursing documentation is used to support the severity of illness and quality of care provided for a patient that is documented as charges by the provider (ANA, 2010). This is important for billing and payment recovery.

Research (ANA, 2010)

The data collected in the EHR, for either individual patients or groups of patients who fall into a similar population, may be used in a research study (ANA, 2010). Medical records can be used for research without patient consent, assuming that the research has undergone review by an institutional review board, is deemed to be of no more than minimal risk, and the study could only be conducted with the waiver (Kass et al., 2003). You will likely never know that your documentation was reviewed to conduct research. In the future, if you decide to pursue graduate study and, as part of your final project, you would like to use the medical record data from your unit, you must strictly adhere to the formal processes for requests for medical information at your healthcare organization and your program. Because you have login access to the medical record as part of your employment, it does not mean that you can access the data without permission for other purposes.

Quality Processes and Quality Improvement (ANA, 2010)

Many hospitals have adopted organizational models that support quality and safety improvement through formal processes that might include designated staff (Children's Hospital Association, n.d.). EHR documentation can be used to analyze variance from established guidelines and measure and improve processes and performance related to patient care. All nurses must have thorough, evidence-based knowledge of the impact of the care they provide on the outcomes that patients experience and data on the nursing-sensitive measures such as data available through the National Database of Nursing Quality Indicators® (ANA, 2010).

Event Reporting

Due to potential threats to the patients' and staff's safety, Anna could have used her organization's event reporting structure to report deviations from standard practices. To improve the quality and safety of health care, actual or potential incidents and adverse events that could harm a patient, a caregiver, or other individuals should be reported through formal organizational processes (Patient Safety Company, 2024). Sometimes healthcare workers do not report events for fear of blame, retaliation, embarrassment, or disciplinary action (Duffey et al., 2019). *To Err Is Human* (IOM, 2000) increased awareness of medical errors and called for collaboration among all stakeholders.

> However, not all the costs can be directly measured. Errors are also costly in terms of patients' loss of trust in the system and diminished satisfaction by both patients and health professionals … . Health care professionals pay with loss of morale and frustration at not being able to provide the best care possible. (IOM, 2000, p. 2)

These reports, often called *incident reports*, are voluntary patient safety event reports that rely on front-line staff to provide detailed information (Agency for Healthcare Research and Quality, 2019). They should be completed as quickly as possible, generally within 24 hours, and are not part of the patient's medical record (NSO, 2024). The report should objectively capture essential information, such as the dates, time, and location of the event; names of people affected and witnesses; names of those notified; the condition of the person affected; and any actions taken in response (NSO, 2024). Once the report is made, a root cause analysis (RCA) is completed by an individual with the training to investigate adverse events and help those closest to the event brainstorm solutions, learn from errors, and improve safe nursing practice (Abreu, 2021). In this case, having a staff member outside of Anna's unit complete the RCA may have helped the team gain insight into opportunities to value all team members and maintain a safe environment. It also demonstrates professional accountability by her.

Accessing Medical Records

We briefly mentioned earlier that you should be accessing patients' medical records only when they are directly under your care. There are times when this is less obvious, such as when a charge nurse is planning for an admission, and while you will not be directly caring for that patient, your decisions are based on critical patient information that may not be obtained other than in the EHR. You leave a digital footprint of what pages of the EHR you access and how long you view them. Under no circumstances can you access an individual's medical record unless your workload authorizes you to do so.

Should I Get My Own Nursing Malpractice Insurance Policy?

That question is asking for legal advice. I am not a lawyer; as you know, I am a nurse. I will give you information that you may find helpful as you make your own decision. When new nurses consider this question, it usually regards their questions of potentially being named in a lawsuit for reasons such as medication error, failure to follow errors, practicing outside of their scope, failure to recognize an order error, failure to monitor and assess patients adequately, failure to communicate pertinent patient information, and wrongful delegation of a nursing function (O'Neill, 2021). Under the legal doctrine of *respondeat superior* (let the master answer), employers remain responsible for acts employees perform within the scope of their employment. Nurses can become involved in legal action, even when they follow the standard of care (NSO, 2024). Some nurses are told that obtaining an individual professional liability policy increases the potential sources of money for a claim settlement or jury award at trial, making them more likely to be named in a lawsuit. Literature supports that attorneys decide who to sue based on the facts of the case, not whether someone has an individual policy. Also, the plaintiff's attorney will not know if a nurse has a policy until the nurse is named a defendant and discloses that fact during the discovery process (NSO, 2024).

One important consideration is that your employer's policy will not cover legal representation before the state board of nursing, the agency with disciplinary authority over nurses and their licenses (Massachusetts Nurses Association, 2023). Some policies also offer coverage if you suffer from personal injury or become a victim of violence in the workplace (NSO, 2024).

If you are called by someone identifying as an attorney representing either side of a patient case with which you were involved, do not speak with them until you receive more information from your supervisor and legal affairs office. Suppose that you do have your own individual professional nursing insurance policy. In that case, you may be able to speak to an advocate about your situation, even if you are not formally named in the claim. Get your facts and consider all the options. If you decide to pursue your own policy, consider policies endorsed by professional nursing organizations, such as the ANA (2024).

YOU MATTER: TO ERR IS HUMAN

You have worked so hard to become a nurse, and the thought of potentially harming a patient because of something that you did or did not do is terrifying. Over the past 25 years, healthcare organizations have come a long way in recognizing that any one error is the result of multiple system failures. You may feel marginalized and fear punishment. Take accountability for your role and become part of the solution, because you matter!

Book Club Questions

1. How should the manager have addressed the medication error while working in a just culture?
2. What are some best practices you have seen in the clinical setting regarding nursing documentation? In what areas do you need to improve?

About This Chapter's Authors

Anna Mulac, BSN, RN

Anna was born and raised near Pittsburgh. She attended Fairfield University, where she received her Bachelor of Science in Nursing while playing for the women's tennis team. After graduating in 2021, she moved across the country and worked at a community hospital's medical-surgical/telemetry floor. She then moved out of the hospital into a dermatology/aesthetics specialty. During this time, she has been pursuing her family nurse practitioner master's degree from United States University. Outside of work, Anna loves to be with family and friends as well as cooking, reading, working out, and doing anything active in nature.

Laurie Nolan-Kelley, DNP, RN, CNL, CEN, TCRN, EMT-P

Dr. Laurie Nolan-Kelly is a passionate advocate for the professional development of nurses and advancement of the nursing profession. She brings the clinical nurse leader perspective to her work, pursuing excellence in delivering safe, high-quality, and equitable health care. She welcomes any opportunity to mentor nurse leaders and drive continuous interdisciplinary care improvement. Laurie lives with her husband, Barney, in coastal Connecticut, where they often (and noisily) gather their four daughters, sons-in-law, grandchildren, and grand-pets. She is an avid sailor and describes her sailboat, *Bikini*, as her happy place.

References

Abreu, T. (2021). *Adverse event reporting and root cause analysis*. American Nurse. https://www.myamericannurse.com/adverse-event-reporting-and-root-cause-analysis/

Agency for Healthcare Research and Quality. (2019). *Reporting patient safety events*. https://psnet.ahrq.gov/primer/reporting-patient-safety-events

American Association of Colleges of Nursing. (n.d.). *Personal, professional and leadership development*. https://www.aacnnursing.org/essentials/tool-kit/domains-concepts/personal-professional-and-leadership-development

American Association of Colleges of Nursing. (2021). *The essentials: Core competencies for professional nursing education*. https://www.aacnnursing.org/Portals/0/PDFs/Publications/Essentials-2021.pdf

American Health Information Management Association. (2022). *Revenue cycle management: Connecting technology, people, and processes*.

American Nurses Association. (2010). *Principles for nursing documentation: Guidance for registered nurses*. https://www.nursingworld.org/globalassets/docs/ana/ethics/principles-of-nursing-documentation.pdf

American Nurses Association. (2024). *Personal benefits*. https://www.nursingworld.org/membership/member-benefits/personal-benefits/

Boysen, P. G. (2013). Just culture: A foundation for balanced accountability and patient safety. *Ochsner Journal, 13*(3), 400–406.

California Department of Public Health. (n.d.). *L&C program home*. https://www.cdph.ca.gov/Programs/CHCQ/LCP/Pages/LandCProgramHome.aspx

Children's Hospital Association. (n.d.). *The next phase of quality in children's health*. https://www.childrenshospitals.org/news/childrens-hospitals-today/2022/02/the-next-phase-of-quality-in-childrens-health

De Groot, K., De Veer, A. J. E., Munster, A. M., Francke, A. L., & Paans, W. (2022). Nursing documentation and its relationship with perceived nursing workload: a mixed-methods study among community nurses. *BMC Nursing, 21*(1), 34. https://doi.org/10.1186/s12912-022-00811-7

Duffey, P., Oliver, J., & Newcomb, P. (2019). Evaluating the use of high-reliability principles to increase error event reporting. *Journal of Nursing Administration, 49*(6), 310–314. doi:10.1097/NNA.0000000000000758.

Everhart, D., Neff, D., Al-Amin, M., Nogle, J., & Weech-Maldonado, R. (2013). The effects of nurse staffing on hospital financial performance: competitive versus less competitive markets. *Health Care Management Review, 38*(2), 146–155. https://doi.org/10.1097/HMR.0b013e318257292b

Institute of Medicine. (2000). *To err is human: Building a safer health system.* National Academies Press. https://doi.org/10.17226/9728

Kass, N. E., Natowicz, M. R., Hull, S. C., Faden, R. R., Plantinga, L., Gostin, L. O., & Slutsman, J. (2003). The use of medical records in research: What do patients want? *Journal of Law, Medicine & Ethics, 31*(3), 429–433. https://doi.org/10.1111/j.1748-720x.2003.tb00105.x

Labrague, L. J. (2021). Influence of nurse managers' toxic leadership behaviours on nurse-reported adverse events and quality of care. *Journal of Nursing Management, 29*(4), 855–863.

Lancaster, R. J., Vizgirda, V., Quinlan, S., & Kingston, M. B. (2022.) *To err is human, just culture, practice, and liability in the face of nursing error. Nurse Leader. 517- 521. https://doi.org/10.1016/j.mnl.2022.06.010*

Massachusetts Nurses Association. (2023, June 8). *Why you need your own liability insurance and common misconceptions.* https://www.massnurses.org/2023/06/08/why-you-need-your-own-liability-insurance-and-common-misconceptions/

Nurses Service Organization. (2024). *Incident reports: A safety tool.* https://www.nso.com/Learning/Artifacts/Articles/Incident-reports-A-safety-tool

O'Neill, S. (2021). *Individual nurse liability insurance.* Nursing Service Organization. https://www.nso.com/Learning/Artifacts/Articles/Incident-reports-A-safety-tool

Ozeke, O., Ozeke, V., Coskun, O., & Budakoglu, I. I. (2019). Second victims in health care: Current perspectives. *Advances in Medical Education and Practice, 10,* 593–603. https://doi.org/10.2147/AMEP.S185912

Patient Safety Company. (2024). *Reporting incidents in healthcare.* https://www.patientsafety.com/en/incident-reporting

Reason, J. (2016). *Organizational accidents revisited.* CRC Press.

Reason, J. (2017). *The human contribution: unsafe acts, accidents, and heroic recoveries.* CRC Press.

Schmidt, A. A. (2008). *Development and validation of the toxic leadership scale.* University of Maryland, College Park.

The Joint Commission. (n.d.). *Who we are.* https://www.jointcommission.org/who-we-are/

CHAPTER 7

Out of Our Element

Floating to Another Unit as a New Nurse

Katherine (Katie) Knapik, BSN, RNC-MNN; Erin McMahon, EdD, CNM, FACNM; and Linda Roney, EdD, RN-BC, CPEN, CNE, FAAN

Learning Goals

1. Describe Katie's strengths and challenges in getting floated to another unit as a new-graduate nurse.
2. Reflect on personal beliefs and attitudes that affect one's decision to communicate in new situations.
3. Design your strategy for success for when you are floated or redeployed to another unit.

'Irrevocably Intertwined'

By Katherine (Katie) Knapik, BSN, RNC-MNN

The maternal-newborn world at my hospital is, in theory, one big happy family. The labor and delivery unit (L&D), the postpartum unit, and the neonatal intensive care unit (NICU) all collaborate to give the same pool of patients the quality care to which they are entitled. No single unit could even pretend to operate without the support of the other two. As a nurse on the postpartum unit, not a day goes by when I'm not regularly communicating with the nurses working in L&D and the NICU. One minute I'm getting report from L&D on a new delivery, and the next I'm calling down to the NICU to ask when my patient can visit her 32-week preemie.

What's more, not only do the three units share patients, but we also share staff. Most of us nurses can float to at least one of the other two units. We regularly shuffle around bodies to ensure that each unit is adequately staffed for the day. I daresay that no one enjoys being floated, but we learn to grin and bear the occasional trip to a sister unit when that means our fellow nurses can practice in safer conditions and our patients receive better care as a result.

In short, the three units are irrevocably intertwined. Our ultimate goal is the same. Day in and day out, we all show up to work with the hope that we can make a positive difference in the lives of mothers and newborns alike. And we certainly could not achieve this goal without the special contributions of each branch of the family tree.

Naturally, as is the case with all families, we don't always get along. Such close collaboration between the three units—especially given the inherently stressful and demanding nature of the maternal-newborn field—inevitably lends itself to conflict. Each unit has its unique set of needs, and almost without exception, each unit tends to think its needs are more pressing than the others.

One of my earliest and most memorable experiences with interpersonal conflict in the healthcare setting occurred a mere week after I got off orientation. I waltzed into the breakroom at 7:00 one morning, prepared to take on another glorious day on the postpartum floor. A glance at the whiteboard on the wall suggested that this would not be the case today. Next to my name, scrawled in bright-red dry-erase marker, was the word *FLOAT*, indicating that I would need to grab my things and head downstairs to the L&D floor. I had only just wrapped up my two-week orientation on learning how to care for the high-risk pregnant women to whom I would be assigned, so being floated was, admittedly, quite jarring. I was still very much getting used to the idea of being a nurse on my home unit. Now, I was expected to adequately care for a different patient population in a different environment with different colleagues around me. A daunting prospect, to say the least.

"Don't worry," the night charge nurse on my unit reassured me. "I've already worked it out with the girls downstairs. You'll be the second nurse caring for the antepartum patients from 7:00 to 3:00. Kristine will be with you. It should calm down in L&D by this afternoon, so you'll come back up here at 3:00 with the scheduled C-section once she's delivered. Libby will be in charge up here, so keep in touch with her in case anything changes."

This was a game plan I could get behind. I had only been at my hospital for a few months, and I was meeting new faces every single day, but I had gotten along well with the labor nurses I'd met so far. Kristine, the other nurse alongside whom I'd be working, had even trained me to care for these antepartum patients during a few of my orientation shifts. While training me, she was both enjoyable company and a helpful teammate, so given the circumstances, I figured that I would survive.

The day started like any other on the unit. I said hello to my patients. I did my head-to-toe assessments. I passed my medications. I completed my nonstress tests. I filled water pitchers and fetched crackers. I relished the time I had to talk with my patients. I enjoyed listening to them divulge their excitement, nerves, and every other emotion one could imagine when expecting a baby. As the day progressed, the idle chit-chat with patients and the almost lazy way I sauntered around the hallway to complete my tasks became things of the past. A steady stream of new admissions and the hurdle of a few unexpected patient complications meant that the morning passed in a flurry of movement and excitement. We became busy, but Kristine and I were managing to get through the day.

"You know," Kristine directed to me as we were both catching up on some mid-morning charting at the nurse's station. "It's honestly unfair to you that you're being asked to go back upstairs later today after working so hard down here."

"I don't mind," I replied as I continued clicking away on the computer. "Makes the day fly by, you know?"

"If Libby were really your friend, she wouldn't make you give up your entire assignment so late into the day. I would be upset if I were you."

The sound of Kristine typing filled the silence as I processed what she had just said. *"If Libby were really my friend?"* As far as I was concerned, the plan for me to float back to the postpartum unit had nothing to do with our friendship. Rather, it had everything to do with what made the most sense staffing-wise for everyone. I didn't feel slighted by the decision to float back to the postpartum unit at all. But then again, should I have felt troubled by this plan? I was still becoming familiar with the complex dynamic between postpartum and L&D. Was floating back more than halfway through the day truly that heinous of an act? No, I decided—not to me. My easygoing nature gave me the clarity to understand that although it was a minor inconvenience to take on a new assignment, it wasn't going to kill me to pick up a few couplets on the postpartum floor for the remainder of my shift.

Kristine swiveled in her chair to look me straight in the eyes and said, "I think you should text Libby and let her know you'd rather stay down here. It's really not fair."

Understanding that there was a clear disconnect between our perceptions of the current events, I assured Kristine that I would text Libby, and I carried on with my work.

It didn't take long for Kristine to badger me again. "What did she say when you texted her?"

"Oh, uh, just that the plan is still for me to come up at 3:00," I fibbed on the spot. I hadn't texted Libby.

Kristine's voice took on a slightly more acidic tone when she replied, "I would just be so frustrated about this situation."

As another nurse walked past the nurses' station, Kristine piped up. "Meg, don't you think it's unfair that Katie's going back upstairs? She's worked so hard all day, and it's still so busy. This'll leave me with all six patients, which is just unacceptable."

A-ha. The motive was revealed. It became evident as the two nurses conversed about staffing ratios that Kristine's zeal to see me remain in place was never about me. Kristine didn't want to be left alone with my patients.

Kristine and Meg, who had now gotten roped into the situation, both urged me to text Libby again. To implore her to see reason. To help her understand that I felt wounded by her decisions. The more they continued to talk at me, the more I wanted to get back to the safety of the postpartum unit. In fact, at this point, I was simply giddy to get a whole new assignment upstairs. Although I had not texted Libby initially, when Kristine indicated that she was heading to the break room to call Libby herself, I did shoot off a brief warning text. "Kristine's calling. It's mayhem down here." *Send*. I didn't await a reply as I continued with my patient care in the hope that I could avoid facing the inevitable drama that was coming my way.

Whether Kristine liked it or not, 3:00 rolled around, and I gathered my belongings to go upstairs. Before I could make it off the unit, Kristine managed to sneak in a final spiel about loyalty, knowing who your friends are when the going gets tough, and the importance of teamwork—an ideal the girls on the postpartum unit, Kristine believed, seemed to lack.

My eyes prickled as I tried to hold back the hot tears that threatened to spill over. I felt like my own loyalty was being tested during this lecture. Do I speak up and defend my coworkers or keep quiet and nod in agreement to maintain my reputation in the eyes of the L&D nurses? I chose the latter, my heart aching as I listened to the virtues of my coworkers be called into question.

When I walked into the break room on the postpartum unit, I locked eyes with Libby, who was sitting at the head of the room's large table. She, too, looked on the verge of crying. Upon seeing each other, we both let a few tears drop. The situation was, in all honesty, utterly ridiculous and almost comedic. "What a mess of a day. Why are you crying?" I laughed through the tears.

"Kristine called up here no less than five times to tell me how upset you were about being floated back. We desperately need you up here, but Kristine said that you weren't happy at all about the situation. I thought you were mad at me," Libby revealed.

"What?" I was beyond shocked to hear this. "I never said any of that." We compared our respective sides of the story and realized that Kristine had played both of us. Kristine was using our friendship against each other to influence Libby into letting me stay downstairs.

Although we had nothing to be truly sorry about, as a testament to our friendship and respect for one another, Libby and I both apologized profusely for the misunderstanding. We carried on with our day as if nothing had happened, but I know both of us were still reeling from the emotional manipulation that we had experienced. We reported the events to our nursing leaders, and Libby eventually received an apology from Kristine. I did not.

This was an extremely challenging situation for me to navigate. As a new graduate, I was very conscious of my newness through every step of this ordeal. When you work in such a team-oriented field as health care, it behooves you to build and maintain positive relationships with your coworkers. I didn't want to destroy my budding rapport with the nurses on L&D. I was wary of disagreeing with or contradicting anything Kristine or the others said out of fear that I would be labeled as difficult to work with. I was convinced that if I spoke up, then I would be met with cool glares and not-so-sneaky whispers behind my back the next time I floated down to L&D. Better to do and say what I needed to fit in, I figured.

At the same time, however, I felt fiercely protective over my sisters upstairs. They were, after all, the ones who had supported and guided me through four tumultuous months of orientation. None of them had a mean bone in their body as far as I was concerned, and I was confident that they would never act in a way that was intentionally "unfair" to anyone, let alone one of their own. I so badly wanted to articulate all of this and more to Kristine, but I was halted by my own fear of retaliation.

What I've come to realize, though, is that it was OK to feel conflicted and unsure about how to proceed. It was perfectly acceptable to feel uncomfortable in an objectively uncomfortable situation. I didn't win any awards for attempting to manage this conflict alone. Life, not just work, is riddled with conflict, and it's unrealistic to believe that you'll always have the right answers. What's essential to learn, however, is whom to call when trouble is afoot. Charge nurses, clinical leaders, nurse supervisors, and nurse managers are available as resources to guide nurses through whatever difficult situations may arise. In my story, there was simply no reason for so many staff nurses to intervene in staffing decisions for two separate units. The charge nurses should have communicated with each other and with our manager as a mediator if need be. Firmly proclaiming that I deferred any decision-making to the charge nurses would have taken me out of whichever game was being played while still protecting the various relationships I was working so hard to build.

Conflict resolution takes practice. As I've encountered conflict and seen how others have navigated difficult situations, I've built a toolbox from which I can draw from past experiences to guide future choices. It still isn't easy to manage conflict at work, especially when it involves the other two units. Remember, we're a family, and all families have their good and bad days together. I don't have all the answers (again, no one does), but with each passing day, I grow more confident in myself and my ability to keep my branch of the family tree running smoothly.

'You Can Go Back for a Do-Over'

By Erin McMahon, EdD, CNM, FACNM

I have been a nurse for 31 years. I come from a family of nurses. My aunt is a nurse, my cousin is a nurse, and my daughter is a nurse. I have been a nurse-midwife for 25 years. I have practiced in a variety of clinical settings, and stories like the one above make me so angry. I want to jump into nurse-manager mode and confront the nurse who exhibited such hurtful and unprofessional behavior. However, that would not have fixed this problem and may have made things worse. So, let's take a deep breath and analyze this situation.

The truth is the situation described is not uncommon. L&D, postpartum, and the NICU are deeply intertwined. They care for overlapping patient populations, and patients move back and forth between the three units. It is also very common for there to be strong feelings between the units. L&D nurses have unique skills, including maternal and fetal surveillance, labor progress assessment, labor support, assistance with birth, and responding to complications and emergencies. Postpartum nurses are experts in postdelivery maternal and neonatal assessment and support families in the transition to parenthood, provide lactation support for newborn care, and respond to complications and emergencies. The NICU nurses provide assessment and critical life support to some of our smallest patients. They provide intense care to premature infants and medically compromised babies. They also offer emotional support to parents and families. Each group of nurses has a unique set of skills; they work in high-stress environments and support each other as needed. The problem occurs when each nurse identifies with their "home unit" and sees themselves as separate from the other two units. Over the years, I have heard comments such as the following:

- "Those L&D nurses are prima donnas; they think they are better than everyone else."
- "Those postpartum nurses just feed babies and change diapers all day; anyone can do that."
- "Those NICU nurses only have one patient to take care of for 12 hours; how hard can that be?"

Katie described how she had respect and admiration for her colleagues on the other units. What happened over time that caused the nurses to segregate, isolate, and treat each other in such unprofessional ways? We do have some insight into why this happens. Contributing factors include being overworked, being understaffed, working in a high-stress environment, having compassion fatigue, and experiencing burnout. If these factors take hold in a hospital unit and are not addressed by leadership, the culture becomes toxic. In a perfect world, the nurses would truly see themselves as one team, collaborating to provide excellent patient care. Everyone would float seamlessly between the three units, and the barriers would be broken down. The problem is that each of the three areas requires a unique set of nursing skills, and it is very difficult to be an expert in all three areas simultaneously. Since we cannot create a perfect shared unit, let us turn our attention back to the new-graduate nurse. How could we help her going forward?

First, here are the strengths that the new nurse brought to the situation. She was enthusiastic about coming to work and eager to start her day providing high-quality care to her postpartum patients. She was shocked that she would be floating when she was newly off orientation. To her credit, she decided to stay positive. The other unit needed help, and she knew the nurse with whom she would be working. We can relate this to the *theory of mattering and marginalization* and the idea of *ego extension* (Flett, 2018). Remember that *ego extension* happens when an individual sees another person emotionally invested in you (Flett, 2018). Katie knew Kristine; they had worked well together in the past, and it would be a good day. She arrived on the new unit and went to work. Even as the workload picked up, she stayed positive and worked as a team with Kristine.

Where did this shift go wrong? First, the night charge nurse told the new nurse that L&D "should" quiet down in the afternoon, and then she could return to postpartum. This was the wrong thing to say. L&D, much like the emergency department, is unpredictable. You can have an empty unit one minute and 30 minutes later be full of patients in active labor, needing to be triaged or awaiting labor induction. Postpartum and the NICU will fill up as L&D decants, only to fill up again. Truly the circle of life. Sending the newest nurse to float when the units are very busy is not the best plan. The best float nurse has some experience and can call on those prior experiences to provide care in a new environment with a new patient population. Floating new nurses to a unit, when there is less pressure and stress, is what I would recommend to gain experience for the future.

Let us turn our attention to Kristine, the nurse on the high-risk antepartum unit. First, Kristine attempts to influence Katie. "*I would be angry if I were you.*" "*If she really were your friend, she would not make you give up your assignment.*" We do not know for sure, but Kristine seemed concerned that she would have to take over the full assignment of six patients from 3 to 7 p.m. Given her language, we can tell that she did not think it was fair. Kristine was focused on herself, not on the needs of all three units or on the needs of her patients. To get what she wanted, Kristine attempted to manipulate the situation by encouraging the new nurse to stand up for herself, preying on the fear of a new nurse that she was not advocating for her patient or herself. *Be brave, be strong, and speak up.* If Kristine was concerned about the assignments, she should have communicated that concern to the charge nurse herself. Formulas and patient-to-nurse ratios are used to make these decisions. If Kristine believed that the assignment was being applied unfairly and the charge nurse disagreed, there was a chain of command to activate until the issue was resolved. That may have involved communicating with the nurse manager or shift supervisor. Attempting to manipulate the situation, taking advantage of a new nurse, and publicly speaking disparagingly about the charge nurse to another nurse were unprofessional behaviors that warranted education and counseling from the supervisor. Unprofessional behaviors that are tolerated create emotional contagion and that can spread through hospital units like wildfire. Establishing champions to role model effective communication, negotiation, and problem-solving can also help improve a unit's culture.

Now, for our new nurse, what advice can we offer her for the future? Every situation is new and creates an experience that we learn from and can apply to future experiences. Our new nurse could not have seen this coming because she took all communication at face value and trusted her colleagues. A bit of situational awareness can be helpful, considering the impact of being pulled back to your home unit at 3 p.m.

Things to think about:

- How did the move affect our new nurse?
  She was glad to be back in a familiar setting and looked forward to meeting new patients.

- How did this affect Kristine?
  She would have been left alone with the six pregnant patients and was worried about how she would manage for the next four hours.

- How would this affect the other units?
- What was happening on L&D and the postpartum unit? Did they just receive five new admissions?
- Did postpartum have some late discharges?
- Most importantly, how did this affect the patients on all the units?

Even though you are not the charge nurse, it is helpful to understand what is happening on the other units so that we can support each other as a team. This makes it easier to understand our colleagues under stress, trying to make decisions about what the next few hours will hold and how to best staff all the units.

Responding to Kristine's comments will take some consideration. Let me be honest—my natural impulse would have been to challenge Kristine and say something sarcastic, such as, *"If you disagree with the assignment, why don't you call the charge nurse yourself? Or are you questioning my loyalty to you or the patients on this unit?"* **THIS IS NOT THE CORRECT RESPONSE. IT WILL NOT END WELL.** Please take a deep breath and use our best nursing reflective communication. Here is a better script that you might want to try if you are in this situation: *"You sound very worried about managing this assignment by yourself from 3 to 7 p.m. I wonder what is happening on the other units. Maybe we should check in with the charge nurse and ensure they have our correct census and acuity levels."*

I would encourage the person concerned to address the issue with the charge nurse directly rather than trying to manipulate other people to get the outcome they wanted. A conversation with the charge nurse may have revealed an error in the calculations and that it would have been better to leave the new nurse on the original unit to complete the shift with Kristine. Alternatively, the conversation may have revealed that the postpartum unit had received five new couplets from L&D and the new nurse was needed more urgently on the postpartum unit. A brief explanation could have helped increase understanding and promote teamwork versus mistrust and an assumption that you get help only when you have a friend in the charge nurse. I have observed charge nurses effectively manage staffing resources, and I have also witnessed bullying and an abuse of power in the role. If the final decision was still for Katie to return to her home unit, she could have offered additional support before leaving—for example, asking things such as, *"Is there anything that I can help you with before 3 p.m.?"* and *"Do you need help positioning or completing a nonstress test before I go back to the postpartum unit?"* These would present a good-faith effort to acknowledge Kristine's concern while supporting the plan that was the best for all three units.

Kristine again pressured Katie by asking, *"What did she say when you texted her [the charge nurse]?"* The new nurse, wanting to be accepted and trying to avoid conflict, felt pressured to lie that she had texted the charge nurse and that the plan was to stay the same. Feeling pressure that you cannot speak the truth in a situation is always a red flag for dysfunctional communication. First, we must consider the patient assignment that is best for patient care, and then the nurses' preferences may be considered. Direct, clear communication could have avoided this entire scenario.

Kristine could have told Katie, *"I am worried about managing this assignment when you go back to postpartum."*

Katie, using her best therapeutic communication, could have replied to that response from Kristine by saying, *"I hear that you are worried about managing this assignment alone. I will go wherever I am needed most; let's talk to the charge nurse."*

Katie, Kristine, or both nurses could have communicated that to the charge nurse.

Based on the new information, the charge nurse could have either reconsidered the assignment or explained that the plan had to stay the same due to events of which Kristine and Katie were unaware. In nursing, it is critical to establish boundaries, especially when colleagues exhibit unprofessional behavior. Katie could have responded to the continued badgering by drawing a clear boundary. An example would be by stating:

> *"I understand that you are upset, but do not question my integrity or loyalty. I am here to take care of patients wherever I am needed most. I had a good shift working with you as a team and appreciated your support while orienting to this unit."*

If Kristine was not mature enough to respond to this boundary professionally, it may still have been necessary to escalate to the supervisor. Consistent expectations for professional communication must be maintained to avoid a culture of bullying and retaliation.

Know yourself, understand your why and what motivates you to do this work. Then identify what are your values and what is important to you. This will help you stand firm when you need to apply boundaries. You can be a new nurse who is still learning and growing, committed to providing high-quality, patient-centered care and maintaining your boundaries within the collaborative team. If you are grounded in your values as a nurse, it is easier to stand up for yourself when someone is falsely challenging you or trying to manipulate you.

Another hint: Sometimes we do not handle a situation in the best way the first time around. Sometimes our colleagues can shock us with an attack in a high-stress situation. This is even worse if it occurs publicly. After you have time to reflect and gather your thoughts, you can go back to that individual for a do-over and say something like this:

> *"Kristine, I need to talk with you. I am very uncomfortable with our last conversation. I felt like you were questioning my loyalty to you and our patients. I am a new nurse trying to navigate the role of floating and doing my very best. Please do not speak to me that way in the future. I want to do what is best for our patients and our team of nurses. If you have concerns about how staffing decisions are being made, then you should bring that up to the charge nurse and our supervisor."*

This was a challenging situation for a new nurse to deal with. Being floated to a different unit can be scary when you are just starting to gain your confidence on your primary unit. Being manipulated, bullied, threatened, and having your loyalty questioned is very stressful. This could bring tears and a strong emotional response to anyone. I am so sorry that any new nurse would be put in this situation. We have identified some of the clear unprofessional behaviors and possible alternative responses that may have produced a different outcome. Let us consider some other concrete actions that speak to **Domain 10 of the American Association of Colleges of Nursing (AACN)** essentials (2021): Personal, Professional, and Leadership Development.

1. **Make a commitment to personal health and well-being** (AACN, 2021). Nursing schedules are long and can take a physical and emotional toll on the individual. Being serious about getting adequate rest before and after shifts is vital. When we are overtired and sleep-deprived, it is the same as working under the influence of alcohol. Nutrition is also essential. Having some protein snacks on hand for quick meals will improve your functioning. Identifying what refills your cup of resilience is important. Is that exercise, music, yoga, meditation, gardening, art, dancing, hiking, or spending time with friends? Find it and build it into your schedule.

2. **Demonstrate a spirit of inquiry that fosters flexibility and professional maturity** (AACN, 2021). I think of this as trying to understand

those around us. I mentioned *situational awareness* earlier in our conversation. For example, try to understand why someone is acting the way they are, what could be bothering them, or what are they stressed about? We can always ask them, but sometimes they need to figure out why they are acting so poorly. Operating from a spirit of inquiry helps mitigate a conflict before it erupts. As an example: *"Hey, Libby, Kristine seems very worried about being down here alone with all six patients. Is there any chance I can stay, or can we offer any other support? Do we have any patient care associates or another nurse who might come in early for the night shift? Just wondering if we have any other options."*

3. **Develop the capacity for leadership** (AACN, 2021). This begins with seeing beyond my patient assignment, looking around the unit, and having *situational awareness*. There is that term again, which means being aware of what is happening around me, my group of patients, offering to help when I can, and asking for help when needed. I advocate for my patients, my colleagues, and myself. Being a team player and willing to take on additional assignments is not ideal, but it is what is best for the patients—these small steps toward developing your leadership also role-model leadership for others. We have discussed how emotional contagion can allow negative attitudes to spread from person to person. We can also use emotional contagion to spread a culture of respect, admiration, and teamwork.

Floating, a.k.a. 'Redeployment'

By Linda Roney, EdD, RN-BC, CPEN, CNE, FAAN

There is one word that can evoke intense emotion in nurses, and that is the word *float*. When looking at the definition of the word, *float* sounds like something pleasant, including "to rest on the surface" and "wander." In nursing, *floating* is a form of cost-effective resource sharing among patient care units to address fluctuations in the patient census (O'Connor & Dugan, 2017). While *floating* is a more common term among nursing staff, recently, the term *redeployment* is more commonly used, especially when speaking of nurses going to areas of higher census or acuity since the COVID-19 pandemic (Karim et al., 2023). Mandatory floating can be used to address staff call-outs or increases in patient acuity or census (Lafontant et al., 2019). Some of the reasons that floating can evoke such emotion in nurses are fear of making a mistake in an unfamiliar patient care area, feeling overloaded with work, and being unable to care for patients and answer questions at the level of expectation (O'Connor & Duggan, 2017). Literature supports that new-graduate nurses should not be expected to float, but the definition of the period for this limitation is unclear (O'Connor & Duggan, 2017).

One of the hardest things about floating to another unit is that you need to know these temporary coworkers on whom you rely for support during your shift. The ideal situation is that you have oriented to the unit ahead of time to learn the basic flow of the unit and what is expected of you; however, for most of us, that does not happen. This is when you must get past the disappointment of working for some time on another unit. An emotional reaction to your redeployment will not help you retain the new information that you must learn quickly. If you have a specific reason, you believe working on the other unit is impossible due to safety, contact your supervisor immediately.

So much of the tone of the floating experience is set by the charge nurse with whom you will be working on the new unit. They *should* lead the team in welcoming you and provide you with an assignment with lower acuity and smaller patient assignment than regular staff on the shift. There are many reasons why this might not happen, so although that might be our expectation of what would be reasonable, be prepared that this might not be the case. Remember, on many units, being assigned the role of charge nurse on many units is purely a promotion of attrition, meaning that they have been there the longest or are rotating among the staff eligible for the unit's role. I still find it shocking that some units put some nurses in charge when they have been on a unit for a long time but do not have the skill to care for higher-acuity patients.

As you walk on the unit, take a deep breath and know that you can determine the tone of your shift. Choose to have a good day. *Smile.* Professionally greet the staff and identify yourself as the nurse assigned to help them that day. Use verbal cues throughout the day to remind the staff that you are there to help them during that time. At this point, the charge nurse should take the lead in supporting your transition to this new unit. I will proceed as if they do not so that you are prepared.

Ask to meet the charge nurse and ask for an orientation to the unit. If you arrive during report, which is what usually happens, delay asking for a unit tour until after you get report on your new patient assignment. Someone should identify the nurse who will give you report. Ask this off-going nurse for assistance in setting up your clinical context in the electronic health record (EHR) so that you can see the correct panel of patients on the unit and choose yours for the shift. During report with the off-going nurse, ask how many patients the other nurses have and whether your assignment is a heavy or light assignment to gain perspective and context for this new unit. Review all the orders and ask clarifying questions with the off-going nurse. If you are facing an order for something that you've never done before, now would be a good time to ask the off-going nurse to introduce you to the incoming charge nurse.

Greet the charge nurse warmly and communicate clearly, including whether or not you have been there before. Ask for a unit tour, including the essential areas such as the restroom, breakroom, medication room, and supply rooms, ensuring that you write down all door codes. If there is identification badge access to these areas, check whether yours works. If it does not, the unit should have a process for temporary staff to use to gain badge access to critical areas. Request the identification of a point person to serve as a resource for your shift and request an introduction to that individual. If you feel that any patient on your assignment is outside of your scope, give factual reasons why this is so and ask for consideration of reassignment of this patient. If this is not needed or not possible, circle back to the task about which you identified concerns during report, as it is not part of your usual workflow on your home unit and ask the resource person if they can complete the task at the appropriate time for the patient. What exactly this task entails will determine whether you need to escalate this to a supervisor. If this person will not complete the task for you and it is something you have been signed off on but have not recently done, ask the resource nurse to supervise you in completing the task. Again, how you frame this request depends on the task.

Ask the off-going nurse to help you organize your shift, including any workflows in the EHR or other devices. I forgot to ask this question when I recently floated to another unit. I was so focused on the tasks of caring for the patients outside of my regular work area during report that I never asked where I could find the Mobile Heartbeats (hospital-issued smartphones) we log on to during our shift. About halfway through my shift, one of the nurses asked me if I was reviewing and documenting all the monitor events going to my Mobile Heartbeat. When my patient alarmed, I immediately responded to their bedside and took appropriate clinical nursing action. I had no idea that I needed to do something in the EHR. While no one had told me to do this, it became a lesson learned, and I could complete this for the rest of my shift.

Take your time with your work and give yourself grace as you are working in a new area for your shift. Speak with yourself and the others with whom you are working positively. If you notice that you are consumed with caring for your patients and the regular staff on the unit is sitting or engaging in nonwork conversations for prolonged periods, ask for their assistance and even delegate some of your tasks to them. Nothing feels worse than when you are working somewhere you were not planning to work and, in addition to feeling like an outsider, you feel like you are working the hardest. Perhaps you misunderstand the situation but make it clear to the regular staff that you are open to receiving help, especially when they have time. Letting your feelings fester is not helpful to you, your patients, or your temporary team. When you have a few moments, socially interact with the nurses who usually work on the unit. You may meet a new friend or mentor but also find a new clinical area in which you might have interest.

At the close of your shift, be sure to debrief with the charge nurse. Thank them and the resource nurse during the shift. Offer feedback if anything was challenging as someone who did not regularly work on that unit and provide constructive feedback for a solution if you can foresee one. Importantly, remind them that if they float to your unit, you will provide the same degree of kindness and support that they offered you. While this guide is written from the perspective that you are the one floating, keep these points in mind if you receive help from a redeployed nurse on your unit. Offer them the same support you would hope for if you were in their shoes.

Let's look at Table 7.1 to see how Katie provided person-centered care and demonstrated personal, professional, and leadership development.

TABLE 7.1 Examples of Domain 2: Person-Centered Care and Domain 10: Personal, Professional, and Leadership Development in This Exemplar

Domain 2: Person-Centered Care	
2.1 Engage with the individual in establishing a caring relationship.	Katie showed empathic and compassionate care on her temporary unit.
2.2 Communicate effectively with individuals.	Katie strived to communicate with her patients and her new team to do what she felt was right.
Domain 10: Personal, Professional, and Leadership Development	
10.2 Demonstrate a spirit of inquiry that fosters flexibility and professional maturity.	Katie was flexible in floating to the new area and wanting to help promote safe patient care.
10.3 Develop capacity for leadership.	Katie was involved in a messy situation that was complicated by dishonesty. She took the high road even when it was awkward, which demonstrated authentic leadership.

When outside our comfort zone, letting our emotions take over is very easy. This is not helpful to us, our patients, or our team. Walk into new situations with the assumption that the nurses receiving you are grateful for your help and will support you with any challenges that come your way. If they do not demonstrate this behavior on their own, communicate your needs clearly and allow them to support you.

YOU MATTER: GOING OUTSIDE YOUR COMFORT ZONE

Situations where you are forced out of the comfort zone of your home unit can be uncomfortable but, with support, also a positive learning experience. You should not be in a position where you feel marginalized and unsupported at the beginning of your shift. Those who are receiving you should welcome and support you, but if they do not, remember to advocate for yourself, because you matter.

Book Club Questions

1. Have you ever floated to another unit? What did it feel like? What was helpful and not helpful in that experience?
2. What is your comfort level with confrontation? How do you handle difficult conversations in and out of the clinical setting?
3. Katie demonstrated her accountability and commitment to her relationship with Libby. What would you have done if you were in Katie's position? Libby's?

About This Chapter's Authors

Katherine (Katie) Knapik, BSN, RNC-MNN

Katie was born and raised in Westfield, Massachusetts. She received her bachelor's degree from Fairfield University's Egan School of Nursing and Health Studies in 2021. Following graduation, Katie moved to Boston and began her nursing career as an emergency management nurse at a local hospital. She aided in the hospital's response to the COVID-19 pandemic by administering vaccines and tests in a bustling clinic setting. She soon transitioned to an inpatient role on a postpartum floor and has now been there for over three years. Katie has stepped into several leadership roles on her floor. She regularly acts as the unit's charge nurse, enjoys precepting new nurses and nursing students, and is a member of her unit's practice-based council. She is also proud to have recently earned her NCC Certification in Maternal Newborn Nursing. Katie spends her free time traveling with friends, running around Boston, doing crossword puzzles, and reading at the beach near her apartment.

Erin McMahon, EdD, CNM, FACNM

Dr. Erin McMahon has been a certified nurse-midwife for 25 years and was first called to midwifery work 30 years ago. Serving birthing persons and families and providing reproductive care in various settings have been the joys of her life. She is the founding program director for the Midwifery Specialty at the University of Arizona College of Nursing. She has taught in the classroom for more than 13 years and precepted midwifery students and resident physicians for more than 20 years. She is passionate about the use of simulation as a teaching strategy. Erin is an American College of Nurse-Midwives (ACNM) fellow and pastAmerican Midwifery Certification Board (AMCB) member. She has served on national committees to revise the ACNM Core Competencies of Basic Midwifery Practice and the International Nursing Association of Clinical Simulation and Learning (INACSL) standards of best practice.

References

American Association of Colleges of Nursing. (2021). *The essentials: Core competencies for professional nursing education*. https://www.aacnnursing.org/Portals/0/PDFs/Publications/Essentials-2021.pdf

Flett, G. L. (2018). *The psychology of mattering: Understanding the human need to be significant*. Elsevier Academic Press.

Karim, H. N., Groom, P., & Tiu, M. (2023). Intensive care unit staff perceptions of redeployment to other clinical areas: A mixed method approach. *SAGE Open Nursing, 9*, 23779608231196401. https://doi.org/10.1177/23779608231196401

Lafontant, M., Blevins, D., Romer, C., & Ward, P. G. (2019). Exploring nurses' feelings on floating: A phenomenological study. *Nursing & Health Sciences Research Journal, 2*(1), 21–29. https://doi.org/10.55481/2578-3750.1025

O'Connor, K., & Dugan, J. L. (2017). Addressing floating and patient safety. *Nursing, 47*(2), 57–58. https://doi.org/10.1097/01.NURSE.0000511820.95903.78

CHAPTER 8

The First Goodbyes

New Nurse Experiences With Death and Dying

Kathryn (Katie) Magennis, BSN, RN; Eileen R. O'Shea, DNP, APRN, PCNS-BC, CHPPN; and Linda Roney, EdD, RN-BC, CPEN, CNE, FAAN

Learning Goals

1. Describe Katie's strengths and challenges in caring for patients at a cancer hospital's emergency department (ED).
2. Understand the nurse's role as a patient advocate.
3. Reflect on your support community both in and outside of work.
4. Identify your strategies for self-care in the physical, psychosocial, emotional, and spiritual domains.
5. Select actions and reactions to challenging encounters with patients and families as their emotions run high.

'Their Stories Are Part of My Life Now, Too'

By Kathryn (Katie) Magennis, BSN, RN

People fail to tell you that nursing can be absolutely miserable. It can be beautiful and fulfilling, but there are days that I go home and question every decision I made that led me here. When I chose to become a nurse at age 17, not truly knowing what that meant, I dreamt of working in Manhattan and in a fast-paced environment where no two days would be alike. I did not know I would be working in the ED at one of the best cancer hospitals in the country. I did not know that I would feel like I was doing more harm than good. I did not know that I would have more ethical questions than practical ones. Working in oncologic emergencies is different from working in other EDs. EDs at medical hospitals handle issues such as broken bones, skin infections, chest pains, respiratory infections, and other nonspecific ailments from the general public. In our hospital, working in the ED means that we treat only patients who have a cancer diagnosis.

Patients come to us with a wide range of complaints, from allergic reactions to chemotherapy, neutropenic fevers, neurological problems, or obscure and specific oncologic emergencies, such as graft-versus-host disease or superior vena cava syndrome. We also see patients for all the reasons they may present to a general medical ED. We have to know how to treat what regular people can identify as an emergency as well as manage that treatment for patients with complex medical histories and comorbidities. Shortness of breath (SOB) is never just SOB; it is new metastasis to the lung or a pulmonary embolism (PE). Abdominal pain is never just abdominal pain; it is either small bowel obstruction or constipation from the diverse cocktail of pain medications the patient is taking. At this point in my career, I often know which symptoms lead to which diagnosis. One thing I do not know, however, is at which point I am doing more harm to my patients than good.

During summer 2020, I worked as a nursing assistant at a long-term rehabilitation facility. It was the worst job I have ever had. There are so many people and not enough staff, things would fall through the cracks, people would not care enough, and the residents would often become sicker at that facility. Any time a patient comes in from a rehab facility, it is bound to be a multifaceted case. So, when an 87-year-old non-English-speaking patient came into our ED from rehab, I was not surprised to hear that she had been walking two weeks prior and was now completely bedbound with a stage 2 pressure injury on her sacrum. She came in for altered mental status on top of general failure to thrive. Her son met her at the hospital, but he had not seen her in a week, so I had no details about when her condition had changed.

When she came in, her vital signs were abnormal in triage, including a blood pressure of 82/46 mm Hg and a heart rate of 121 bpm. We brought her to an open room and started some bloodwork before immediately hanging a liter of normal saline. Her white blood cell count was indicative of infection, with a result in the 20s. When her labs came back, the liter was done, and her pressure was exactly the same. I obtained a second access, gave another liter, and grabbed the provider. The plan was to see how she did after the second liter, and if no progress was made, we would give her albumin and reassess her condition. With her blood pressure now 79/40 mm Hg, I hung the albumin.

As I was in the process of doing this, she grabbed my arm and said one of the few English words she knew: *pain*. Her son pleaded with me to give her something, anything for the pain. Her last dose of hydromorphone had been over six hours ago, and the pressure injury was becoming further irritated. I explained that she was not allowed to take anything by mouth because of her altered mental status as well as the fact that she physically could not sit up to swallow a pill and posed aspiration risks. I also reasoned that pain medications could decrease blood pressure, and hers was already very low and not responding to our interventions. They verbalized their understanding but begged that as soon as it became possible, I must give her something for the pain. The albumin failed to touch her blood pressure, so we decided to call the intensive care unit (ICU) team regarding her hemodynamic instability. By the time they got downstairs, she had tried to roll onto her side to alleviate the pain, and the movement caused her heart rate to elevate further. Her blood pressures were now reading in the 50s/30s. She grabbed me again, repeating "*Pain, pain, pain*" over and over. It became clear that she had also soiled herself. She would not let me move her to clean her out of fear that it would cause more pain, and I truthfully was fearful to move her and somehow drop her blood pressure more. Speaking with her son in their native language, the patient continuously said that all she wanted to was to *be out of pain*, to help *put her out of her misery*, to *stop the pain*, to *stop the pain*, and to please do anything to *stop the pain*. This patient had a full code status, and we could not take away her pain and treat her blood pressure at the same time without getting the ICU involved. As nurses, we are supposed to care for people. While that includes healing them when possible, is prolonging life really the same thing? If the most caring thing I could have done for this woman was give her pain medications, should I have done it despite the fact that it would likely have made her medical condition worse? The ICU team immediately started vasopressors, and we brought her up to the ICU. While I do not know the details of what happened in the end, I know the team had a goals-of-care conversation with the family. She ended up on a fentanyl drip along with the pressors, and she remained a full code status until she died later that week.

Despite advocating for this patient, communicating closely with the doctor, and pushing to involve the ICU, I do not feel that I helped this woman. When I was first starting my job and someone would ask how my day was, I would sometimes respond with "*Well, no one died, so I must've done something right.*" I was partially trying to make light of things, but I also meant it. If I was keeping people alive, I must be doing things the way I should be doing them. I no longer believe that to be true. Just because someone is still alive does not mean that they are being taken care of, does not mean that they have any quality of life, and does not mean that I did my job "right."

The beautiful and horrifying thing about the human body is that everything is connected. When one system fails, another mechanism often picks up the slack until we sense that something is wrong. Or, when one system fails, it causes the downfall of an adjacent system. A generally well-presenting 63-year-old woman came to us after going to our outpatient clinic earlier that day for chemotherapy treatment. While there, she began reporting some heart palpitations. After getting an electrocardiogram (ECG), she was found to have a new presentation of atrial flutter. Because of this finding, they were unable to administer the chemotherapy and instead sent the patient to us for a further cardiac workup. During our assessment, she reported a productive cough that had started about a week ago. We obtained a chest X-ray, and she was diagnosed with pneumonia. Her oxygen saturation (SpO2) was on the low side of normal, with a reading of 93% on room air, while her baseline was around 97%. She was placed on 2 liters (L) of oxygen via nasal cannula, to which she responded well. Her mother and sister were in the room with her, and they told me they were going to go home and get some rest, left me a phone number, and said their goodbyes. I gave the patient her nighttime medications, helped her walk to the bathroom, and settled her in for the night. Because of the atrial flutter and new supplemental oxygen requirement, we kept her on the telemetry monitor and left the pulse oximeter on her finger throughout the night. Around midnight, I saw her oxygen drop to the mid-80s. I went into the room, assuming that it was a problem with the monitor, and found the patient with increased work of breathing and saying that she was feeling short of breath. I bumped up the oxygen to 6 L and messaged the provider, who told me that a similar episode had happened earlier while she was in the room. She suggested leaving her on 6 L and putting in an order for Optiflow, a form of supplemental oxygen that offers a higher concentration than the nasal cannula. She told me to use it if I thought the patient would benefit from it, but I did not think that it was indicated at that time. The patient seemed far more comfortable since increasing the oxygen, so I let the Optiflow order sit for a bit before reassessing. About an hour later, the patient's SpO2 dropped back to mid-80s. I called the respiratory therapist, informing them that we would need a setup for the Optiflow and asking if they had any further suggestions. The patient did not appear to be using accessory muscles or have labored breathing, so I messaged the provider to update her. Not long after, I called the respiratory therapists back to the bedside to increase the provided oxygen as her SpO2 would not come up. The respiratory therapist and I spoke about how this patient had come in less than 10 hours ago, and in that time, her supplemental oxygen requirement increased from 2 L by nasal cannula to 60 L high-flow. I messaged the provider, asking whether now would be an appropriate time to involve the ICU team. I explained to the patient that a critical care team would be coming to assess her just so that we could get their recommendations, but not to worry. It was mostly routine. At this point, the patient still looked relatively comfortable, and she blamed her dropping SpO2 on falling asleep with her mouth open. After digging through the patient's chart, the ICU physician came to the bedside and decided to follow the case but that the patient would not require admission to the unit. She gave us some suggestions about nebulizers and which antibiotics to try.

About 20 minutes later, the ICU physician returned to the ED and informed me that they had changed their minds; they would take the patient. I never got a chance to ask what made them change their mind because, at the same time, our unit assistant called me to tell me the patient had hit the call bell and sounded like they were in distress. I grabbed some of the equipment needed for an ICU transfer, asked one of my friends to grab the rest, and walked into the patient's room. I found her on her side with her head in the space between the slats on the side of the stretcher, diaphoretic, repeating, "*I can't breathe,*" more to herself than anyone else. Her SpO2 was 67% on 100% fraction of inspired oxygen (FiO2) and 60 L via high flow. My friend met me in the room with the rest of the transport equipment, assessed the situation simultaneously, and moved to grab the ICU physician while I placed a nonrebreather on top of the Optiflow device. This patient was now on 200% FiO2 and 75 L of supplemental oxygen hours after being on room air. My friend returned with the ICU admitting physician and a nurse from the rapid response team (RRT). I called the respiratory therapist back to the bedside for their expertise. At that point, the only other thing we could do is intubate, which the physician suggested. The patient protested, stating, "*I don't want a tube down my throat. I can't live like that. I don't want to see a tube down my throat.*" I often forget that the general public lacks the medical knowledge we do. Someone on the street may mistake a seizure for a stroke. People do not always know that being intubated means being heavily sedated. Instead of explaining this reality to the patient, the doctor nodded, unsure of what to say next. It was me who grabbed the patient's hand, saying something along the lines of "*I understand it is scary and uncomfortable, but breathing like this is unsustainable. You won't survive like this. When they put the tube down your throat, they sedate you first so that you don't fight against it. You won't see it in your mouth.*" I didn't even know if I was qualified to explain intubation to a patient, but the physician clearly was not going to do it, and someone else had to. She nodded, understanding my explanation.

The RRT registered nurse (RN) jumped in, asking if there was anyone we should call. The patient was adamant that we not call her mother or sister; she did not want to wake or worry them. Still holding her hand, I looked her in the eyes and said that now would be a good time for them to worry. We called both of them, but neither answered. It was 5:03 a.m. on a Wednesday. Anesthesia came to the bedside; we pushed the etomidate and rocuronium while I held her hand. Based on her reaction, both medications burn while going through the vein. The certified registered nurse anesthetist intubated. Immediately, the respiratory therapist pulled away from the patient, and blood started coming out of her new endotracheal tube. He yelled the phrase "flash pulmonary edema" with urgency in his voice. From my understanding of what happened, by placing the nonrebreather on top of the high-flow oxygen, we essentially overhyperoxygenated the patient, causing the capillaries in her lungs to burst and create the textbook pink frothy sputum I remember learning about in college. The respiratory therapist used the suction within the ventilator to help clear the airway and then hooked up the patient to the portable ventilator until we could get to the ICU. Because of the pulmonary edema, the ventilator could not provide the necessary amount of oxygen, leaving her SpO2 at around 85%. We brought her to the ICU while manually bagging her, a task that was passed between the respiratory therapist, RRT RN, and myself.

On December 5, this woman had hopes of chemotherapy being the answer to her cancer treatment. On December 6, she was brought to the ICU for respiratory failure. Over the course of two weeks, she failed attempted extubation twice. Her code status was changed to do not resuscitate (DNR) on Christmas Day, and on December 26, surrounded by her mother, sister, and daughter, she was terminally extubated. She had not understood the plan, and while it was an emergent situation, someone with more knowledge on the matter should have explained what being intubated meant. Should we have asked whether she wanted to be on life support? Should she have had that conversation in an office months prior instead of at the bedside as it was happening? Should I have tried to call her family a second time? Should I have been more proactive in giving nebulizers and antibiotics? And should I have advocated for her to have these things done? I still cry when I think about her.

On a busy day over the summer, I cared for a beautiful young woman with a slight accent that I could not place. She came in for SOB, not requiring supplemental oxygen, and was found to be tachycardic during triage. After an unchanged ECG, she remained in the hallway because the high volume of patients ensured that no rooms were available. During my assessment, I asked about her accent. She informed me that she had been receiving care at a hospital in Spain, but her husband had pushed her to come back to New York City for care as her condition worsened. After hearing the story of her successful career in public health and how she had fallen in love and left it all behind to follow her husband to Europe, I knew that she would be my favorite patient of the day. The workup ordered for her included computed tomography (CT) to rule out a PE. After getting notified that she had returned from the CT, I saw that the doctor had put in an order for continuous telemetry monitoring, a cardiac consult, and an echocardiogram. While she did not have a PE, the CT revealed a tumor pressing on her heart so hard that her ejection fraction was a mere 10%. She was to be admitted to the hospital for radiation. I approached my charge nurse, explaining that we would have to find a room to initiate the telemetry order, and informed the patient of the plan of care. She immediately looked to her husband, and they started rearranging their travel plans and canceling flights back to Spain. Not long after, I wished her well and sent her to the inpatient floor, where her care would be continued. Two weeks later was Labor Day, my summer holiday to work. I saw this patient's name on our board and let my charge nurse know that I would care for her, already knowing her history and excited to see how she was doing. That day, however, she was brought in on a stretcher by emergency medical services. There was no sign of that spirited 40-year-old woman whom I had previously met. She was unresponsive, on a nonrebreather, with bilateral pitting edema so severe that I could barely fit our 3XL socks on her feet.

Unable to answer any of my questions, I turned to her husband, who filled me in on deterioration since discharge and how he had found her unable to awaken from sleep this morning. Because she had been primarily treated in Spain, we did not have any of her advance directives on file. Because she was unresponsive, we did not know what her wishes were. Once again, turning to her husband, our doctor asked about her wishes. His face crumbled, understanding the meaning behind those words. There was nothing we could do to cure her illness. Her heart was failing. She had walked around the unit two weeks prior, joking with me and teasing her husband. Now, with all the same characters present, she was actively dying. Knowing that she would rather be comfortable than kept alive with no hope for a cure, her family chose to make her code status DNR. She died later that day.

EDs often get the same patients repeatedly with the same chief reports. Every time a specific name populates on our board, we know he is coming in with a small bowel obstruction and to ask for an order of intravenous (IV) Dilaudid as it is the only medication that alleviates his abdominal pain. I have had patients come back and ask about family trips because that is how often I see them. Forming friendly relationships with patients is not something I had expected in emergency medicine. Although it is not the same as having patients for weeks at a time, the bonds between nurses and patients during their visits to an ED shape their opinions of the staff, the hospital, and the care they receive. I pride myself on remembering patients and their care.

There are days when walking through the doors to the hospital takes every ounce of sheer will in my body. I was scheduled to work the shift after my first code, and I cried the entire way in, unable to cope with the fragility of life. I would only be able to do my job with the support systems I have in place. Nurses are the backbone of all hospitals, and my peers offer that same stability for me. Some of my coworkers have become my best friends. They are the only people who understand what it is like to be in my position. I was able to work after my first code only because I did not have to explain the horror I had endured—they experienced it with me. Specifically, when the world is quiet on the night shift, I am grateful for my colleagues, whom I can call my friends. You learn who to call if someone is a hard stick, you need extra hands for a Foley, or you just want someone to walk to the pharmacy with you. One of the relationships for which I am most grateful is that of my preceptor, Grace. Grace has shaped me into the nurse and young woman I am today. She is the first person I reach out to for personal and professional matters. After starting the night shift, I began to experience severe compassion fatigue accompanied by feelings of hopelessness within the nursing profession. It felt like the hospital's four walls were converging to trap me between them. Grace listened to my grievances and expressed that she had the same problem. As she put it, we are not supposed to be surrounded by this much death. The hospital we work at is unique in that we never see patients getting better; our patients leave the hospital only to return a few weeks later with more severe ailments. In other hospitals, patients have an actual shot at getting better. Over the past year, our hospital has seen an increase in patient volume beyond what we have in previous years. Unfortunately, for the ED, we have no max capacity. We may see an alert on our screens that the hospital is at 112% capacity, but we must accept, treat, and make room for any patient. There have been nights when nurses who work from noon to midnight stay until 4 a.m. because handing off their patients to the night shift would mean remarkably unsafe nurse-to-patient ratios. There have been nights when our charge nurse acts as triage and takes a full patient load. We thrive on camaraderie and teamwork, knowing that it is the only possible way to succeed at our jobs.

I accepted my job offer in June 2022, but my start date was not until September of that year. During the summer, I worked to pass my National Council Licensure Examination (NCLEX) and set myself up for success as I entered the workforce. The first thing I did was make sure that I started seeing a therapist. Unaware of how badly I would need to talk about the happenings in my workplace, I was not naive enough to think that I could brave this job on my own. Certain parts of being a nurse are impossible to share with even your closest friends and family. It is not comfortable talking about the loss of life, the futile attempts to revive it, and the dark ordeals to which I have become numb. I sometimes find myself telling a "funny" work story only to completely kill the conversation because only a nurse would understand. My weekly therapy sessions have become a place to unpack these occurrences and reflect on my personal life and how the two intertwine. Of course, having the support of my family and friends is irreplaceable. Spending days off with them reminds me that although I may feel isolated in the strange nature of my job, I am not truly alone. As nurses, we are often so busy caring for other people that we forget that we must first take care of ourselves. The times I feel myself starting to burn out at my job directly correlate with not using my free time to do things I know will make me feel better, such as going for runs, spending time with loved ones, and talking with my therapist.

Working at one of the most prestigious cancer institutions in the world sometimes makes me want to rip my head off. Whenever I tell someone where I work, it is as if they are reading from a script, responding with, *"Oh, wow, what a great hospital. My [insert friend or family member] was treated there, and it saved their life. You must be really tough and good at your job."* I don't want to be tough. I don't want to be expected to be some superhero. I don't want to look at the freckle on your back and tell you if it is suspicious. While I take pride in my work, it is unfair when people dismiss my grumblings about my job by saying, *"But you're saving lives."* Everyone else is allowed to complain about work. What is wrong with me doing the same? Becoming numb to the realities of cancer care and treatment is one of the requirements of my job. I did not expect that numbness to extend to the care of the patients as people. I reflect on the cases shared here and keep those people, their families, and their stories in my heart. Their stories are part of my life now, too.

'Discerning What Brings You Meaning and Purpose'

By Eileen R. O'Shea, DNP, APRN, PCNS-BC, CHPPN

As I reflect on the above scenarios, I can relate immediately. To echo Katie's initial beginnings, when I graduated with my baccalaureate degree, I too dreamed of working in a major metropolitan area and cutting-edge medical center, Boston. I did not know I would work in a neurological medical-surgical unit, caring for adult patients at one of the country's most prestigious acute care hospitals. Patients came from all over the world for this facility's provider expertise. The population spanned all socioeconomic levels and cultures, ranging from the rich and famous to the underserved and unhoused.

I can also relate to Katie's challenges and emotional state. My first year of nursing was the best of times and the worst of times. With much support from nursing colleagues, grit, and perseverance, I cared for adult patients for one year until I was ready to take the next step and move onward professionally. But first, I want to highlight the gravity of an initial nursing position. Envision that you are 21, and after enduring rigorous studies in nursing school, attaining your baccalaureate degree, and then passing the NCLEX, you begin your first nursing position. As a novice nurse, you may feel elated, accomplished, or fearful (or other emotions). There is so much to learn, and the pace is extremely fast. These feelings are normal; managing your feelings and expectations is the first challenge.

Similar to Katie's stories, at times, I questioned myself—did I know enough to care for so many patients with such grave conditions? What comfort can I offer a dying patient? Why must I learn about serious illness care by trial and error? I am seeing so much anguish; in most cases, there is no silver lining. These patients are not all going home to return to their prior living state; they will be forever changed. I witnessed suffering.

One of my earliest recollections on this adult neurologic medical-surgical unit was caring for a female older adult who was dying from cancer. The primary cancer site was in her bones, but she also endured widespread metastasis. In the report, my colleague told me about her medical diagnosis and social background. She was a wonderful pediatric nurse by profession and had a loving husband and family. Aspiring to become a pediatric nurse, I imagined that the patient in the bed must have provided stellar nursing care to many ill children and their families. However, she is no longer a care provider—she is now a nursing care recipient. When I met her, she looked cachexic, and she was nonverbal, perhaps in a transitioning state, waiting to die. She was on comfort measures and receiving a continuous morphine drip for pain. As a night nurse, the protocol was to turn patients every two hours to prevent skin breakdown. Yet, as I turned this actively dying, frail woman (who was a wife, mother, and pediatric nurse), she would moan loudly, and her face had a furrowed brow, which indicated a significant amount of pain. Thankfully, I had an order set allowing the titration of IV morphine to be increased as needed to establish a level of comfort. So, every two hours, I would increase the rate of the infusion as she continued to moan with every turn. I began to wonder, is this too much morphine? Will she stop breathing due to the increased amounts of morphine and the cumulative effect of the drug? Will I be the cause of her ultimate death? Will I cause harm, or is this considered good nursing care? I was confident in my pain assessment skills, and I never had the intention of causing harm. My professional responsibility was to provide compassionate care and alleviate pain, so I cleared my head of the self-doubt talk and continued with the appropriate nursing interventions. I recall during the change-of-shift report that my colleagues were appreciative of my addressing this woman's ongoing pain and promoting a comfortable transition into death. My colleagues would continue with the plan of care, focused on alleviating pain and promoting a dignified death. This patient died within the next shift.

During that first year, I witnessed countless patients who endured a serious illness. There were patients with rare neurological diseases, such as Creutzfeldt-Jakob disease and Guillain-Barré syndrome, as well as patients with brain tumors, aneurysms, chronic back pain, cervical spine issues, amyotrophic lateral sclerosis, head injuries, strokes, and seizures. The patient narratives were all so moving and, at times, shocking. Can you imagine taking care of an unhoused person who sustained a random act of violence (a brutal beating) from another human, resulting in a shattered skull, brain bleed, and castration? Or a young woman in her 30s who was addicted to cocaine? She snorted the drug frequently and acquired a brain abscess due to the erosion of the nasal cavity and direct exposure of cocaine to the brain. One of the most challenging days for me was seeing an old friend from junior high school walk down the hallway to say hello. However, as he greeted me, I could not mistake that he was a patient because of the cloth hospital gown he was wearing. He was awaiting treatment (proton beam therapy) for a large brain aneurysm. Unprompted, he shared with me that he had a large brain aneurysm, which was at high risk of ruptur-ing. I realized that meant a potential bleed could result in a massive brain injury, altering his life forever. As Katie noted previously, the fragility of life was apparent daily. Finding myself lost for words (and being scared for this 22-year-old), I shared that he was in the best place for the treatment and the follow-up care. By the end of this first year of nursing, I realized it was time to move toward achieving my dreams and professional goals: to become a pediatric nurse.

In my second year as an RN, I moved to a new setting within Boston to work with a population about whom I was passionate and to whom I was excited to provide care. At first, I felt a sense of joy and as if I was in the place I was called to be. Yet, as my journey unfolded, I encountered similar feelings of being a novice nurse (caring for children and their families [family-centered care] versus an adult nurse) and witnessing hardships and suffering. The unit I began on was a school-age surgical and solid organ transplant unit. Although I was elated to be with children and their families, I experienced many challenging cases. One such case was with a preschool-aged boy. He was admitted with an ear infection. I thought to myself, *Oh, this will not be too challenging because this is not a child with complicated organ failure (such as other children on this unit)—I will prepare to administer IV antibiotics, and then he will go home.* Strangely, this was not a simple case; it was not a bacterial infection. Instead, this beautiful child endured a fungal ear infection. At the time, the initial medication regimen did not eradicate the infection. Over a few months, he would come in and out of the hospital, trialing various treatments and medications to rid the fungal ear infection. Unfortunately, the fungal infection spread from his ear and entered his brain. Despite IV antifungal medications, the brain infection worsened. Devastated by the lack of curative treatments, the parents, in collaboration with the eye, ear, nose, and throat team, decided to return home with support and provide their young child with comfort measures and love. I wondered, could there be a miracle or possibly a new treatment to save this child's life? Would a new (or experimental) drug come to market? What else could the healthcare team provide this child and their parents? I thought to myself, just over one month ago, this child was well, and now he may die. How do we, as nurses, process the devastation and tragedies yet stay strong to support and provide comfort to children with serious illnesses and their families? For survival as a nurse, I wondered if developing a hardened exterior shell is necessary and not allowing these patient cases to impact us. Is that even possible? Do we become devoid of emotions and feelings over time? Is burnout inevitable?

Sadly, this precious child did die. The available treatments were not effective in curing the disease. As a young nurse, this child and family greatly affected me. In addition, I wondered about my role in the aftermath. Do I attend funeral services? Should I contact the family, or would that be considered crossing professional boundaries? I cared for this child and developed a trusting relationship with him and his family. Now, what is my role in his care? I decided to attend the funeral services together with a group of nurses who had also taken care of this child. Watching his mother walk down the central aisle of the church, following the tiny white casket, was unforgettable. Two men, one on each side of the mom, needed to support her; her face was so pale, lifeless, and her legs buckled as she walked down the aisle to the very first pew. The parent's sadness, grief, pain, and suffering were palpable; it was completely overwhelming for me to process. After the ceremony, I learned that my colleagues felt the same way. We shared a sort of communal grief because of this shared work experience. Somehow, my colleague's presence provided me with a sense of solace. I was glad that I attended the service and came to appreciate that this child would no longer suffer. I hoped the parents felt supported that day by those of us who attended the service. However, little did I realize that this would not be the only child's funeral that I would participate in as a pediatric nurse. Attending other funeral services would be a part of my future. I had to learn how to cope with illness, tragedies, suffering, loss, and grief. I had to learn how to find a healthy work-life balance. How will you take care of yourself?

Developing a Community of Support: You Are Not Alone

Again, I agree with Katie. Nurses need to find a trusted circle of healthcare colleagues to confide in—to help debrief from a long shift of patient care and intense family dynamics. Strive to develop healthy professional relationships in your work environment. We need help to process. Sometimes we may need something simple, such as a colleague who is an excellent listener or can read your nonverbals and intuitively offer a hug. At other times, a professional is needed, such as a therapist or counselor. Colleagues in the healthcare field can relate to you because of similar experiences. In contrast, your friends and family do not understand your struggles in the professional environment, and you cannot share details because you are bound to ensure patient confidentiality. Therefore, find yourself a group of nursing mates (start with the nurse residency group) and schedule fun things to do outside of work to create a bond. The social gatherings can be simple, such as meeting after the night shift for breakfast (before going home to sleep) or signing up for an exercise class together. Try something new!

Family and friends are also a great support to round out your community of replenishment. Stay connected despite your working unusual shifts, weekends, and holidays. You will need to schedule "connection times." You may have to be the scheduler of event planning because your circle may not understand your need to sleep during your days off. Do not let that be a barrier; provide alternate dates and weekends. For families, offer to plan holiday celebrations outside of the actual dates. Be creative! For example, in my family, we celebrate "Baby (Little) Christmas" when my daughter, who is a pediatric ICU nurse, has to work on December 25. Baby Christmas may occur before or after the actual holiday. The important part is to come together with family and spend time with one another.

Additionally, professional organizations can support your connectivity to the profession. When you attend professional conferences, you will see just how many nurses are interested in the same area or specialty in which you are interested. I guarantee you will not feel alone if you connect with them. Professional organizational websites typically contain links explaining how to get involved as well as education and events. Some of the organizations offer mentoring programs and leadership development.

Lastly, don't forget about your faculty and classmates. We are here to offer continued connections, support, and mentorship. Your classmates may be going through similar challenges, and your professors have probably endured identical struggles. They can lend a listening ear or provide perspectives and advice. Reach out to us—you are not alone!

Professional Development

Don't become complacent. Seek out coaches and mentors. Coaches will partner with you to foster inspiration and motivation. It is a thought-provoking and creative process to maximize your personal and professional potential (International Coaching Federation, 2024). A mentor tends to be a different type of relationship, one that is longer-term. You may select several mentors who have varied professional experiences. Mentors will offer you wisdom and advice as a junior employee and will be interested in your development over time, taking a more holistic approach to career and development; it is common for mentees to seek mentors outside of the organization (Zust, 2017). Coaches and mentors can offer you an extra layer of support.

Self-Preservation/Self-Care: Physical, Psychosocial, Emotional, Spiritual

Self-care is a critical component to sustaining a long career in nursing. As we profess to provide holistic care for the patient, we must walk the walk to nurture our bodies, minds, and spirits. There is so much that we can do daily to balance our busy lives with all we experience in work environments. For your consideration, below are a few ideas on how to care for yourself. The first steps are setting a goal, managing your time, and developing a schedule. The following questions may trigger new ideas to consider, when caring for your whole person:

Body:

- Do you work out regularly? How much and how frequently?
- Do you belong to a gym? Are there classes that you are interested in taking?
- Can you find an exciting place to walk/hike/run/ski and connect with nature?

Mind:

- How can you best empty your busy mind and seek quietness?
- Have you tried meditation? Body scan? Yoga? Journaling? Breathwork? Prayer?
- When do you turn off your electronics and detach from social media?
- Have you tried counseling or therapy for mental health support?

Spirit:

- I strongly encourage individual reflective time to explore your sense of spirituality. Discerning what brings you meaning and purpose in life will help you through the long days and days of deep sadness and the days of joy in which your heart feels light. Reflect on the broadest sense of the definition as described below in *"On Improving the Spiritual Dimension of Whole Person Care: The Transformational Role of Compassion, Love and Forgiveness in Health Care,"* (Puchalski et al., 2014, p. 646):

> Spirituality is a dynamic and intrinsic aspect of humanity through which persons seek ultimate meaning, purpose, and transcendence and experience relationships to self, family, others, community, society, nature, and the significant or sacred. Spirituality is expressed through beliefs, values, traditions, and practices.

For me, my personal beliefs, religion, and faith have been a guiding light through many dark personal and professional struggles, especially when bearing witness to human suffering. Developing a spiritual, moral, and ethical compass may help you navigate this profession in the long run, providing a sense of security and direction. I encourage you to take time to know where your north star is. What is your purpose in life? What brings you meaning? What relationships/connections matter to you? Does your career contribute to what is meaningful to you, personally? Does this work contribute to your purpose? How do you make sense of human suffering?

Man's Search for Meaning (Frankl, 1984) is a well-known personal account of Viktor Frankl's time as a prisoner of war in Auschwitz during World War II. Frankl, a neurologist, psychologist and philosopher, shares his experiences and observations in this book, focusing particularly on the importance of finding meaning in life, even in the most challenging circumstances. He states that through the book's writing, he wanted to convey a "concrete example that life holds a potential meaning under any conditions, even the most miserable ones" (preface). Throughout his imprisonment, he took note of the experiences of the suffering prisoners who struggled for survival each day. He writes, "The prisoner who had lost faith in the future—his future—was doomed. With his loss of belief in the future, he also lost his spiritual hold; he let himself decline and became subject to mental and physical decay" (p. 95). He reiterates this message: "Woe to him who saw no more sense in his life, no aim, no purpose, and therefore no point in carrying on. He was soon lost" (p. 98). Frankl emphasizes that it is not a general question of what the meaning of life is, but rather an individual's responsibility to discover the *why* for his existence. He explains (p. 101):

> A man who becomes conscious of the responsibility he bears
> toward a human being who affectionately waits for him, or to
> an unfinished work, will never be able to throw away his life.
> He knows the "why" for his existence and will be able to bear
> almost any "how."

As nurses, we can learn a great deal from Frankl's experience. What is the *why* for each of our existences, and how will we assist others (e.g., patients) if they have not uncovered the *why* for their existence? You will struggle to make sense of many tragic patient scenarios. However, by delving into your spiritual beliefs and developing your authentic self, you can help yourself as well as your patients. There will be times when you will have no adequate response to a patient's questions, such as *"Why is this happening to me, or why my child?"* You may even avert difficult questions because you are uncomfortable with the topic. Please take the time now to know your beliefs, develop an interior life, and cultivate humility. This self-discovery journey will not only benefit you but also enhance your ability to provide compassionate care to your patients. Might you be willing to meet with a spiritual advisor on campus or reach out to a faith-based organization with which you may have a connection? The time you spend now will help you when you do not fully understand why bad things happen to good people.

Palliative Care Education/Death/Dying

As another resource, I recommend spending time with palliative care teams. In my first case, the patient who had a terminal cancer diagnosis, I feared that increasing the IV morphine drip would hasten her death. If I had a palliative care team to consult with, they would have provided me with advice related to her pain management. Palliative care teams provide expert counsel on pain and symptom management. Maybe there were adjunct medications or other comfort measures that we could have provided had there been a palliative care team to consult. In the case of the child who had a fungal ear infection, I struggled with my role after his death. Again, had I had a palliative care team available for support, so many of my questions could have been alleviated. It would have been ideal to know that this family would receive bereavement services for the year after the death of their child, if he had received hospice care. Also, a palliative care team would have supported the child's healthcare team members attending his service. I was unaware that research shows that families feel supported and not "abandoned" when the medical team continues the professional relationship after leaving the acute care setting. A palliative team could have eased my worries.

Related to developing our authentic self and interior life (which takes work and contemplation), we must come to terms with living out our lives, recognizing that alongside joy and awe, there will be times of tragedy, suffering, grief, and death. Reading *On Death and Dying* by Elisabeth Kübler-Ross (1969) is foundational. In this book, Dr. Kübler-Ross writes about her experiences working with dying patients over two and half years. She explains that she uses patients' perspectives to refocus healthcare providers on the patient as a human being and reports her understanding of "the final stages of life with all its anxieties, fears, and hopes" (preface). Dr. Kübler-Ross concludes the book with the following (p. 276):

> Watching the peaceful death of a human being reminds us of a falling star: one of the million lights in a vast sky that flares up for a brief moment only to disappear in the endless night forever. To be a therapist [healthcare provider] to a dying patient makes us aware of the uniqueness of each individual in this vast sea of humanity. It makes us aware of our finiteness and our limited lifespan. Few of us live beyond our three score and ten years [70 years], and yet in that brief time, most of us create and live a unique biography and weave ourselves into the fabric of human history.

Each of us will need to build our capacity to continue living fully and balance the demands of our chosen profession, serving humanity with compassion in times of wellness and illness. Can you find mutual moments of graciousness and kindness to extend to another human each day, whether small or large? How will you remember the patients and families who will touch your lives forever? Will they become a thread in the fabric of your life story? How will you honor them, and how will you integrate these experiences into your interior life?

'I Tried for Years to Push the Sadness Aside.'

By Linda Roney, EdD, RN-BC, CPEN, CNE, FAAN

As we read Katie and Eileen's reflections, it is clear that they are both passionate patient advocates and have left an indelible mark on countless patients and their families. Similarly, it is also clear that many of their special patients have left a memorable impression on them. The American Nurses Association's (ANA) *Code of Ethics With Interpretative Statements* (2015) guides the profession's ethical obligations and responsibilities for quality nursing care. Specifically, it states that the nurse promotes, advocates for, and protects the patient's rights, health, and safety (p. v). We will talk about this more in Chapter 9. In our minds, these concepts were reinforced through countless hours of classes, clinicals, and labs. However, our response to the shift in the professional practice turns from curative to symptom management, or when death is inevitable, it can feel like treatment failure and an unnatural order of life by nurses who care for specific populations of patients (Chew et al., 2021). Eileen has opened our minds to learning from palliative care teams to help us learn many things about supporting our patients and their families through the multifaceted challenges of time. In 2019, it was reported that 72% of U.S. hospitals with 50 or more beds report having a palliative care team (Center to Advance Palliative Care, 2020). We hope that this number continues to grow worldwide.

Katie demonstrates aptitude in the American Association of Colleges of Nursing essentials' (2021) domains 2 and 10 competencies and subcompetencies.

TABLE 8.1 Examples of Domain 2: Person-Centered Care and Domain 10: Personal, Professional, and Leadership Development in This Exemplar

Domain 2: Person-Centered Care	
2.1 Engage with the individual in establishing a caring relationship.	Throughout the stories of caring, it is clear that Katie demonstrated qualities of empathy, compassionate care, and mutual respect with her patients.
2.2 Communicate effectively with individuals.	Katie demonstrated tremendous emotional intelligence in her communication with patients and families, showing her ability to have difficult conversations.
2.3 Integrate assessment skills in practice.	Katie provided high-level, holistic nursing care for her patents.
2.7 Evaluate outcomes of care.	Due to the complexities of these situations, Katie recognized the need to modify the care plan for her patients.
2.8 Promote self-care management.	Katie demonstrated leadership skills in respecting individuals self-determination in their healthcare decisions.
Domain 10: Personal, Professional, and Leadership Development	
10.1 Demonstrate a commitment to personal health and well-being.	Katie took time to reflect and seek resources for personal support.
10.3 Develop capacity for leadership.	Katie demonstrated leadership in the situations she described to us. She led with an authentic leadership style.

The other day, I spoke on the phone with a nurse who had just graduated from her prelicensure program five months ago and was on orientation. Like Katie, I knew her well as an undergraduate student. She is also, like Katie, intelligent, compassionate, hard-working, and kind. During a recent shift, her patient's mother returned to the bedside to find her adolescent child incontinent of stool. The mother called this new nurse into the room, screaming at the nurse that her daughter was soiled, and questioned whether she had checked on her while she was gone for nearly an hour. One major problem:

The mother had not told the new nurse that she was leaving her daughter's room. The new nurse did not answer (it felt like a rhetorical question), ran feverously, grabbed new linens, and helped clean her patient. Once the teen was clean, the mother fell to her hands and knees and was sobbing hysterically. It was clear that she was not just upset about her daughter's incontinence but about something more significant. As the new nurse rubbed the mother's back, as she, too, was on the floor, the mother shared that the medical team had met with the mother and told her the news that her 15-year-old child now had just over a year to live.

The medical team had called the mother into the meeting without telling the nurse that the patient was alone. They also did not invite the new nurse to be part of this critical family meeting. Yet, the new nurse, who had now cared for the patient and her family for several shifts, was the recipient of this tremendous emotional release by the mother. Any compassionate person—especially the new nurse—understands that this outpouring had to do with the mother's loss of control and news of the mortality of her previously healthy daughter. For the rest of her shift and days after, the new nurse had a heavy heart and a sense of tremendous guilt over the situation. *Should she feel guilty? What should she do?*

PRN (PLEASE READ NOW)

Imagine that you were the new nurse seated with the patient's mother on the floor as she told you the news that the medical team shared with her daughter.

- How would you react? What would you do while you were in the room?
- Would physical touch be appropriate?
- How would you manage your time in this situation, knowing that you had other patients on your assignment who might have needed you, as you had been in the room for a long time?
- How do you address the medical team of whom you were not aware at this meeting?

Reactions are feelings or actions responding to a situation or event (Merriam-Webster, n.d.). The first step for the new nurse in this situation is to acknowledge their feelings about the situation silently. It does not help to offer to the mother how you feel about her child's prognosis or relate her story to that of another experience. Acknowledging your feelings can help you be aware of your emotional response to the situation, which is essential. Still, it reminds you that now is not the time to put your response in the middle of the mother's reaction to the situation. You might feel embarrassed that you did not check on the patient while the mother was in the meeting, angry that the medical team did not tell you about it, or overwhelmed with the experience of hearing this sad news about an adolescent. This moment is not about you but rather about her grief. These are all essential items to follow up on, but she needs you to be present with her now. Use the space of silence to reflect on your feelings and give her the space for hers. Silence has critical benefits, including encouraging active listening, reducing tension and emotions, promoting thoughtfulness, and signaling openness (Patterson et al., 2021).

Saying less is more in this situation. Brief questions or statements that might be appropriate in this situation and will give you more time to make sure you are making the shift from your reactions to hers include the following:

- Can I stay with you?
- Is there anyone you would like to call to be here for you?
- Would you like me or another staff member to stay with your child so that you can have a few moments?

Touch is very personal, and nurses should always ask a patient or family member's permission before touching them. There is strong evidence that social touch between the nurse and their patients can reduce stress and have a calming effect, conveying security, presence, trust, and relationship with the patient (Sandnes & Uhrenfeldt, 2024). However, culture and past experiences with trauma can affect whether a person receives a nurse's social touch warmly (Pepito et al., 2023). Always ask permission before touching another person when offering comfort, as it gives them a choice and empowers them to control their body and physical space (Fleischman et al., 2019).

You do not want to seem distracted from the conversation in this situation. However, at some point, you must use your judgment when considering your responsibilities with your other patients. Asking your charge nurse or other coworkers to support a time-sensitive task might give you the time you need to help the family members identify the resources that they need for support. Resources are unique to each person's situation and might include outreach to social workers, other family members or friends to be with the family, and the chaplain. Maybe right now is not the best time to complete a spiritual assessment on your patient, which is part of most patient admission assessments; however, this is valuable insight to help support the patient and their family. The FICA (Faith, Importance, Community, and Address in Care Tool) Spiritual History Tool is a helpful tool for nurses and healthcare providers to use and ask questions to address their spiritual concerns (Borneman et al., 2010). Table 8.2 provides a list of questions that can be part of this assessment. This information can help you support the family members in identifying their next steps to feeling supported.

TABLE 8.2 FICA Spiritual History Tool

	Questions to Consider Asking
Faith	Do you consider yourself spiritual or religious? Do you have spiritual beliefs that help you cope with stress?
Importance	What importance does your faith or belief have on your life? What role do your beliefs play in your healthcare decision-making?
Community	Are you part of a spiritual or religious community? Is there a group of people who are important to you?
Address in care	How can your health-care providers best support your spirituality?

Source: Adapted from Puchalski (2006)

Now, let us get to some of the professional issues that need improvement in this case.

The child was alone in the room without the nursing staff's knowledge. The medical team came into the room and invited the mother to the meeting; however, from her perspective, it was implied that the nurses would directly supervise her daughter in her absence. That handoff communication did not happen between the medical team and the nurse. When the nurse has the chance, they need to follow up with the provider to ask for an update on the meeting about which the mother advised you. Discuss opportunities to improve the handoff if they had taken the mother out of the room and the patient was alone without the nursing team's knowledge. Finally, discuss the opportunity to include the patient's primary nurse, if possible, in team meetings to offer support and nursing insight when possible.

Colleagues are often cited as the most valuable source of support for new nurses, and facilitated debriefing sessions and reflections are a strategy to build resilience after a death experience (Chew et al., 2021). If you are considering taking a position in a unit that supports patients with serious illnesses and their families, ask what types of resources and supports are available to staff. Consider asking about the initiatives the unit includes to assist staff with processing emotionally laden patient care, and what the organization offers to promote self-care of the nursing staff. Caring for seriously ill and dying patients has a significant emotional impact on the healthcare team and, if it is not addressed, may have negative consequences (Eng et al., 2015). Because patients are living longer with serious illnesses and co-morbidities, there exists significant emotional impact on the healthcare team (not just during the dying phase). For example, think about a family who learns that their child has a genetic condition that will limit the child's life span. Although the child is not actively dying, the bedside nurse bears witness to the breaking of bad news and the family's psychologic/spiritual/physical pain, suffering and grieving over the loss of their hopes and dreams for a well healthy child and their future.

Due to the nature of some settings, such as emergency care, we may have different relationships with patients and their families. Receiving a patient from the pre-hospital team that you have never previously met with CPR in progress sets a very different tone for communication. We do not have insight into past conversations and the wishes of the patient and their families. As Katie describes, we may quickly assess that there were missed opportunities for discussions with healthcare providers in different settings. We may or may not know the patient's medical and surgical history. There may be complex circumstances around the patient's cardiac arrest, and until we are told otherwise, we continue with advanced life support and work as a team to try to restart their heart and breathing. When the code is over, either ending with a successful resuscitation or patient death, we have new tasks to complete.

For many years, I tried to convince myself that my patient's death did not impact me because I did not know them before I met them during the code. Unconsciously, I told myself I was not permitted to have a personal reaction to their death because I only briefly cared for them. Yet, as I shared with you earlier in this book, as someone who cares deeply, the cumulative impact of caring for patients has impacted me. I changed as a person the first time a mother placed her lifeless infant's body in my arms and begged me to save them. The image of a car stopping in front of our department's doors with two people lifting and tossing a lifeless teen's body in front of my triage desk after he was fatally shot is never too far away from me when I hear someone talk about gun violence. I still have not forgotten the beautiful red-haired baby, Sydney, who came in as a full code in the middle of the night, and her father held her tiny right hand the entire time we tried to resuscitate her.

We need to advocate for practice settings that promote the time, space and support to address our reactions to caring for patients. Debriefing with the team following potentially intense situations can help provide individual support and improve team culture and resilience. Nurse scientists need to continue working with bedside nurses to identify additional supports that can best support our reactions to caring.

Emotional Burdens of Caring

We read the examples of how Katie and Eileen showed empathy for their patients and their families, a mode of understanding another person and being moved by that person's experience (Hilas, 2020). It is a highly valued attribute and an essential indicator of high-quality care (Neumann et al., 2009). It is important to distinguish the term *empathy* from *empath*; an *empath* is someone who uses empathy and may detect unspoken feelings, moods, and energy and subsequently can absorb other people's energy, emotions, or feelings, leading a nurse to feel depleted by their patient care interactions (Hilas, 2020). *Empathic accuracy*, the ability to understand others' emotions accurately, is typically viewed as beneficial; however, it may be problematic if an individual assimilates another's feelings or emotions as their own (Brown et al., 2023).

Many empaths go into helping professions such as nursing because of their desire to help others, but it is critical that we take care of our energy and do not absorb our patients' stress (Kennedy, 2019). While empaths are among the kindest and most compassionate healthcare providers as a result of their connections with others, they need to set boundaries and practice self-care as they can become overwhelmed, overstimulated, stressed, and exhausted if they continuously absorb the physical symptoms and emotions of others (Hilas, 2020, p. 334). We will talk more about this shortly.

Understanding your patient's situation (and, possibly, the pain, frustration, and anxiety) may help you connect deeply with them and their families. However, it can also put you at high risk for developing compassion fatigue (Wolters Kluwer, 2018). *Compassion fatigue* is a negative response to caring for others, composed of burnout and secondary traumatic stress (Stamm, 2010). *Burnout* is exhaustion, frustration, and anger in response to a nurse's work as a carer. *Secondary traumatic stress* (STS) is a negative feeling driven by fear and work-related trauma (Stamm, 2010). One cause of burnout in nursing is *workload*, which refers to the type of skills and effort needed to perform work tasks or the amount of work to be done and the speed at which it has to be performed (Diehl et al., 2021). Nurses who experience STS are described as suffering emotionally as a result of shared traumas with their patients and experiencing recurrent thoughts or distressing dreams, sleep disturbances, and even flashbacks of difficult patient experiences (Bock et al., 2020).

I became interested in studying the idea of compassion fatigue in nurses because of my own experiences with it. In Chapter 2, I described my first experiences with it. Looking back with a lens of more life experience, why did I think it was necessary to deny my reactions to such significant losses of patients at work? How could I possibly quickly have moved on from (*try to forget*) the trauma of losing these patients for whom I cared so much? Reacting emotionally to such significant professional trauma in such a short time was not a sign of weakness but, instead, a sign that these experiences truly mattered and that I am, in fact, human. *So is Katie. So is* Eileen. *So are you.*

I did not know how to address my reactions to caring for the patients on the inpatient pediatric unit, so I changed my practice setting. I felt more protected from my responses to caring for patients in the pediatric ED. Meeting children and families on what could be the worst day of their lives did not intimidate me because I did not know them. Our introductions are often very brief, especially if the child is critically ill or, even worse, has no vital signs. *"Name? Date of birth? Allergies? Any health problems? Do you know their weight?"*—sometimes these questions contain all the information I need to know to get started with the team on trying for the miracle the parents of my patient are hoping for. As a new nurse in the pediatric ED, I studied whenever I had downtime, often jotting little notes to myself on a brown paper towel or an alcohol swab as a reminder to look things up when I had more time.

I tell you that I am not tough or emotionless. I cry at commercials, cannot watch a movie about a dog dying, and tear up at the sound of young children singing at a holiday concert. What is the disconnect within me? How can I be two completely different people inside of the same body? I assure you that I am not. Katie's story resonated with me, especially when she said earlier in this chapter, "*I don't want to be tough. I don't want to be expected to be some superhero. I don't want to look at the freckle on your back and tell you if it is suspicious.*" There is a lot of meaning in those three sentences. I will share what they mean to me.

'I Don't Want to Be Tough. I Don't Want to Be Expected to Be Some Superhero.'

In our day-to-day work, nurses commonly witness the extremes of human lived experience, substantially more so than the average person may see throughout their lifetime (Roney & Acri, 2018). Some of us are privileged to witness life when it is most fragile. Some of us would say it is a blessing and a curse. If you have taken care of a very sick patient or one with many needs of end of life needs, you know how this goes. You are trying to juggle it all: outstanding, holistic patient care for all your patients, not the only one with the most needs. With so many balls in the air, there is no time for you to take a sip of water or use the restroom. By the afternoon, you realize you have yet to have a morsel of food or a moment to gather your thoughts. Challenging clinical situations are often accompanied by those equally burdensome on an emotional level. By now, you are emotionally and physically depleted, but due to the demands of patient-centered care, you have to keep going. Hospitals do not often get the guessing game right to project how many nurses a shift will need and now, more often, are short-staffed (Hilgers, 2022).

If our patients receive palliative care or wish to have no life-sustaining interventions, we feel a profound duty to keep them comfortable, as Katie did in her narrative. As nurses, we often receive situations created by situations that should have taken place a long time ago. Katie shares with us, "*She did not understand the plan, and while it was an emergent situation, someone with more knowledge on the matter should have explained what being intubated meant.*" That takes a lot out of us. The conversation would have been challenging, but it would certainly have been less demanding than the one Katie and the team had to have with the patient on the brink of making this decision. An excellent, free resource for you to be aware of is The Conversation Project (theconversationproject.org; Institute for Healthcare Improvement, n.d.). It provides accessible resources for starting conversations about people's wishes for care through the end of time. It also includes specialized guides for choosing and being a healthcare proxy as well as guides for caregivers of special populations (e.g., children with serious illnesses). Reading these materials can help you become more comfortable with this topic as you speak with patients and families.

If our patient requires life-saving interventions to try to resuscitate them and the efforts are not successful, we then transition to supporting the family and following our organization's protocols for the next steps. That also takes a lot out of us. We often do not have time to process this as we move on to the next thing. This does not set us up for success when we are likely already depleted. However, more often than I'd like to admit, I've both been asked by a charge nurse—and I have also been the charge nurse to ask a colleague—who has just experienced a patient death or transferred a patient to the ICU to take the next admission because they were next in line. This requires the nurse who just experienced the challenging event to put aside their own reactions and push through.

Your heart will react to these emotionally and intellectually charged experiences that are not part of most people's day-to-day lives. When Katie said that she did not want to be tough, it made me think of the times when I was forced back onto the unit, much like an injured soldier goes back to the battlefield. One time, after an extended code for a pediatric patient, followed by preparing the child's body to be transported to our private family bereavement area of the ED, I went back to work on the *battlefield*. As much as we try to maintain the privacy of each event on the unit, the change of the milieu on the unit changes when there is a code that ends in death. As I was walking back to the unit from the bereavement area, a patient's mother whom I had never met stopped me and asked me for a ginger ale. I went to the refrigerator, grabbed one can, and passed it to the mother as I tried to resume my work. Instead of thanking me for the beverage, she said, "*No ice?*" "*No, ma'am, no ice,*" I said in my head. She got no response from me. My eyes were filled with tears, my own heart rate was elevated, and I felt my flushed face. It took every ounce of my fortitude and resilience not to walk off the unit.

What did *I need* in that moment? It certainly was not the next patient who was now in my newly deceased patient's bed space. I needed time away from the unit to reflect on the situation and care for myself. After these intense professional events, you will need time away from your work as a nurse. Nurses gain in-the-room insight by spending prolonged periods at the bedside with patients and families, which gives us an intimate understanding of the patient and family experiences as they interface with the rest of the healthcare organization (Broden et al., 2024). While these are some of the most professionally gratifying experiences, they are emotionally and physically exhausting.

When interviewing for a new position, ask what support nurses on the unit receive when they have difficult patient transitions (e.g., prolonged care of a critically ill patient or death). If you are in your position, advocate for yourself and your coworkers. Has your coworker's patient just died? Offer to cover their patients or ask the charge/resource nurse for support so that they can recover from the event. Ask for the same for yourself. If you have this experience, be clear about what you need and ask for the time away from patient care to recenter yourself before you return to patient care. Accumulated stress, inability to process experiences, and piled-on tasks will negatively affect your mood and fatigue in the short term (Martínez-Zaragoza et al., 2020). Cumulative stress can lead to compassion fatigue (Roney & Acri, 2018). Signs of compassion fatigue are listed in the following box. Structured debriefing sessions immediately after critical events may reduce compassion fatigue by providing social support and increasing job satisfaction (Beres et al., 2022).

PRN (PLEASE READ NOW)

What are some signs of compassion fatigue?

- Anger
- Irritability
- Tearfulness
- Difficulty concentrating on tasks
- Annoyance
- Skepticism
- Anxiety
- Lapses in memory or forgetfulness
- Anger
- Cynicism
- Irrational fears
- Negative self-image
- Intolerance
- Mood swings
- Sadness/numbness
- Addictions (including smoking, alcohol, drugs, and gambling)

Source: Stoewen, 2020.

Helping Yourself Through Challenging Times

The first step is for nurses and the organizations that they work for to implement strategies to prevent compassion fatigue, including regular self-care practices (Paiva-Salisbury & Schwanz, 2022). We will discuss integrating self-care practices into your daily life in Chapter 12. This is not something optional for us as nurses. Find your community of support and plan activities to make yourself happy, as Eileen describes in this chapter. Perhaps you have heard that planning a vacation directly affects your happiness, possibly even more so than the trip itself (Nawijn et al., 20210). Anticipation of future positive events has shown on magnetic resonance imaging (MRI) that the bilateral medial prefrontal cortex was activated during anticipation for positive events relative to neutral events, and the enhanced brain activation in MPFC was associated with a higher level of well-being (Luo et al., 2018). We all need to have things to look forward to.

For some of us, our healthcare colleagues are our second family; for others, we appreciate relationships outside of work more. Our schedules make planning a little more complicated, but the benefits are tremendous. Finally, consider seeking out mental health resources at work through occupational health/employee assistance or privately to support you as you process these experiences and integrate them into your life experience. Katie shares the positive impact of regular therapy sessions on her personal and professional life. You are worth the time to invest in yourself.

'I Don't Want to Look at the Freckle on Your Back and Tell You if It Is Suspicious.'

OK, with the weight of everything else Katie shared with us, this might feel like it is just a comment, but I would like to highlight how important it is to discuss this with you. My husband, also in health care, and I are usually the first call for many of our friends and family members who encounter health care. We have been on many dinner dates, airplanes, church services, and more when there is an announcement that asks, *"Is there a health care provider that can help us with a medical emergency?"* While we do not mind helping our close friends and family in any way, it has taken me until very recently to realize that I do not have the bandwidth to help everyone whom I encounter navigate whatever healthcare situation they face. These conversations often take place in social environments when we should be relaxing and having fun, but instead, one of us is cornered by a new acquaintance who hears we are in health care and does not appreciate that we might not want to talk with them for 70 minutes about their knee pain, upcoming MRI, and treatment options offered by their surgeon. It is usually followed up with requests for a phone call and unsolicited text messages including screenshots of their MRI images. These situations drain me and in no way fill my cup. I used to feel bad not listening and offering free advice to acquaintances, but if I were at a party and a person I had just met were a financial advisor, would I feel comfortable taking their uncompensated 70 minutes to ask them how to invest my money? *Of course not.* The same goes for you. You also are putting yourself at risk of facing litigation if something goes wrong (Boyce, 2023).

When you started nursing school, your community "saw" you as a nurse even before you took your first lab or clinical course. Family members might have called you for medical advice. Friends might have started to disclose health information they never would have told you if you weren't on your path to becoming a nurse. At first, it is flattering, but soon, it becomes exhausting. Your bandwidth as a caregiver needs to have limits. Some caregiving roles, including those we have in addition to our nursing role, are ones we can't give up, such as for your child, parent, and partner. Be aware of your time and be cautious about requests for the nurse role when you are not on shift. It is your choice whom and when you help others in these types of situations. There are responses that I have learned over time that have helped me in conversations that become requests to blur the lines and slip into my nursing role in nonclinical, such as, *"I'm off duty tonight! I am here to have fun"* or *"I cannot give medical advice outside of work, but if you are concerned, you should talk with your provider."* Giving all the time takes away from the time during which you should replenish yourself. It is your choice how to respond in these situations, but be aware that if your compassion is already maxed due to a combination of professional and personal situations, continuing to give nursing care off the clock when you feel that it would be impolite not to offer advice can make you feel worse.

My brilliant coworker and friend Siedah often reminds me, *"Remember, Lin, we match energies."* We can easily jump into every situation with our holistic nursing lens and help everyone and everything in our personal lives. We make great friends and family members because we are empathetic, supportive, and great listeners. We are excellent at person-centered care, so we often put the needs of others before our own, even in our personal life. Of course, in many of our personal roles, we frequently have to put others' needs before our own, but we must be aware that it does not need to be *every person in your life.* This, too, will contribute to burnout and fatigue. No one ever told me this, and I have found myself giving of myself too often and ending up in personal relationships that were not reciprocal. Perhaps this might upset some readers when I say this, but it is okay to pull away (even if it is just a little) from personal relationships that drain you and never offer you anything in return. Having awareness and boundaries in our personal lives can give us some of our energy back.

In Chapter 12, we will focus heavily on the need for nurses to incorporate self-care into our daily lives. As someone who still regularly works 12-hour shifts, I know what that does to your free time on your scheduled days. Here are a few tips that I have found to have a tremendous impact on my sense of well-being daily, especially on my busy days.

PRN (PLEASE READ NOW)

- **Book-end your day.** Always start with something for you and end with something for you. My two things are usually movement and a bath. This might mean in my especially busy days my movement is a five-minute walk outside and a five-minute bath at the end of the evening. Both feel decadent to me.
- **Habit stack.** I meal-prep my lunches for the week; sometimes, it feels like a real chore. Add something fun at the same time. I used to get upset because I didn't have time to read as much as I would like. I started borrowing audio-books from the library using the Libby app (https://libbyapp.com/interview/welcome#doYouHaveACard) and saving them for when I do chores that I am not crazy about doing. I also listen to podcasts I like when cleaning the house or folding laundry. It suddenly makes everything more fun.
- **Earthing.** *Earthing* is having direct skin contact with nature, which physically rebalances our energy when stressed (Cleveland Clinic, 2024). This might mean walking to the mailbox through the grass and pavement without shoes or crushing a fallen, dry leaf in my hand. I started this practice without knowing what earthing was; I felt compelled to do these things. As I took more time to reflect, I often did this when most stressed. Give it a try.

YOU MATTER: CARING FOR PATIENTS AT THE END OF THEIR LIFE

Katie and Eileen shared insight into their important work caring for dying patients. While some new nurses start their careers with personal experience caring for friends or family members, most begin with minimal familiarity with this new experience. Clinical rotations and work experience may have provided a little exposure. However, as a licensed professional responsible for their patients' holistic needs, this new role can cause a range of emotions to surface. Use the strategies discussed in this chapter to find support, and always remember that you matter to your patients, their families, your colleagues, and those in your personal life.

Book Club Questions

1. Have you observed nurses manage their emotional responses while caring for patients facing end-of-life decisions? What was the situation, and what did they do?
2. How do you see the nurse's role as a member of the interdisciplinary team providing holistic care to patients at end-of-life?

3. What signs might you have if you are experiencing negative responses to caring for others, and how can you address them?

4. What strategies can you employ to practice self-care as you work in a demanding and emotionally intense clinical setting?

About This Chapter's Authors

Kathryn Magennis, BSN, RN

Kathryn (Katie) Magennis was born and raised in northern New Jersey. After graduating from Fairfield University Egan School of Nursing and Health Studies in 2022, she moved to New York City to pursue her dreams of working in an ED. Katie has maintained the same place of work since graduation and is always seeking a fast-paced environment that both her job and life in the city have to offer. Katie's days off are spent reading, traveling, running through Central Park, and hosting dinner parties for friends.

Eileen R. O'Shea, DNP, APRN, PCNS-BC, CHPPN

Dr. Eileen R. O'Shea, professor at the Egan School of Nursing and Health Studies, Fairfield University, is the founding director of the Kanarek Center for Palliative Care Nursing Education. She holds a BSN from Boston College, an MSN from the University of Pennsylvania, and a DNP from Case Western Reserve University. With extensive pediatric nursing experience, Dr. O'Shea has worked in several leading U.S. children's hospitals and holds national board certification as an advanced practice nurse and national certification in hospice and palliative pediatric nursing. Her passion and clinical expertise have been in caring for children with serious illness and their families.

She received additional education in palliative care through the End-of-Life Nursing Education Consortium, the Harvard Program in Palliative Care Education, and the Interprofessional Spiritual Care Education Curriculum. Most recently, she founded the first Pediatric Palliative Care Coalition for the state of Connecticut, serving as the president, and was a Panel member to the Palliative and Hospice Nursing Professional Issues Panel convened by the ANA and the Hospice and Palliative Nurses Association.

Dr. O'Shea's research interests include enhancing nursing education and practice, simulation, and curriculum development, specifically focusing on palliative care. As a leader and educator, Dr. O'Shea has widely disseminated outcomes via publications and presentations at local, national, and international levels.

To recharge, Dr. O'Shea enjoys traveling, reading, skiing, walking half-marathons, and caring for her new grand-puppy, Murphy!

References

American Association of Colleges of Nursing. (2021). *The essentials: Core competencies for professional nursing education.* https://www.aacnnursing.org/Portals/0/PDFs/Publications/Essentials-2021.pdf

American Nurses Association. (2015). *Code of ethics with interpretative statements.* https://www.nursingworld.org/practice-policy/nursing-excellence/ethics/code-of-ethics-for-nurses/coe-view-only/

Beres, K. E., Zajac, L. M., Mason, H., Krenke, K., & Costa, D. K. (2022). Addressing compassion fatigue in trauma emergency and intensive care settings: A pilot study. *Journal of Trauma Nursing, 29*(4), 210–217. https://doi.org/10.1097/JTN.0000000000000663

Bock, C., Heitland, I., Zimmermann, T., Winter, L., & Kahl, K. G. (2020). Secondary traumatic stress, mental state, and workability in nurses—Results of a psychological risk assessment at a University Hospital. *Frontiers in Psychiatry, 11*, 298. https://doi.org/10.3389/fpsyt.2020.00298

Borneman, T., Ferrell, B., & Puchalski, C. M. (2010). Evaluation of the FICA tool for spiritual assessment. *Journal of Pain and Symptom Management, 40*(2), 163–173. https://doi.org/10.1016/j.jpainsymman.2009.12.019

Boyce, H. (2023, May 16). Nurses: What to do when friends and family ask for medical advice. *The Atlanta-Journal Constitution.* https://www.ajc.com/pulse/what-to-do-when-friends-and-family-ask-for-medical-advice/QLCSQYIW5FFNZPP4AAL6VPQP5E/

Broden, E. G., Eche-Ugwu, I. J., DeCourcey, D. D., Wolfe, J., Hinds, P. S., & Snaman, J. (2024). "At least I can push this morphine": PICU nurses' approaches to suffering among dying children. *Journal of Pain and Symptom Management, 68*(2), 132–141.e2. https://doi.org/10.1016/j.jpainsymman.2024.04.018

Brown, C. L., Grimm, K. J., Wells, J. L., Hua, A. Y., & Levenson, R. W. (2023). Empathic accuracy and shared depressive symptoms in close relationships. *Clinical Psychological Science, 11*(3), 509–525. https://doi.org/10.1177/21677026221141852

Center to Advance Palliative Care. (2020, May 11). *Palliative care report card.* https://reportcard.capc.org/

Chew, Y. J. M., Ang, S. L. L., & Shorey, S. (2021). Experiences of new nurses dealing with death in a paediatric setting: A descriptive qualitative study. *Journal of advanced nursing, 77*(1), 343–354. https://doi.org/10.1111/jan.14602

Cleveland Clinic. (2024, April 19). *Is earthing actually good for you? Here's what we know.* https://health.clevelandclinic.org/earthing

Diehl, E., Rieger, S., Letzel, S., Schablon, A., Nienhaus, A., Escobar Pinzon, L. C., & Dietz, P. (2021). The relationship between workload and burnout among nurses: The buffering role of personal, social and organisational resources. *PLOS One, 16*(1), e0245798. https://doi.org/10.1371/journal.pone.0245798

Eng, J., Schulman, E., Jhanwar, S. M., & Shah, M. K. (2015). Patient death debriefing sessions to support residents' emotional reactions to patient deaths. *Journal of Graduate Medical Education, 7*(3), 430–436. https://doi.org/10.4300/JGME-D-14-00544.1

Fleishman, J., Kamsky, H., & Sundborg, S. (2019). Trauma-informed nursing practice. *Online Journal of Issues in Nursing, 24*(2), Manuscript 3.

Frankl, V. E. (1984). *Man's search for meaning*. Pocket Books.

Hilas, O. (2020). Empathy or empath? Increasing self-awareness for healthy patient-provider interactions. *Senior Care Pharmacist*, 35(8), 334–335. https://doi.org/10.4140/TCP.n.2020.334

Hilgers, L. (2022, February 15). "Nurses have finally learned what they're worth." *The New York Times*. https://www.nytimes.com/2022/02/15/magazine/traveling-nurses.html

Institute for Healthcare Improvement. (n.d.). *The conversation project*. https://theconversationproject.org/

International Coaching Federation. (2024). *All things coaching*. https://coachingfederation.org/about?gad_source=1&gclid=CjwKCAjwmrqzBhAoEiwAXVpgouWaKHARPQMoymmVTmNs_s8zrV2P5kT8rlj360FMMqa_AqDYPmQDMxoCGA8QAvD_BwE

Kennedy, R. (2019). *Is it healthy to be both a nurse and an empath?* kennhttps://www.wolterskluwer.com/en/expert-insights/when-empathy-turns-harmful

Kübler-Ross, E. (1969). *On death and dying*. Macmillan Publishers.

Luo, Y., Chen, X., Qi, S., You, X., & Huang, X. (2018). Well-being and anticipation for future positive events: Evidence from an fMRI study. *Frontiers in Psychology*, 8, 2199. https://doi.org/10.3389/fpsyg.2017.02199

Martínez-Zaragoza, F., Fernández-Castro, J., Benavides-Gil, G., & García-Sierra, R. (2020). How the lagged and accumulated effects of stress, coping, and tasks affect mood and fatigue during nurses' shifts. *International Journal of Environmental Research and Public Health*, 17(19), 7277. https://doi.org/10.3390/ijerph17197277

Merriam-Webster. (n.d.). Reactions. *Merriam-Webster Dictionary*. https://www.merriamwebster.com dictionary/reaction

Nawijn, J., Marchand, M. A., Veenhoven, R., & Vingerhoets, A. J. (2010). Vacationers happier, but most not happier after a holiday. *Applied Research in Quality of Life*, 5(1), 35–47. https://doi.org/10.1007/s11482-009-9091-9

Neumann, M., Bensing, J., Mercer, S., Ernstmann, N., Ommen, O., & Pfaff, H. (2009). Analyzing the "nature" and "specific effectiveness" of clinical empathy: A theoretical overview and contribution towards a theory-based research agenda. *Patient Education and Counseling*, 74(3), 339–346. https://doi.org/10.1016/j.pec.2008.11.013

Paiva-Salisbury, M. L., & Schwanz, K. A. (2022). Building compassion fatigue resilience: awareness, prevention, and intervention for pre-professionals and current practitioners. *Journal of Health Service Psychology*, 48(1), 39–46. https://doi.org/10.1007/s42843-022-00054-9

Patterson, K., Grenny, J., McMillan, R., & Switzler, A. (2021). *Crucial conversations* (*3rd ed.*). McGraw-Hill Contemporary.

Pepito, J. A. T., Babate, F. J. G., & Dator, W. L. T. (2023). The nurses' touch: An irreplaceable component of caring. *Nursing Open*, 10(9), 5838–5842. https://doi.org/10.1002/nop2.1860

Puchalski, C. M. (2006). The FICA spiritual history tool. *The Journal of Palliative Medicine*, 9(1), 16-17. https://doi.org/10.1089/jpm.2006.9.16

Puchalski, C. M., Vitillo, R., Hull, S. K., & Reller, N. (2014). Improving the spiritual dimension of whole person care: Reaching national and international consensus. *Journal of Palliative Medicine*, 17(6), 642–656.

Roney, L. N., & Acri, M. C. (2018). The cost of caring: An exploration of compassion fatigue, compassion satisfaction, and job satisfaction in pediatric nurses. *Journal of Pediatric Nursing, 40,* 74–80. https://doi.org/10.1016/j.pedn.2018.01.016

Sandnes, L., & Uhrenfeldt, L. (2024). Caring touch as communication in intensive care nursing: a qualitative study. *International Journal of Qualitative Studies on Health and Well-Being, 19*(1), 2348891. https://doi.org/10.1080/17482631.2024.2348891

Stamm, B. (2010). *ProQoL manual.* https://proqol.org/proqol-manual

Stoewen, D. L. (2020). Moving from compassion fatigue to compassion resilience. Part 4: Signs and consequences of compassion fatigue. *Canadian Veterinary Journal, 61*(11), 1207–1209.

Wolters Kluwer. (2018). *When empathy turns harmful.* https://www.wolterskluwer.com/en/expert-insights/when-empathy-turns-harmful

Zust, C. (2017, July 5). *Know the difference between coaching and mentoring.* Center for Corporate and Professional Development, Kent State University. https://www.kent.edu/yourtrainingpartner/know-difference-between-coaching-and-mentoring

CHAPTER 9

Heartfelt Decisions

Ethics in Caring for Patients Who Need Us the Most

Iris Johnson, BSN, RN; Aaron Carpenter, DNP, MDiv, APRN, CPNP-PC, NEA-B; Sarah E. Wawrzynski, PhD, RN, CCRN; and Linda Roney, EdD, RN-BC, CPEN, CNE, FAAN

Learning Goals

1. Describe Iris' successes and challenges in caring for a critically ill infant as a new-graduate nurse.
2. Value the nurse's role as a patient and family advocate.
3. Reflect on your beliefs and attitudes that affect your influence as an ethical leader in practice.
4. Apply the American Nurses Association's (ANA, 2015) code of ethics in providing ethical patient care.

'Who Are We, I Suppose, to Deny a Family's Child a Chance?'

By Iris Johnson, BSN, RN

To be a nurse is to know ethical dilemmas. Whether you are working at the bedside, in outpatient, in emergency, or in primary care, it is inevitable that you will find yourself facing an ethical challenge within the healthcare system. There is nothing to do in order to prepare yourself for the gravity of bearing witness to these situations and the feelings that follow. Yet, at times, these conditions feel preordained to the healthcare system's operation. Thus, it is important to know how you will act in the face of adversity, advocate for the issue at hand, and, most importantly, identify what morality means to you and how to apply that to your practice.

As I began my nursing career, I knew I was starting in a difficult specialty, but I would be a hypocrite if I did not admit I was naive to the gravity of the role I was going to be playing in the cardiac intensive care unit (CICU) at a world-renowned children's hospital. Grappling with the responsibility and the nursing autonomy of my unit was a steep learning curve. In the CICU, the nurse is responsible for titrating various intravenous (IV) drips, administering sedation, understanding an array of anatomy and physiologies as well as the implications of various modes of ventilation, and using their critical thinking and clinical judgment to send important labs based on the patient's condition. With time and acclimation, I learned the nuances of the unit. I understood what the fellow meant when they requested volume; this typically meant Albumin 5%. Or when my resource nurse asked if I had made a long line, which essentially was a saline flush with a 2cc tubing line attached to my push port, that was used to administer procedural or emergent medications. I knew my CVP (central venous pressure) could be referred to as *filling pressures*, that T_{max} meant simply the maximum temperature of my patient that shift, and that allowing a patient to breathe on pressure support ventilation based on the patient's goals and needs was a *sprint*. It can be a lot. Needless to say, the physicians and nursing leadership expect you to be three steps ahead of them before you call to address a patient's clinical status. This can be distressing and overwhelming for any nurse—let alone a new nurse—and it makes you question how your scope of practice is being applied in this clinical setting and possibly infringed upon.

When I think of why I became a nurse, I reflect on the principles of compassion, empathy, and healing. These principles were challenged more often than not, and it is difficult not to be overcome by pessimism and defeat when I reflect on my first years as a nurse. Yet, those years have taught me invaluable lessons that I continue to carry on, which are lessons on humility in the face of adversity and the knowledge that ethical challenges are inevitable; however, the moral distress of nursing does not have to overcome you. It is easier to do the work we do every day when we acknowledge the humanity of it all, that it does serve a purpose, and that there is strength in hope. I reminded myself of this often in my first years as a nurse.

Furthermore, let me offer a glimpse of a challenging moment in my practice and how I applied these principles to sustain my passion for nursing. Imagine that it was February 2023, and I had been a nurse for just over a year, already having experienced two significant patient losses. I was feeling overwhelmed by the daunting task of walking into work and acknowledging the unknown of how my shift may pan out. I remember that I had just come back from a long stretch of being off. I felt refreshed and a little more at ease than I typically did walking onto the unit. As soon as I rounded the corner to my patient's bed space, I could see from the nurse, Ellen, who I was receiving report that this would be a tough night. I stood at the entrance of my bed space and saw an open-chested newborn with multiple lines and tubes exiting his body. He had a cute little sign at the end of his crib that displayed his name and tiny feet, which, to me, always serves as a friendly reminder that there is, in fact, delicate life in that crib. This was not an uncommon sight to walk into, yet I always pause for a moment to acknowledge what a challenging start to this baby's little life.

As I sat for the report, I learned more about this sweet baby boy's story. His name was Isaiah, and he was born with hypoplastic left heart syndrome (HLHS). There are various formations of HLHS. For Isaiah's heart, this consisted of HLHS with mitral atresia, aorta atresia, and an intact atrial septum. Moreover, babies born with HLHS have a significantly smaller left side of their heart, which results in the underdevelopment of the left-sided heart structures and the dependence of the right side of the heart to pump blood flow to the lungs and the body. Specifically, these babies are dependent on having some form of communication within their heart to ensure that they receive oxygenated blood to their body, so an atrial communication, typically a patent foramen ovale (PFO) in fetal circulation and a patent ductus arteriosus (PDA), are a necessity. Yet, at birth, these are at risk of closing imminently as they are fetal circulation structures; thus, a baby born with this defect must be started on prostaglandins (PGEs) to maintain a patent PDA, and hopefully, they have an atrial septal defect in addition to their PFO, which may close and compromise their body's efforts to receive oxygenated blood.

Nonetheless, this anatomy is critical and life-threatening at birth, and for Isaiah, he lacked any ability to have oxygenated flow. Therefore, he was rushed to the catheterization laboratory after delivery to create an atrial septostomy, which can be accomplished via a balloon atrial septostomy (BAS) or, in Isaiah's case, by placing an atrial stent, along with pulmonary artery (PA) bands. Now Isaiah can receive oxygenated blood flow with his PDA maintained with PGEs, an atrial septostomy so that the blood from the left can flow to the right, and PA bands to protect his lungs from all the extra flow they will now receive. Typically, these newborns affected by this heart defect are extremely ill and require the first-stage surgery of a three-stage palliation within the first week of life. Yet, prior to any intervention, they usually live on room air, attempt to bottle or breastfeed, receive cuddles, and remain on PGEs, all of which are dependent on how the severity of HLHS compromises their circulation. But, for Isaiah, he required an open chest, three vasopressors, and significant resuscitation to sustain life. At this point, Ellen said to me, "Yesterday evening, he cardiac arrested, requiring CPR [cardiopulmonary resuscitation] and multiple rounds of code medications, and it was uncertain what the etiology of the arrest was."

At that moment, I knew that Isaiah was one of the sickest babies I had ever cared for, and I knew from that moment this would be one of the toughest challenges in my early nursing career.

Isaiah's few weeks of life were critical enough that our medical and surgical teams held thorough discussions with his mother, Celia, conveying that he would not be a surgical candidate for the typical HLHS palliation and that he was not an extracorporeal membrane oxygenation (ECMO) candidate. By specifying ECMO candidacy, the team clarified that despite the fact his heart and lungs may fail, they would not provide the highest level of life support to fully assist his heart and lungs because, in Isaiah's case, even when providing the rest that this machine could provide for his body, it would not be enough. I remember talking to Celia about how this information made her feel and acknowledging the gravity of how heartbreaking this whole experience must be. Celia always remained hopeful and believed in her deep faith that Isaiah would get better. She had never held Isaiah. He was always too labile to be safely held, something that would be a typical act if he was not born in such a critical state. Despite this, Celia would sit by his side day in and day out, reading to him, saying prayers, and singing. She never gave up on her faith or hope.

From my nursing perspective, I agreed with the surgical plan not to operate. Isaiah was critically ill and barely tolerated his initial intervention, and as an interdisciplinary team, we all struggled to advance his care to a more stable state. I believed this already fragile baby did not deserve to endure an open-heart surgery that would not result in a positive outcome, nor did his mother need to experience the extended pain of watching her son live in a paralyzed and sedated state, which, in most cases, we can refer to as a *coma*. Months passed, and he required more resuscitation, new IV drips, and ventilation modifications. Isaiah tolerated being awake for stretches of time but eventually required more sedation and was chemically paralyzed. Despite the team's efforts to keep him alive, he was struggling, and he lived most of it in a deep coma. It was only a matter of time. Then, as the end of the week came around, a new perspective entered the discussion as a new attending who had yet to care for him came on service. Isaiah's plan of care changed, and the decision was made that he would be a surgical candidate and go for the stage one operation, which he would now receive at age 4 months, a procedure usually completed during the first week of life. It was risky and controversial, but the physician pushed, and the surgical team agreed. For his mother, this felt like her faith prevailed and he would be better. However, for nursing, this created a spiral of ethical concerns and dilemmas that would persist for months to follow, creating a tense and distressing environment.

Naturally, I did not always care for Isaiah because our unit was large, and there were other patients in between. I can say that when I did, there were always significant moments in his care. I knew Isaiah from the start, when he was denied interventions to not too soon after his first true surgical intervention. He was the same, yet awake. But his little blue nose and persistent agitation showed me that he still was not compatible with his repair or the life we were offering him. It begins to be morally distressing when you must sedate a baby with sedation boluses large enough for a full-grown adult to make them comfortable. That was what Isaiah required. He would have profound hemodynamic changes, and that became the norm for him. But, if these changes occurred in another patient's bed space, this would have been cause for alarm and constant code bells. If you know anything about an HLHS baby, their oxygen saturation should be 75%–85%. Isaiah lived in a hypoxic state of 40%–60%, which could be relieved with vent changes until, eventually, his ventilator became maxed out or, at times, sedation, which still did not seem to be relieving enough. Nothing that I did felt like it was enough—he would be in the deepest coma and he still shed tears, and I felt helpless. Isaiah always made me question myself, asking, *"What am I doing? What are we doing as a team? There has to be something else for him."* I have always firmly believed in the power of hope and refuse to deny a patient or family that; however, for the first time, I struggled with knowing how to preserve it.

Another factor important to Isaiah's care was the fact that he was a Black baby. Before I elaborate on the reason why it was important that he was Black, I must pause to acknowledge that as unfortunate as it is to have to address the color of a patient's skin, nonetheless a baby's, this is a persistent issue plaguing health care and society that I hope one day we can all overcome. Regarding Isaiah's care, I feel strongly that the team provided him with all the options possible and available to him regardless of his race. Yet, I do feel there was often judgment passed on how his family responded to his plan of care, their parenting style in the capacity they could, and their choices. I saw judgments passed on families often because it's ethically challenging to watch a family go through the inevitable. I will admit that it could be challenging to care for Isaiah when his parents were not always fully present at the bedside. I could make biased comments based on how I presume a parent should behave at the bedside, yet who am I to say that they should be there 24/7? It was distressing enough to watch Isaiah for 12 hours a shift, let alone be his parent, who watched him every day at all hours. I cannot even fathom the emotional or mental strain. Yet, in this circumstance, I felt that the other comments were more escalated, and I believe that was because of the family's race. When eavesdropping on neighboring conversations or receiving report myself from another nurse, specifically more senior nurses than I, it was not uncommon for a negative family remark to be made. The comments consisted of judgments on their intentions of having Isaiah in the United States versus their home country, whether that was intentional or by chance, and why they would push for more interventions when they should understand his prognosis at this point. Many nurses felt his parents pushed for more life-preserving interventions because they were seeking an opportunity to qualify for U.S. residential benefits, such as a visa, which I felt was a careless assumption to make and deeply concerning. It was a frightening claim to be made because not only it could not be true, but it also shed light on the scarier notion that there are some deep-rooted unconscious biases and prejudices against Black families in the CICU. On the unit, it was not rare to have an international family in your care, yet this was never a comment I intercepted referencing Caucasian international families. It made me worried about how Isaiah's family was being supported by nursing and concerned me that they would feel the prejudices translate through the care. It is not uncommon to hear and not the first time this has happened to a Black family encountering the medical profession, but it is shameful and scary that despite efforts for inclusion and acknowledgment of disparities, these opinions still carry weight. There was enough ethically inapt with Isaiah struggling to hold onto his life, but that did not have anything to do with his race and certainly did not need to play a part.

Unfortunately, the burdensome implications of racism marred the intentions of his care because the rumor of the reason for preserving his life for immigration purposes prevailed rather than just because of his parents' love, which broke my heart. However, if you held a bird's-eye perspective in this case, you would appreciate that Isaiah's family had developed an immense amount of medical mistrust. They would communicate this often, and I understood why because he began his life as a candidate for nothing, and then months passed, and he was allowed an intervention. To the nonmedical mind, this seems good and sounds like progress. Nevertheless, his parents were faced again with the inevitable that despite all the efforts, some progress, and then a few steps back, Isaiah was dying. Rather than them seeking immigration opportunities, a prejudiced assumption to make, I believe they were preserving their hope and advocating for their baby, who, to them, was defying all the odds of what they were initially told. I believe Isaiah's parents felt obligated to advocate extensively for him after everything they endured because our team dismantled any rapport that we were genuinely seeking out what was best for him. It was so much more than a ticket to the United States.

In the final months of Isaiah's life, it brought me peace of mind to know that he had about a month of time where he was able to be the closest thing to a baby as possible. Celia would help give him a bath, perform tracheostomy care, and perform his gastrostomy and jejunostomy (G/J) tube dressing changes. She could hold him. If he was having a good day, his nurses would place him in a high chair and have him sit at the front of his bed space to watch the many people go by in the busy intensive care unit (ICU). He eventually weaned off his sedation and was ready to go to an outside hospital where he could have a non-ICU long-term care solution, yet he became septic, which led to him experiencing a life-threatening ventricular arrhythmia, resulting in a ventricular tachycardia arrest, from which he never truly recovered afterward. His hemodynamics worsened, the parameters set by the medical team got wider, and, for nursing, the stress of fearing cardiac arrest occurred every day while caring for Isaiah. His critical status became normal even for his parents, who became frustrated, and the bedspace became depressing and difficult to manage. I began to feel as though I was doing more harm by keeping this child alive by giving anesthetic-worthy boluses of sedation and keeping a baby paralyzed for more than half of his life. The number of times I was able to preserve Isaiah's dignity and make him feel safe were far and few in between when I was challenged with preventing his imminent death.

I knew I felt unsafe in his bed space when he would become desaturated to 40% oxygen saturation, and instead of being able to give him an oxygen boost on the ventilator, he was already set to 100% with the addition of nitric oxide, which in theory should work as an adjunct to his oxygenation support as a more potent pulmonary vasodilator. I cannot explain the number of times I would call the team to explain that he was desaturated, significantly hypotensive, bradycardic, and severely hypertensive or crying through his paralytic despite being still and sedated. More often than not, I would be met with the response "He does this; ride it out for now," which was correct; Isaiah did do this often, but that did not make it right or safe. It was evident that Isaiah was suffering and in pain.

We learn in nursing school the ABCs (airway, breathing, circulation), for which the interventions are typically self-explanatory; however, for me, I lost my ability in this space to do the usual interventions that would work for a desaturated HLHS baby because, clinically, my only options were limited. There were limitations to managing Isaiah's hemodynamics since there were only so many ways to support a baby's circulation, the ventilator did not have room to increase, and his sedation became the only thing that changed, and in excess. Although the sedation was meant to keep him safe and painless, this usually involved providing boluses, in which the dosages could be significant even for an adult to require. I felt that my care delivered more malfeasance than benevolence at times because, despite my options to relieve pain and keep Isaiah comfortably sedated, he would still cry; although he was motionless, you would see a single tear stream down his face. His current state made him unsafe for the activities he used to do for his development, and his mom could no longer safely hold him. Where was the benevolence in any of this? I still find myself trying to answer this question.

The harm of Isaiah's care was ultimately challenged in the final month of his life. It was understood from weeks of hypoxia, nonreassuring echocardiograms, hemodynamic lability, and team discussions with no positive outcome that Isaiah's life would end soon. The team started having more family meetings to discuss Isaiah's status and the option to not perform an ECMO cannulation if he were to arrest; however, the team would still perform a full code per his family's wishes. For nursing, even the thought of carrying out a code on this fragile baby felt cruel, yet who are we, I suppose, to deny a family's child a chance? With that in mind, it felt negligent not to acknowledge the elephant in the room that he was dying and that there was nothing we could do. There was not a surgical intervention willing to be offered, and Isaiah's medical support was nearly maxed out.

Then, again, an attending decided to present the need for a catheterization lab intervention to evaluate Isaiah's true hemodynamic status more invasively. This was controversial because the team and beyond knew this could be a life-threatening trip for him, that he may not tolerate it, and that this could result in cardiac arrest, for which the team deemed ECMO would be indicated in this event since it would be triggered by a procedure. Nurses felt outraged by this. We are taught to do no harm, provide healing and compassion, preserve dignity, and protect our patients. This catheterization lab trip felt ethically compromising; therefore, after a lot of escalation, the ethics committee started rounding on this case. The team met for honest, ethical meetings to discuss the complexity of Isaiah's case, and nursing offered the perspective that it felt morally distressing to allow this intervention to happen when the results do not change the inevitable result of death. The overseeing providers listened but did not back down, and nursing started to be uninvited to family meetings. This was explained to nursing as a parental choice, which possibly could have been the truth; however, it felt malicious toward nursing, who spends the most time at the bedside with Isaiah and knows him best. Ultimately, this created animosity between the doctors and Isaiah's nursing team, who felt helpless when it came to providing him the care he not only deserved but protecting him from being subjected to one last poke and prod. For nursing, caring for Isaiah felt isolating because most of the time it was just you and him, endless sedatives, and watching him cry. Doctors cannot be at the bedside since they have a plethora of patient responsibilities; therefore, in cases like this, it was frustrating to feel nurses were being undervalued for their role in care but not respected for their opinion. In spite of that, Isaiah would go to the catheterization lab, avoid ECMO cannulation, and continue on the same health trajectory, which led to his death not too soon after. I suppose now that it may have brought his family closure that they did everything for him and for the providers that they offered them all the options, but for me, I felt shattered for him and that he was subjected to one last invasive and painful procedure. It felt malevolent and unfair.

Patients such as Isaiah challenge your values as a nurse. They frustrate you because you feel like you are causing more harm than healing. Yet, who am I to claim to know what it feels like to watch their own child endure a life like Isaiah's? Celia exhibited a strength like no other mother I knew, and I believe, despite the pain and loss, that she did get a small piece of Isaiah that allowed her to truly feel like his mother without all of the CICU interference. Isaiah taught me humility and the importance of preserving yourself in this all-consuming and high-stress specialty, let alone the field of nursing. Humility aids you in practicing more empathy and compassion for all: the patient, the family, the team, and yourself. I would remind myself after a tough day that I could leave my work at the door, but for Celia, this was her baby, and this was her life. Despite this all, I recognize how my time at the bedside can be impactful for families, the patients, and myself. For Isaiah, it was the comforting banter with Celia that I would always do his curls for him during his evening bath, even when his hair started to fall out, or put on his special oil so that his skin wouldn't dry. Because of these moments, I can acknowledge that in this vulnerable space, we can still celebrate the small wins and milestones, maintain hope in the darkest hour, but, above all, recognize the power of offering self, making humility the most powerful tool in nursing. Humility would be nothing without vulnerability, and I put that at the center of everything I do in my practice. Although I felt at times this wavered, if Isaiah still were alive and required the same care today, I would be there for him, his mother, and their family without question. Because that is the essence of nursing.

"As We Watch Suffering, Our Distress Accumulates."

By Aaron Carpenter, DNP, MDiv, APRN, CPNP-PC, NEA-B, and Sarah E. Wawrzynski, PhD, RN, CCRN

We read and reflect on Iris's experience with compassion, empathy, and a shared clinical experience. Aaron currently serves as the chief nursing and patient operations officer of a freestanding level-one pediatric trauma center and quaternary referral hospital in the mid-Atlantic region, following a clinical career as a registered nurse and pediatric nurse practitioner in cardiac intensive care, pediatric emergency medicine, and pediatric primary care. Sarah is a nurse scientist and registered nurse with a clinical specialty in pediatric and cardiac intensive care. We have walked the proverbial mile in these shoes, and both of us share a passion for supporting and developing the next generations of nurses, realizing the challenges that face nurses in our ever-changing healthcare landscape. We have learned that listening to the stories of new nurses allows us to respond, with the best available evidence, in a way that builds our nurses up and provides safe places for them to fall when faced with moral distress and its inevitable and monumental impact. To Iris, we are so grateful for your courage and willingness to share your experience and for your willingness to bring this very difficult conversation to light.

Moral distress, burnout, and compassion fatigue are each unique concepts; however, they are closely tied to one another in nursing and healthcare literature and play upon each other creating a complexity of interrelated distress among nurses (Cherny et al., 2015). This is especially prevalent in new nurses entering acute and critical care settings such as the CICU, where high levels of moral distress and burnout have been reported in as many as 77% of nurses working in critical care (Giannetta et al., 2022; Matsuishi et al., 2021). As nurses, we experience moral distress when we believe we know what "should" or "could" be done to support a family but feel our hands are tied because of patient loads, system structures, policies, and perhaps the clinical inertia of "wait and see," which continues as days turn into weeks and the on-call team defers to the day team, who defers to next week's team.

As we watch suffering, our distress accumulates; we begin to protect ourselves by detaching from our patients and feeling a diminished sense of caring toward our patients, known as *compassion fatigue* (Cavanagh et al., 2019).

Further complicating our frustrations at work, beyond moral distress, are issues common in nursing that leads to burnout syndrome. *Burnout* is caused by limited resources and poor management, which leaves nurses feeling overloaded, detached, and disengaged (Cherny et al., 2015). Individually experiencing any one of these three factors can heighten our risk of developing another, perpetuating a cycle of distress that can lead some to abandon a career they once loved and were passionate about (Karakachian & Colbert, 2019; Matsuishi et al., 2021).

Iris's experience is shared by nurses in hospitals and healthcare facilities across the country. The motivating factors that drive us to the profession of nursing are noble and often closely aligned with personal values and belief systems. When those values and beliefs are challenged by deeply difficult ethical scenarios, the ensuing conflict between personal values and contradictory decision-making occurs, and nurses face moral distress. Atashzadeh-Shoorideh and colleagues (2021) identify that lack of institutional support, hierarchical power structures in health care, and legal and policy constraints contribute to moral distress in nursing. In their systematic review, they identified a shortage of nursing staff, nurses' inexperience in decision-making, lack of support from organizations and colleagues, and lack of educational classes as leading causes of moral distress. Added to these contributing factors for nurses is the critical role nurses play at the bedside, spending the longest periods of time in family interaction. In a mixed-methods study of a pediatric CICU team, Broden et al. (2024) explain that nurses' rating of the family experience of quality of death and dying (QODD) was lower than other team members, noting that, importantly, the time nurses spend with families and their forced position as intermediary between family and medical teams likely contribute to their lower rating of the QODD.

Communication or lack thereof is another important factor contributing to moral distress. As a CICU nurse herself, Sarah recalled a similar experience to the one Iris describes. An infant on her unit had severe hydrops fetalis and several cardiac diagnoses. She had been on continuous renal replacement therapy and high-dose pressors for weeks without improvement. It seemed clear that the infant wasn't going to survive; however, the communication regarding this fact was vague and put the decision of withdrawal in the parents' hands. The mother refused, and the team frustratedly left the room. Later, the nurse caring for the infant was changing drips and assessing the baby when the mom was tearful on the phone, saying that she felt it was a mortal sin to withdraw support for her child and describing her pain in watching her child suffer. The nurse was heartbroken that no one had explored this mother's feelings, beliefs, or goals and that she felt she was responsible for what was happening to her child. After the mother got off the call, the nurse asked if she would like the chaplain to come and sit with her or if she could contact the mother's priest. The mother took the nurse's hand and kissed them in the sincerest thank-you. After talking with the priest, there was a productive care conference during which the priest and parents asked the team questions and reached a place where they understood and accepted that the outcome was out of their hands. While the infant did not have the outcome that anyone hoped for, the nurse felt like she effectively advocated for her patient and embraced the privilege of caring for this family and their child at the end of her life.

Advocacy has been shown to remediate some of the distress nurses experience. Research has shown that when nurses feel that they have the autonomy to advocate for palliative care and see that families are getting honest and helpful communication, they are less distressed. Iris described what she felt was a loss of empowerment, which led to an erosion of respect between the nurses and the medical team. Communication is a simple yet delicate skill that can both help and harm in these complex situations. Many issues, such as cultural beliefs, competing priorities, and timing, may clash or not be fully explored. This can lead to distrust, resentment, and poor resolution of the problems that present and need to be addressed by both families and the healthcare team (Dill & Gumpert, 2012; Kwame & Petrucka, 2021).

We receive fulfillment in our jobs as nurses when we can adequately meet the needs of the patients for whom we care (van Diepen et al., 2020). At the bedside, nurses become intimately familiar with the needs and emotions of the parents and families for whom they care. Nurses can become distressed when they sense that the care provided is not meeting their patients' needs due to hectic assignments, unresolved plans of care, or not preparing families for the challenges that may lie ahead of them. When we listen, speak, and question, our teams can come to a shared mental model. We can better understand and ensure that we keep the family and their needs centered in our care. This can reduce distress among all parties and provide a common goal. This type of communication is a skill that takes practice and courage but that can help us effectively advocate for ourselves and our patients in addition to bringing a sense of meaning into our work.

Distressing feelings at work can become entangled and associated with the job or the institution, leading us to seek greener pastures. It is critically important to explore the feelings we have regarding our patients and our distress. If we begin to pull the threads of distress apart, we are likely to identify specific issues that can be addressed and changed. In this process, we need to show ourselves and others grace. Iris recounted how she saw racism and judgment seep into staff conversations, which likely influenced Isaiah's care. However, she was also able to recognize the limitations of her own understanding. Nurses have the opportunity to serve vastly different people every day, and sometimes our beliefs will be in contrast with those of our patients. One study of clinicians demonstrated that mindfulness improved patient-centered care and fostered a less judgmental attitude (Dobkin et al., 2016). If we believe we know best, we limit our ability to understand and connect with others. This also limits our ability to advocate effectively for our patients. Ultimately, care that aligns with the patient and families' values can lead to greater satisfaction, reduce trauma and secondary trauma, and increase trust, healing, and post-traumatic growth (Dill & Gumpert, 2012; Stewart & Ryan, 2024). As nurses, we can develop resilience and deepened compassion for our patients as we cultivate the skills that promote mindfulness and cultural humility.

While the contributing factors of moral distress in nurses can seem overwhelming and acutely threatening to the profession, these data are encouraging as they identify actionable interventions nurse leaders can implement to decrease the burden of moral distress on new nurses. Nurse leaders and professional governance structures are key change agents who, when appropriately empowered, can improve the experience and satisfaction of nurses in difficult practice environments. Adequate staffing for safe care delivery must be nonnegotiable. When rounding with our bedside teams, we hear this concern. In the most recently published Health Resources and Services Administration *National Sample Survey of Registered Nurses* (2024), burnout and inadequate staffing were identified as the top two most commonly cited reasons for nurses leaving their primary nursing positions. Creating systems, structures, and processes that support the recruitment and retention of nursing staff, thereby stabilizing the nursing workforce and maintaining appropriate staffing levels, can contribute to decreasing moral distress experienced by bedside nurses. Much focus has been directed toward the nursing workforce and the national efforts to stabilize the pipeline. Nursing has a history of ebb and flow with nursing workforce supply and demand, most recently disturbed by the COVID-19 pandemic. In 2021, 100,000 registered nurses (RNs) left the workforce, many more than were predicted for that year. While that statistic is troubling, we can find hope in the fact that by the end of 2022, data suggested that the workforce had restored itself and that the replacement of retiring RNs and the new positions required for maintaining the workforce through 2035 looks favorable (Buerhaus et al., 2023). Encouraging as this may be, contributing factors to moral injury and distress must be addressed through a partnership between nurse leaders, professional governance teams, and the nursing workforce.

Recognizing the impacts of burnout and moral distress and the effect of the hospital environment on nurse well-being, the American Association of Critical Care Nurses (AACN) launched the Healthy Work Environment (HWE) initiative in early 2024. The HWE initiative is an innovative program that allows a two-year collaboration with interprofessional team members that focuses on quality improvement initiatives, retention, and outcomes (https://www.aacn.org). Peers and coworkers can also play important roles in both supporting us or perpetuating our distress. Identify like-minded coworkers whom you can talk with, debrief, and problem-solve with. Engaging and participating in initiatives such as the HWE is another tool nurse leaders can use to support their teams, improve the experience of bedside nurses, and improve patient outcomes.

> If we could change ourselves, the tendencies in the world would
> also change. As a man changes his own nature, so does the
> world's attitude change towards him. This is the divine mystery
> supreme. A wonderful thing it is and the source of our happi-
> ness. We need not wait to see what others do.
>
> —Mahatma Gandhi

The Nurses' Commitments Need to Be to the Patient Without Assumption. Period.

By Linda Roney, EdD, RN-BC, CPEN, CNE, FAAN

Reading Iris's story, I am grateful for her generosity in sharing this devasting and complex case of her care for Isaiah and the support and wisdom Aaron and Sarah offer through their knowledge and personal experiences. Most nurses have had their hearts broken early in their careers by the overwhelmingly complex challenges of caring for patients like Isaiah, who teaches us to be nurses, and family members like Celia, who trust us with their care. *"Jeremy"* and *"Janessa"* taught me early lessons about how to be a nurse and helped me discover what holistic care means and how to find my voice as a new grad who needed to advocate for the complex needs of my patients in the face of ethical issues.

Table 9.1 outlines Iris' specific actions demonstrating competency in the AACN essentials' (2021) domains 2 and 10 competencies and subcompetencies.

Ethics in Health Care

Since 1992, through its *Comprehensive Accreditation Manuals*, The Joint Commission has required hospitals to provide ethics education and a way to address ethical issues in patient care (Aaron et al., 2022). Each healthcare organization has its process to activate or consult the ethics committee, so ask your preceptor or manager how this is activated in your hospital. Most hospital ethics committees provide staff with educational resources about making ethical decisions, develop policies, and provide case consultations (DiNova, 2020). Some organizations will accept invitations to consult from patients, family members, and any healthcare team member (University of North Carolina [UNC] Health, 2024). A clinical ethics committee may have clinical and nonclinical areas to maintain the principles of autonomy, justice, beneficence, nonmaleficence, confidentiality, and honesty (Mehta et al., 2023). Ethics committees typically do not honor emergency requests, and the process takes time, so it is essential to start the consultation early (UNC Health, 2024). Committees average between 12 and 16 members,

TABLE 9.1 **Examples of Domain 2: Person-Centered Care and Domain 10: Personal, Professional, and Leadership Development in This Exemplar**

Domain 2: Person-Centered Care	
2.1 Engage with the individual in establishing a caring relationship.	Iris clearly demonstrated empathy for her patient and his family, using strategies for mutual respect to deliver compassionate developmentally appropriate care in a critical care setting.
2.2 Communicate effectively with individuals.	Iris demonstrated relationship-centered care with Isiah and his family. She considered their values as individuals and as a family to give them the information in a timely way, when it counted the most, using multiple communication modes.
2.3 Integrate assessment skills in practice.	Iris used her nursing knowledge to gain holistic perspective to caring for this critically ill infant.
Domain 10: Personal, Professional, and Leadership Development	
10.2 Demonstrate a spirit of inquiry that fosters flexibility and professional maturity.	Iris embraced principles of diversity, equity, inclusion, and antidiscrimination. She was reflective about her own practice.
10.3 Develop capacity for leadership.	Iris demonstrated leadership behaviors in all the challenges she faced while working with Isiah.

represent a diverse range of viewpoints, and typically include physicians, nurses, social workers, hospital administrators, clergy, and trained ethicists (DiNova, 2020).

In at least two cases in this casebook, it was noted that nurses were excluded from the ethics consults with their patients. Because we do not have all of the details of the cases from all sources, it is impossible to know what each organization's policy was and if nursing was represented on the formal ethics committee. When the clinical provider team does not hear nurses' concerns, the nurse should always go to their manager for guidance and support. These issues, especially when organ transplantation and groundbreaking and potentially experimental interventions are offered, are incredibly complex and outside of the scope of a new graduate to navigate. One resource for those who want to read more about this area is the Organ Procurement and Transplantation Network (OPTN) Ethics Committee (2024) White Papers (OPTN, 2024).

The ANA (2015) developed the *Code of Ethics With Interpretative Statements* to establish an ethical standard for nurses to use as a guide in ethical analysis and decision-making. The code of ethics is divided into nine provisions to guide nurses with ethical issues (ANA, 2015). Let's consider some of the case details Iris shares based on these critical principles.

Provision 1: The nurse practices with compassion and respect for the inherent dignity, worth, and unique attributes of every person (ANA, 2015).

The patient, their family members, and every healthcare team member deserve high respect and compassion. The nursing staff shifted to a point where they did not feel their opinions were respected by the surgical team, which affected their interactions with Ceila. Some nurses demonstrated a lack of respect for Ceila and her family's strong desire for Isiah to survive and attributed it to the family wanting to stay in the United States. Talking among each other in these ways could only negatively affect their approach to Isiah and his family.

Provision 2: The nurse's primary commitment is to the patient, whether an individual, family, group, community, or population (ANA, 2015).

The nurses' commitments needed to be to Isiah and his family and not make any assumptions about his family. Period.

Provision 3: The nurse promotes, advocates for, and protects the rights, health, and safety of the patients (ANA, 2015).

The details in the story show that the nurses provided outstanding, technically challenging, and heroic nursing care for this patient. Very high standards must be met to care for a patient with this high level of acuity.

Provision 4: The nurse has authority, accountability, and responsibility for nursing practice, makes decisions, and takes action consistent with the obligation to provide optimal patient care (ANA, 2015).

The nurse ensures that care is well thought out and ethical concerns are addressed. The following questions might help a nurse determine whether they are facing an ethical issue (Trillium Health Partners, 2013, p. 4):

- Am I trying to determine the right course of action?
- Am I asking a "should" question?
- Are values and beliefs involved?
- Am I feeling uncomfortable?

The nurse should follow the organization's protocols for obtaining an ethics consultation.

Provision 5: The nurse owes the same duties to self as to others, including the responsibility to promote health and safety, preserve wholeness of character and integrity, maintain competence, and continue personal and professional growth (ANA, 2015).

In this case, the nurses had a high regard for patient care and professional development when working in a clinically challenging area. It is unclear what the organization did to promote self-care in this intense patient care area.

Did nurses receive regularly scheduled breaks? Was their schedule optimized for health and work-life balance?

Provision 6: The nurse, through individual and collective effort, establishes, maintains, and improves the ethical environment of the work setting and conditions of employment that are conducive to safe, quality health care (ANA, 2015).

While the nurses seemed to provide nursing care for these complex patients in a way that complemented the surgical and medical innovations in care, no discussion, education, or exchange of ideas about ethics among team members was mentioned. While this may have happened and Iris was unaware, it was clear that the nursing and medical team did not have an aligned vision and goals. This also occurs in Chapter 11 with Grace. Broden et al. (2024) found that because nurses spend prolonged periods at the bedside, they develop a "proximate lens into patients' and families' experiences" (p. 138). Perceptions of suffering may shift in the context of dynamic goals of care that may differ between families and clinical team members (Broden et al., 2024, p. 133).

Provision 7: The nurse, in all roles and settings, advances the profession through research and scholarly inquiry, professional standards development, and the generation of both nursing and health policy (ANA, 2015).

The nurses likely received education on the principles of ethics in their pre-licensure program, and professional organization membership was likely promoted at this organization. This likely supported the high level of clinical nursing care provided.

Provision 8: The nurse collaborates with other health professionals and the public to protect human rights, promote health diplomacy, and reduce health disparities (ANA, 2015).

Iris and her nursing colleagues found every opportunity to promote Isiah's growth and development with normalcy in a highly unusual setting, which should be recognized. The nurses tried to advocate for the clinical needs of the patient, but some of the nurses failed at holistic patient advocacy when they questioned the mother's motivation for seeking advanced care for her child. Racism contributes to ongoing health disparities and is a violation of fundamental human rights.

Provision 9: The profession of nursing, collectively through its professional organization, must articulate nursing values, maintain the profession's integrity, and integrate principles of social justice into nursing and health policy (ANA, 2015).

Nurses must advocate for social justice in all settings and incorporate these values into our profession. Iris' courage in sharing this story with us to learn from is a high-level example of this provision. In Chapter 10, we will reflect more deeply on discrimination in health care and discuss strategies you can implement in your practice when encountering racism and microaggressions in the healthcare setting.

YOU MATTER: WHEN OUR PATIENTS NEED US THE MOST

This chapter has focused on providing holistic, patient-and-family–centered, ethical care. This work weighs heavily on us, and we should prioritize strategies to ensure that we adhere to Provision 5 to promote our health and safety and preserve the wholeness of our character and integrity. While self-care has been mentioned throughout this casebook, we will focus on it in Chapter 12.

Book Club Questions

1. How would you respond to your coworker's comments about Celia? If you say something, when would be the best time? After you read Chapter 10, can you apply any suggested scripting?
2. Have you seen experienced nurses feel unheard by the rest of the medical team? What did they do? What of their actions feels authentic to you if you are ever in the same situation?

About This Chapter's Authors

Iris Johnson, BSN, RN

Iris was born and raised in Bridgewater, Massachusetts. She received her bachelor's degree from Fairfield University's Marion Peckham Egan School of Nursing and Health Studies in 2021. Following graduation, Iris began her nursing career in Boston on a pediatric CICU. There, she often precepted and fulfilled the role of continuity care nurse for chronic patients. After two-and-a-half years, she transitioned her nursing career to a labor and delivery unit outside of Boston and now is a Doctor of Nursing Practice (DNP) student studying midwifery. Outside of work, Iris enjoys exploring new restaurants, spending time with friends, trying different workouts, and going to the beach on warmer days.

Aaron Carpenter, DNP, MDiv, APRN, CPNP-PC, NEA-B

Aaron joined Nemours Children's Health in 2016 and currently serves as the senior vice president, chief nursing, and patient operations officer for the Delaware Valley. He has worked as an RN in adult cardiac critical care and general and academic pediatric emergency nursing. As a pediatric nurse practitioner, he has practiced in primary care and pediatric emergency medicine for more than 20 years. Dr. Carpenter is board certified in pediatrics through the Pediatric Nursing Certification Board and in executive nursing leadership through the American Nurses Credentialing Center.

Aaron's primary academic interest is in building confidence and competence in novice advanced practice providers. He is the founder and director of the Nemours pediatric primary care nurse practitioner fellowship, the first in a freestanding children's hospital. During his tenure at Nemours, he led the restructuring of advanced practice leadership and the growth of that team and supported the development of a professional advancement program for advanced practice providers and the creation of the Nemours Center for Advanced Practice.

Aaron earned a bachelor's degree from Sacred Heart University, a master's degree from Yale University, a Master of Divinity degree from Trinity School for Ministry, and a DNP from Robert Morris University. He is passionate about developing leaders in children's health and connecting clinicians with opportunities to advance in their careers.

Sarah E. Wawrzynski, PhD, RN, CCRN

Sarah is an assistant nurse scientist in the Center for Healthcare Delivery Science and co-director of nursing research at Nemours Children's Health in Delaware. Her current research is focused on the socioecological factors that influence family members' adjustment and management of pediatric chronic and life-limiting disease. Her interest in this area is informed by her experience caring for medically fragile children and their families in pediatric ICUs and CICUs for many years. Her goals as a nurse scientist are to identify equitable and culturally sensitive ways to support families managing pediatric illness over its varied trajectories and empower nurses to use their expertise and passion to drive change in health care.

References

Aaron, B., Crites, J. S., Cunningham, T. V., Mishra, R., & Lesandrini, J. (2022). Hospital Ethics Practices: Recommendations for Improving Joint Commission Standards. *Joint Commission journal on quality and patient safety, 48*(12), 682–685. https://doi.org/10.1016/j.jcjq.2022.09.004

American Nurses Association. (2015). *Code of ethics with interpretative statements.* https://www.nursingworld.org/practice-policy/nursing-excellence/ethics/code-of-ethics-for-nurses/coe-view-only/

Atashzadeh-Shoorideh, F., Tayyar-Iravanlou, F., Chashmi, Z. A., Abdi, F., & Cisic, R. S. (2021). Factors affecting moral distress in nurses working in intensive care units: A systematic review. Clinical Ethics, 16(1), 25-36.

Broden, E. G., Bailey, V. K., Beke, D. M., Snaman, J. M., & Moynihan, K. M. (2024). Dying and Death in a Pediatric Cardiac ICU: Mixed Methods Evaluation of Multi-disciplinary Staff Responses. Pediatr Crit Care Med, *25*(2), e91-e102. https://doi.org/10.1097/pcc.0000000000003357

Buerhaus, P., Fraher, E., Frogner, B., Buntin, M., O'Reilly-Jacob, M., & Clarke, S. (2023). Toward a stronger post-pandemic nursing workforce. *New England Journal of Medicine*, *389*(3), 200-202.

Cavanagh, N., Cockett, G., Heinrich, C., Doig, L., Fiest, K., Guichon, J. R., Page, S., Mitchell, I., & Doig, C. J. (2019). Compassion fatigue in healthcare providers: A systematic review and meta-analysis. *Nursing Ethics*, *27*(3), 639-665. https://doi.org/10.1177/0969733019889400

Cherny, N. I., Werman, B., & Kearney, M. (2015). Burnout, compassion fatigue, and moral distress in palliative care. *Oxford textbook of palliative medicine*, *5*(1), 246-259. https://books.google.com/books?hl=en&lr=&id=ruCrBwAAQBAJ&oi=fnd&pg=PA246&d-q=Burnout,+compassion+fatigue,+and+moral+distress+in+palliative+care&ots=-JaEf-5xhKr&sig=XsRPG_pPD0XYgapzzau0IYBChRw#v=onepage&q=Burnout%2C%20compassion%20fatigue%2C%20and%20moral%20distress%20in%20palliative%20care&f=false

Dill, D., & Gumpert, P. (2012). What is the heart of health care? Advocating for and defining the clinical relationship in patient-centered care. *Journal of Participatory Medicine*, *4*(1).

DiNova, C.R. (2020). Hospital ethics committees. *Albany Law School Government Law Center.*

Dobkin, P. L., Bernardi, N. F., & Bagnis, C. I. (2016). Enhancing Clinicians' Well-Being and Patient-Centered Care Through Mindfulness. *Journal of Continuing Education in the Health Professions*, *36*(1). https://journals.lww.com/jcehp/fulltext/2016/03610/enhancing_clinicians__well_being_and.3.aspx

Giannetta, N., Villa, G., Bonetti, L., Dionisi, S., Pozza, A., Rolandi, S., Rosa, D., & Manara, D. F. (2022). Moral Distress Scores of Nurses Working in Intensive Care Units for Adults Using Corley's Scale: A Systematic Review. *Int J Environ Res Public Health*, *19*(17). https://doi.org/10.3390/ijerph191710640

Health Resourses and Services Administration. (2024). 2022 National Sample Survey of Registered Nurses Snapshot. https://bhw.hrsa.gov/sites/default/files/bureau-health-workforce/Nurse-Survey-Fact-Sheet-2024.pdf

Karakachian, A., & Colbert, A. (2019). Nurses' moral distress, burnout, and intentions to leave: an integrative review. *Journal of Forensic Nursing*, *15*(3), 133-142.

Kwame, A., & Petrucka, P. M. (2021). A literature-based study of patient-centered care and communication in nurse-patient interactions: barriers, facilitators, and the way forward. *BMC Nursing*, *20*(1), 158. https://doi.org/10.1186/s12912-021-00684-2

Matsuishi, Y., Okubo, N., Mathis, B. J., Masuzawa, Y., Shimojo, N., Enomoto, Y., Inoue, Y., & Hoshino, H. (2021). Severity and prevalence of burnout syndrome in paediatric intensive care nurses: A systematic review. *Intensive & Critical Care Nursing*, *67*, 103082. https://doi.org/10.1016/j.iccn.2021.103082

Mehta, P., Zimba, O., Gasparyan, A. Y., Seiil, B., & Yessirkepov, M. (2023). Ethics committees: Structure, roles, and issues. *Journal of Korean Medical Science, 38*(25), e198. https://doi.org/10.3346/jkms.2023.38.e198

Organ Procurement & Transplantation Network. (2024). *Ethical considerations.* https://optn.transplant.hrsa.gov/professionals/by-topic/ethical-considerations/

Stewart, M., & Ryan, B. L. (2024). Evidence of the Impact of Patient-Centered Care on Clinician Well-Being and Patient Outcomes. In *Patient-Centered Medicine* (pp. 300-309). CRC Press.

Trillium Health Partners. (2013). *IDEA: Ethical decision making framework.* https://trilliumhealthpartners.ca/aboutus/Documents/IDEA-Framework-THP.pdf

University of North Carolina Health. (2024). *Hospital ethics committee.* https://www.unc-medicalcenter.org/uncmc/patients-visitors/hospital-ethics-committee/

van Diepen, C., Fors, A., Ekman, I., & Hensing, G. (2020). Association between person-centred care and healthcare providers' job satisfaction and work-related health: a scoping review. *BMJ open, 10*(12), e042658. https://bmjopen.bmj.com/content/bmjopen/10/12/e042658.full.pdf

CHAPTER 10

From Silence to Action

Finding Your Voice as a Patient Advocate

Janeá Butler, MSN, RN, CMSRN; Laura Conklin, MSN, RN; Danielle Hall, DNP, RN; and Linda Roney, EdD, RN-BC, CPEN, CNE, FAAN

Learning Goals

1. Analyze how patients can be marginalized within the healthcare system and propose strategies nurses can implement to advocate for and support patients.
2. Experiment with the Team Strategies and Tools to Enhance Performance and Patient Safety (TeamSTEPPS®) of Situation, Background, Assessment, and Recommendation (SBAR); closed-loop communication; huddles; and shared mental models to improve the quality of patient care.
3. Evaluate communication tools to address racism and microaggressions in health care.

'I Used to Be Her ...'

By Janeá Butler, MSN, RN, CMSRN

I have faced a lot of adversity in my life, so I advocate for injustices for all people. I stand up for things I do not feel are right because we all have a place on this earth, and we all deserve to be heard and seen. In nursing school, I was in the minority. I was one of three people of color in most nursing classes. It was hard to navigate my way without feeling like I was receiving a handout. For the first two semesters of undergrad, I kept to myself, afraid to ask for help for fear of being seen as underserved. Nursing school was hard, and I failed tests and classes because I did not ask questions.

I did not know how to be my advocate. I grew up with the principle of "What happens in this house *stays in this house.*" My parents did not go to college, and I did not have someone to help me navigate through what I needed to know to survive undergrad. Although I knew they loved me and were happy with my decision, I often felt alone because I did not have a support system. During my college career, I worked three jobs. I did not come from money. It was not until I got to college that I realized that I was poor. I had two jobs on campus and one off campus on the weekends. I did enter college with a scholarship, but that did not cover room and board, so I became a resident assistant to help cut that cost. I am no stranger to hard work and dedication. I put my best foot forward in everything I put my mind to.

Fast-forward to after my graduation from nursing school. I have worked in some of the best medical centers in the country, been recognized for my excellence at work, and been promoted to a supervisor position. I care deeply for all my patients, but let me tell you about one whom I still think about to this day. She could not advocate for herself. My duty was to be her nurse and advocate from the moment I met her. I treat all my patients with the best care I can give. It hurts me to think. *What if it was not me on that night? What if she did not get what she deserved?* Knowing how hard it is to show fear and pain, I related to her so much because *I used to be her.*

My shift begins at 19:00; I work the night shift on a medical-surgical unit. Our unit holds approximately 40 beds. This was the first shift of my four-day stretch, and I felt refreshed and ready to take on the night's duties. The nurse who gave me the report was relatively new, and I had been a nurse for just over three years. She had been off orientation for some months now and was still trying to get her bearings when it came to giving a solid report. Even though I knew that I had a busy night ahead of me, I was very patient with her as I had been in her shoes not very long ago. While she was giving me report, I knew immediately that something needed to be done for one of our patients. The previous nurses had notified the medical team about the decline in the health of one of the patients over the past few shifts. The nurse giving me report passed this on and told me that doctors did not share the same impression that nursing had about the patient's condition. I heard the frustration in her voice, and I could see in her eyes how worried she was that her concerns were not being heard; I felt that she needed a few minutes to vent. I let her do so, and we then continued with report. She told me that this was her third day with this patient and that she had persistently contacted the shift attending physician with her concerns. When she was not heard, the nurse got her nurse manager involved to advocate for this patient as she needed a higher level of care than she was receiving.

This patient had been admitted several weeks ago with hematemesis, fevers, and chest pain. She was a healthy 40-year-old woman with no other comorbidities. After extensive testing, our patient was diagnosed with tuberculosis (TB). While I had never taken care of her, I was generally aware of her through my role as a charge nurse. The week before, I knew that previous nurses had contacted providers on multiple occasions about the patient becoming tachycardic to the 130s–140s. The physician ordered boluses to treat tachycardia. The patient responded to the fluids, and the tachycardia resolved briefly. The nurses contacted the provider about increased temperatures, and acetaminophen was ordered. Two weeks before tonight, the nurses called a rapid response on this same patient due to persistent tachycardia. No additional tests or interventions were added to the patient's care during the rapid response, and the medical team felt she did not need to be transferred to a higher level of care. However, on this particular night, she was *my patient.* I felt in my heart that there was something far worse going on than a bolus of intravenous (IV) fluids and acetaminophen could handle.

In my three-plus years, I have cared for countless patients with different responses to many disease processes, and I have a good grasp of what type of care falls within the scope of practice on our unit. When we are full on this unit, we are very busy. We can go up to caring for six patients, sometimes seven, and our charge nurse cares for up to four hallway patients in crisis. This was one of those busy nights, and as I approached the patient, I could see the patient sweating profusely, shaking, and cool to the touch. She tried to give me a small smile, like one of gratitude that I was there because she could not communicate with me. Using the teleinterpreter who did not speak the exact dialect of the patient's language, I tried to gather the information I needed for my assessment. On the Masimo (monitor), I could see her heart rate was in the 140s, and when I checked her temperature, I saw that she was febrile. I quickly notified the provider of the patient's condition and administered the ordered acetaminophen and fluids as ordered. An hour went by, and the fever and tachycardia did not cease. After a few hours, the patient's heart rate jumped to the 180s–190s. I knew that it was time to call a rapid response.

All the providers came to the bedside quickly, and the first thing that came out of the hospitalist's mouth after I summarized the patient's condition was *"WHY IS THIS PATIENT STILL ON THIS FLOOR?"* These words hit me like a knife. At this moment, I felt like everything we had advocated for this patient had gone unheard. The team had failed to see the big picture for several days and had just responded to symptoms. Without looking for the reason, this was happening. I felt that we had failed this patient and her family. Every nurse was taught to advocate for themselves, their patients, and their colleagues in nursing school. And while we felt like we tried to do our best, things did not improve for this patient. As we were moving the patient to the intensive care unit (ICU), I overheard the hospitalist tell the ICU team that the patient must be intubated when they got to the unit. *What was going on?* I had no idea what they were thinking. They did not share their thoughts with me, and I almost felt like we were not on the same team despite all the nurses' concerns for this patient. I also felt like my heart broke into two as I thought about this mother and her children. I could not help but think about how her daughter had not seen her mom in weeks due to her diagnosis, and now it was going to be longer until they were reunited. Could we have prevented this from happening? I wondered what would have happened if it was not me as her nurse tonight or if I did not trust my gut and advocate for her. Would she have made it through the night?

'Speak Up!'

By Laura Conklin, MSN, RN, and Danielle Hall, DNP, RN

Facing adversity can have lasting effects on an individual. Adversities affect the resilience and well-being of individuals and communities and are followed by elevated levels of distress symptoms (Kimhi et al., 2022). Janeá has illustrated her strength through many challenges and vulnerable situations. As an underrepresented student in nursing at a private university, it was difficult for her to speak up for herself and advocate for her needs. The literature supports that the inability to find their voice also translates to new-graduate nurses (NGNs) beginning practice and navigating from novice to beginner nurses. In an article by Nakatani et al. (2024), a questionnaire survey provided results demonstrating that junior doctors and nurses showed low positive responses to "prompt information sharing," "two-challenge rule," "SBAR," "monitoring and consultation," "check back," and "attitudes toward listening," indicating that they have "perceived barriers to speaking up" and have "negative attitudes toward voicing opinions in the healthcare team" (p. 6).

As seasoned faculty and clinical instructors, we would like to point out Janeá's sentiments about being unable to ask for help. She voiced her fear of not being able to ask questions. *Ask questions!* As a student and nurse, I know that learning is lifelong, so continually ask questions. The question one person asks is usually one that many are wondering about. Hearing that a student suffered silently instead of seeking help is disheartening. Our responsibility and commitment as faculty is to aid our students' academic success. Understanding circumstances and struggles makes it easier for us to be involved and advocate for support on behalf of our students. Many times when a student has approached us with concerns, we guide them with compassion and reach out to resources that may aid in the current situation. It is important to be able to reach out and advocate for needs. Faculty may often be unaware of a student's stressors and struggles. Whether it is emotional stress, such as depression or anxiety, financial challenges, or even just situational circumstances, perhaps with roommates, there is always an ear to be listened to and a path to refer you to find solutions. As you transition to your new-graduate position, the same can be said about asking for your supervisor's guidance or support. "When employees do not speak up about problems, organizations miss opportunities for improvement and learning" (Etchegaray et al., 2020, p. e230). As Janeá stated, she felt afraid to ask for help because she felt she should navigate this alone. All nurses and soon-to-be nurses deserve attention, direction, and guidance to find support for their emotional, physical, or educational needs to help them be the best nurses they can be.

In addition to not feeling able to advocate for her needs in nursing school, Janeá also experienced a lack of feeling unsupported by those close to her because they did not fully understand the extent of her needs. She stayed to herself yet could not have been the only one experiencing these emotions. Speaking up and saying, *"I need some help,"* is not easy, especially if you already feel marginalized. However, it is important to realize that when you feel alone, many more may feel the same and can unite and support each other. Some things in our daily lives, such as social media use, make this less possible. Despite your numerous followers, you may feel you must face your struggles alone (Gill, 2021). There is such power in authentic, in-person human communication. While we know this as nurses, we can forget this in our personal lives.

Janeá persevered throughout the nursing program while working multiple jobs and has already found great success early in her nursing career, which is a feat that is not easily done. While she could not advocate her need for support earlier in nursing school through her mentors, she eventually found her voice and learned to advocate for herself. Her hard work on her personal development was highlighted in her transition into nursing, as she was frequently recognized for her excellent work and promoted by her supervisors. Her determination and resilience in facing challenges facilitated her success as the nurse she has become.

The story she shares with us illustrates advocacy for the patient who could not speak up for herself, and Janeá needed to find a way to help when so many of her colleagues had been unsuccessful in their attempts. While Janeá developed these skills as she progressed through nursing school, they continued to flourish as she became a nurse with the voice and commitment to speak up for her patients.

As a new nurse, you must be able to advocate for yourself to achieve success and learn to advocate for your patient's experience. *Speaking up* refers to "the raising of concerns by healthcare professionals for the benefit of patient safety and care quality upon recognizing or becoming aware of risky or deficient actions of others within healthcare teams" (Etchegaray et al., 2020, p. e230). Often new nurses lack the confidence to speak up. With encouragement and support, they can find their voices to raise concern about a patient, especially when the gravity of the situation has been overlooked or downplayed by others. Janeá had the confidence to speak up and advocate for a patient who could not do so themselves based on her experiences and feelings. *"I used to be her."* The courage and strength in these words cannot be overstated.

Nurses care for patients who are often very different from them, yet they aspire to provide holistic care. Some of these differences are due to patients' illness, personality, socioeconomic class, education, or cultural differences (Galanti, 2020). The life experiences of Janeá and her patient were very different. However, Janeá put herself in the position to draw empathy from her past and use it to empower her to bridge the gap and advocate for her patients. Janeá demonstrates a growth mindset, noting that her ability was acquired through her hard work and effort and that failure, as she presents it to us in this case, is an opportunity for learning and improvement (Theard et al., 2021). Later in this chapter, we will discuss this perspective and its application in our work with patients.

The transition from nursing student to registered nurse (RN) is exciting but stressful. NGNs may face unexpected obstacles as they begin their first nursing job. The environment and culture of the current healthcare setting can be overwhelming. An NGN must be able to take the experience from the classroom and school clinicals and apply their knowledge and critical thinking to the bedside as an independent practitioner (Alharbi & Alzahrani, 2023). There are numerous roles nurses must fulfill in order to have a positive and profound impact on patient care.

Janeá discloses her story of sharing a clinical assessment with her physician colleagues while feeling like her concerns were not heard or addressed. The inability of healthcare disciplines to communicate effectively leads to unintended consequences, referred to as *sentinel events* in the acute care setting (The Joint Commission [TJC], 2023). TJC defines a *sentinel event* as a patient safety event that results in death, permanent harm, or severe temporary harm. Communication failures cause more than 65% of sentinel events (Guttman et al., 2021, p. e1465). Nurses spend most of their work time at the bedside and provide powerful and vital information to help improve patient outcomes.

Unfortunately, there are times when nurses have learned to be cautious when speaking up in the clinical environment. Janeá mentioned that multiple previous nurses voiced their concerns and frustrations to her as the oncoming nurse because they were not making progress with the medical team. Nurses encounter this frequently in the acute care setting. A history and culture of physicians being considered higher in the chain of command has made some nurses feel they have less power than their physician colleagues (Schwappach & Richard, 2018). Subsequently, this can make nurses feel less empowered and sometimes inhibited from speaking up, even regarding safety. In Janeá's story, she and her nurse counterparts experienced this. Even though both nurses had addressed their concerns about the patient's condition, no interventions were initiated, eventually leading to unnecessary complications for their patient.

Throughout this casebook, we continue our conversation about Team-STEPPS®, the evidence-based tools that can be used by anyone who wants to improve communication and teamwork in health care (American Hospital Association [AHA], 2024b). Four tools—Situation, Background, Assessment, and Recommendation (SBAR); closed-loop communication; huddles; and shared mental models—provide a template for communication in the healthcare setting. Standardized language and predictable communication structures enable effective team communication (Armstrong, 2019). Janeá shared with us how she felt unheard when the doctor stated, *"Why is this patient still on this floor?"* Let us apply these four TeamSTEPPS tools (AHA, 2024b) to this case to consider how they could have affected the situation.

Situation, Background, Assessment, and Recommendation (SBAR)

In the case, Janeá shares that while receiving the report, the nurse expressed her frustration that she did not feel heard by the medical team. While Janeá was peripherally aware of some of the longstanding issues for this patient, had the nurse provided the report in the SBAR format (AHA, 2024b), Janeá might have received additional information that would have been helpful to set her up for success at the beginning of her shift. SBAR is a structured communication tool that conveys the Situation, Background, Assessment, and Recommendation between healthcare providers. Studies have shown that this deliberate communication method among healthcare providers can reduce the incidence of adverse events in hospital settings. The SBAR communication method is beneficial during critical events such as patient deterioration (Murphy et al., 2022).

TeamSTEPPS TIP

SBAR is most effective when communicating critical information concerning a patient's condition or another issue that affects the team and requires immediate attention and action.

Source: AHA, 2024b.

AN EXAMPLE OF AN EMPOWERING SBAR AT CHANGE OF SHIFT

An example of report that might have empowered Janeá at the beginning of this shift might have been as follows:

Situation: The patient had a heart rate in the 140s and was febrile, sweating profusely, shaking, and cool to the touch.

Background: A 40-year-old patient was admitted several weeks ago with hematemesis, fevers, and chest pain; she was diagnosed with TB.

Assessment: The patient continued to be tachycardic, and IV fluid boluses were not improving the patient's condition.

Recommendation: The physician came to the bedside to evaluate the patient and consider transfer to a higher level of care.

As Janeá and her nursing colleagues wanted to advocate for their patients, they were able to use resources to gain support in this situation. The nurses first used their nurse manager. Nurses report that supportive leadership helps cultivate a positive work environment, which enhances nursing practice and improves the quality of care provided (Stavropoulou et al., 2022). From the details in this case, it is unclear whether the nurses provided their manager with their recommendation as part of the SBAR or what challenges they faced when they tried to take action for the patient.

Closed-Loop Communication

In closed-loop communication, the person receiving instruction or information repeats a message to ensure that it is understood correctly, and the sender confirms in order to *close the loop* (AHA, 2024b). This communication method can help ensure that information is being relayed and received correctly for carrying out. Three strategies for closed-loop communication include call-outs, check-backs, and teach-backs (AHA, 2024b). *Call-outs* communicate essential information to all team members during a situation, help team members anticipate the next steps, and direct responsibility by name to a person required to complete the task (AHA, 2024b).

A *check-back* verifies and validates the information exchanged; the sender initiates a message, the receiver accepts the message and confirms what was communicated, and the sender verifies that the message was received (AHA, 2024b).

A *teach-back* confirms that the sender has explained information clearly and that patients, family members, or caregivers have a shared understanding of what the sender has told them by conveying their understanding in their own words (AHA, 2024b).

TeamSTEPPS TIP

In closed-loop communication, the person receiving information repeats it back to make sure the message is understood correctly, and the sender confirms to close the loop. This procedure typically saves time and ensures safety.

Source: AHA, 2024b.

We do not have the details of all the conversations between the nurses and the providers on the unit for this example Janeá shared with us. An example of how closed-loop communication, specifically a check-back, could have been implemented in Janeá's situation would be as follows:

Sender (Provider): I have entered an order in the electronic health record (EHR) for you to administer a bolus of IV fluids and acetaminophen 650 mg by mouth once for the patient's tachycardia and fever.

Receiver (Nurse): You entered an order in the EHR for me to administer a bolus of IV fluids and acetaminophen 650 mg by mouth once for the patient's tachycardia and fever. Is that correct?

Sender: Yes, administer a bolus of IV fluids and acetaminophen 650 mg po [by mouth] x1 for the patient's tachycardia and fever, as ordered in the EHR.

This method of communication can verify that information is heard correctly to avoid any miscommunication and adverse effects on the patient.

Huddles

Huddles are a technique for bridging communication between disciplines and assisting in delivering better outcomes for patients. They can address a critical concern (AHA, 2024b). Huddles empower and engage frontline staff in problem identification and build a culture of collaboration that enhances the team's ability to deliver safer care (Shaikh, 2020). In the abovementioned case, describe how the team could have used a huddle.

TeamSTEPPS TIP

Huddles are a tool for dealing with unexpected changes or critical concerns on an as-needed basis. Use the word *huddle* to get everyone's attention and gather your team for a quick meeting to reassess your plan, make any necessary changes, and ensure that you are all on the same page.

Source: AHA, 2024b.

Janeá used to advocate for her patients by calling a rapid response. A *rapid response* is initiated when a patient's health status quickly deteriorates; a group of trained medical professionals is called to rapidly respond and address the patient's condition (Stevens, 2022). This, by definition, is a type of huddle. Janeá used both the resources of her manager and the rapid response team appropriately to help support her in achieving a positive outcome for the patient.

Shared Mental Models

At the end of the case, Janeá shared her surprise when she overheard that the patient would be intubated. The provider did not share their impressions, and the nursing staff on the floor didn't have a shared mental model with the medical team. A *shared mental model* is a process in which a person monitors a situation to gain situational awareness that they can bring to the team with whom they work to improve outcomes (AHA, 2024b). In Janeá's story, an opportunity for the medical team to have used shared mental models would have been when the nurse notified the doctor of the patient's current condition and her prior experiences with the patient's response to treatment, and the doctor considered that information and continued decline of the patient and then intervened accordingly. An opportunity for the physician to have shared their mental model might have looked like the following:

> Janeá reported her concerns about the patient's health status to the physician and advocated for the patient. Not knowing the nurse well, the physician would trust that he must address the nurse's concerns. The physician would see the patient with the nurse and give the nurse his perspective on assessing the patient's status, sharing their mental model. The physician would review his orders with the nurse to see whether there were any questions or concerns.

TeamSTEPPS TIP

A *shared mental model* is a mental picture or sketch of the relevant facts and relationships defining a situation; this model is shared with others through communication. A *huddle* is one way to share mental models. In a shared mental model, the team anticipates and predicts each other's needs; identifies changes in the team, task, or teammates; and adjusts the course of action or strategies as needed.

Source: AHA, 2024b.

Learning to Radically Accept Others (and Ourselves)

By Linda Roney, EdD, RN-BC, FAAN

We can all recall a time in our lives when we were made to feel like we were not part of the group. In the first chapter of this book, we first discussed the ideas of *marginalization* and *mattering*. In this chapter's case, Janeá shares with us that she felt marginalized as a nursing student and how she now thinks that she matters and can extend her reach to those marginalized in her nursing practice. This is a tremendous testament to Janeá's character. She did this even when her nursing voice was muted and she was made to feel as if she did not matter on the interdisciplinary team.

The American Association of Colleges of Nursing (AACN) Essentials' Competencies (2021) in Action

In Janeá's story, we see many of the AACN essentials' subcompetencies in action that we can learn from.

TABLE 10.1 **Examples of Domain 2: Person-Centered Care and Domain 10: Personal, Professional, and Leadership Development in This Exemplar**

Domain 2: Person-Centered Care	
2.1 Engage with the individual in establishing a caring relationship.	Janeá demonstrated qualities of empathy, compassion, and mutual respect toward the patient. She saw her patient as an individual with her unique elements, not just a patient in the bed.
2.2 Communicate effectively with individuals.	Janeá used the interpreter to communicate with the patient, asked questions in report, and reached out to the provider to advocate for patient. She demonstrated emotional intelligence in her communications with the patient and the team.
Domain 10: Personal, Professional, and Leadership Development	
10.2 Demonstrate a spirit of inquiry that fosters flexibility and professional maturity.	While Janeá knew there were many tasks ahead of her on the shift, she took the time to listen to her coworker carefully in report.
10.3 Develop capacity for leadership.	Janeá made efforts to advocate for her patient. She took the time to make the members of her team and her patient feel heard and valued. Janeá approached her work with a focus on diversity, equity, and inclusion (DEI).

Marginalized in Health Care: Patients and Colleagues

The U.S. population is more racially and ethnically diverse than ever before (Jensen, 2023). As nurses, we care for those who might differ significantly from us, and we all want to do our best to communicate with our patients. We know that we often meet our patients at very vulnerable times in their lives, and we all want to do our best to provide patient-centered care with every interaction. However, it is essential to note that everyone who works cross-culturally and cross-linguistically will make mistakes (Centers for Disease Control and Prevention [CDC], 2022). Cross-cultural conversations give us more of an opportunity to misunderstand each other. Healthcare providers and patients may meet under stressful conditions, and there is an excellent opportunity for healthcare providers to miscommunicate in these situations unknowingly.

"Race/ethnicity, gender, sexual orientation, immigration status, physical disability status, and socioeconomic level play a role in representation, acceptance, and progress within and outside the healthcare setting"

(Stanford, 2020, p. 247). While we initially think of how our patients are different from us, it is also very likely that our coworkers may be different from us as well. We must also radically accept others' workplace diversity (Grant, 2022). Tara Brach (2004), a teacher of Buddhist meditation, is credited as first describing *radical acceptance*, which is navigating your emotions in response to stresses around you to practice acceptance. Radically accepting those different from us does not mean we compromise our values or beliefs. However, each employee ensures that everyone feels welcomed and belongs, regardless of their differences (Grant, 2022). Some people mistakenly think that having a setting with individuals with various backgrounds, cultures, and beliefs will lead to more conflict. Still, radical acceptance does not mean that you agree with a person's views but rather you acknowledge that they have the right to have their views, ideas, or feelings (Grant, 2022).

Respect for the dignity of every person, regardless of any unique characteristic, is at the core of *The Code of Ethics for Nurses With Interpretive Statements*, which we first discussed in Chapter 9 (American Nurses Association [ANA], 2015). Nurses are not expected to be experts in every cultural tradition and practice but rather to approach others with a sense of cultural humility. *Cultural humility* is the ongoing process of self-reflection in which individuals gain a more profound respect for cultural differences, reflection, openness to establishing power-balanced relationships, and appreciation of another's community expertise on the social and cultural context of their lived experience (CDC, 2022). Through cultural humility, individuals recognize that they do not have all the relevant knowledge and expertise and show a nonjudgmental willingness to learn from a person about their experiences and practices (CDC, 2022).

We must continue to welcome people from diverse backgrounds into nursing to reflect our patient population's diversity better. Men represent about 12% of the nursing workforce (AACN, 2023) but are 49.49% of the general population (U.S. Census Bureau, 2025). The Black or African American population is 14.4% of people living in the United States (U.S. Census Bureau, 2025) compared with 9.9% of nurses who self-identify as Black or African American (Minority Nurse, 2025). In the general population, 19% of people in the United States are Hispanic or Latino (U.S. Census Bureau, 2025), compared with just 4.8% of nurses who identify as Hispanic or Latino (Minority Nurse, 2025). A small percentage of nurses (1.3%) categorize themselves as two or more races (Minority Nurse, 2025) compared with 10.8% of the U.S. population (U.S. Census Bureau, 2025). There is one area of growing representation in nursing: 8% of RNs identify as lesbian, gay, bisexual, or transgender (LGBT) (Zauderer, 2023) compared with 7.1% of U.S. adults in the general population (Jones, 2022). Healthcare studies support that patients generally have better outcomes when cared for by diverse teams, as they are more likely to focus on innovation and team communication and achieve better financial performance (Gomez & Bernet, 2019). Racism affects patients and healthcare teams, leading to poor quality of care, low morale, stress, burnout, and a feeling of not belonging (Sue et al., 2019).

We can do so much better in nursing. Three out of four nurses in a recent survey stated that they had witnessed racism in the workplace. An overwhelming majority of Black nurses reported that racism negatively affects their professional well-being and that they have experienced racist acts from leaders (70%), patients (68%), and peers (66%; National Commission to Address Racism in Nursing [NCEMNA], 2022). Our professional nursing organizations started important work to acknowledge racism in nursing and, hopefully, commit to strategies to eradicate it someday. The ANA's *Racial Reckoning Statement* (2022) was the nursing organization's first step to acknowledge past actions that have negatively affected nurses of color and perpetuated systemic racism. In the document, the ANA recognizes that from 1916 to 1964, the ANA purposefully excluded Black nurses from the organization, and although by 1964, there were no articulated rules preventing nurses of color from being members, there continued to be exclusionary practices (ANA, 2022). In the statement, the ANA apologizes to nurses of color for causing significant harm to nurses of color. It acknowledges tangible steps toward creating a more inclusive and representative professional nurse organization (ANA, 2022).

Newborns Do Not Have Negative Biases

Bias happens because of our human need to classify information and make sense of the world, and it most often occurs below the level of consciousness (U.S. Department of Justice [DOJ], 2021). We are not born with negative biases toward any group; they come from our experiences (or lack of experiences with others) and the messages we receive during our lifetime (Osta & Vasquez, n.d.). There are two types of bias: *explicit* and *implicit*. With *explicit bias*, people are aware of their prejudices and attitudes toward particular groups, which manifest as positive or negative preferences (DOJ, 2021). Affinity biases or preferences for a group might be shown by a manager who hires only employees from the same ethnic group to work on their team (Vazquez, 2022). Negative preferences for a group might be expressed through a racist comment (DOJ, 2021).

Implicit biases, also known as *unconscious biases*, are "the attitudes that affect our understanding, actions, and decisions in an unconscious manner, that can have both favorable and unfavorable assessments, and are activated involuntarily and without an individual's awareness or intentional control" (TJC, 2016, p. 1). Nurses and other healthcare providers can hold implicit biases against marginalized groups, such as racial and ethnic minoritized populations (Vela et al., 2022; DOJ, 2021). While implicit biases cannot be prevented, we can become more aware of our biases, and slowing down to question our attitudes and beliefs is a crucial step (Vasquez, 2022). Implicit bias is more likely to appear when people make stressful or hurried decisions (Ursery, 2019).

Healthcare organizations should be involved in creating safe, accessible environments for patients and their employees. Your healthcare organization may offer specific training to help you mitigate your implicit biases and provide education to develop leadership skills related to your nursing role. You may have developed knowledge, skills, and attitudes in these areas through personal and professional development. Because mitigating bias is ongoing, reflecting on your interactions with patients and coworkers can help you develop in this area. Using some of the strategies in Table 10.2 can also help you create a habit of nonbiased thinking (Office of Minority Health [OMH], n.d.).

TABLE 10.2 **Creating a Habit of Nonbiased Thinking in Nursing**

Strategy	Description	Example
Stereotype replacement	Take the time to be conscious of the stereotypes you have and find ways to think differently about others.	**Stereotype:** "IT (information technology) professionals are men and do not have good communication skills." **Non-stereotype replacement:** "Computer programmers come from diverse backgrounds and interests. They may be male, female, or nonbinary. Some enjoy working with others, and others prefer to work independently. Their hobbies outside of computer programming can be quite vast."
Counter-stereotypic imaging	Think of a time when a person you met did not fit the stereotype of a particular group.	**Stereotype:** "Nurses are women." **Counter-stereotypic imaging:** Imagine a male nurse caring for children with cancer in an inpatient setting.
Individuating	Each person deserves to be seen as an individual and not as a part of a particular stereotyped group.	**Stereotype:** When, on your shadow day during the interview process, you walk into the breakroom and think that these nurses are all women who look and act exactly the same as one another. **Individuating:** When, on your shadow day during the interview process, you notice that one of the nurses has a water bottle that has the name of a local powerlifting gym that you have been thinking of joining.

Strategy	Description	Example
Perspective-taking	Try to understand another group's point of view.	**Stereotype:** You walk into work only to hear that there has been a sick call and a nurse from another unit is being floated to your unit to help. They don't look familiar to you, so that probably means they have never floated to your unit. What help could they possibly be anyway? Today is going to be awful for you. **Perspective-taking:** You walk into work and hear there has been a sick call. A nurse from another unit is being floated to your unit to help. They don't look familiar to you, so that probably means they have never floated to your unit. This probably started their day differently from how they expected, and they are probably very nervous to be here. They are probably hoping that someone will be kind and show them around.
Contact	Make deliberate effort to meet others who are very different from you.	**Stereotype:** Surgical residents are such arrogant jerks. They run away after they come to see your patients and feel like they are too good to share their thoughts with you before they disappear. **Contact:** I never knew the reason that the surgical residents seem to race from room to room as they preround was that they needed to see all the patients on their service before they scrub into the operating room with their attending. When we played on the hospital's softball team last year, we got to know one another after the games and found out that we had a lot more in common than we thought.
Emotional regulation	Take time to pause and consider any potential negative emotional reactions that you might have to people from social groups that are different from your own.	**Stereotype:** When you look at the clinic schedule for the next day and notice that a patient is coming in who needs a foreign language interpreter, does not have a documented vaccine record, and is being treated for TB. He is coming in with his mother for an appointment—*are they even here legally?*

(Continued)

TABLE 10.2 **(Continued)**

Strategy	Description	Example
		Emotional regulation: When you look at the clinic schedule for the next day and notice that a patient is coming in who needs a foreign language interpreter who is accessible by virtual interpretation. While the child does not have a documented vaccine record and is being treated for TB, it is great that the mother is bringing him in to start the process to protect him from preventable diseases.
Mindfulness	Practice mindfulness by purposefully focusing your attention on what you are doing in the present moment. This attentiveness may stop you from acting on biases or stereotypes.	**Stereotype:** When working at the bedside as a neonatal ICU (NICU) nurse, your patient's mother comes in five hours later than you heard that she was going to arrive. Her hair is curled, and she is wearing a full face of makeup and a dressy outfit. She took a "me day" instead of spending time at the bedside, learning to provide hands on care for her newborn. Is she even cut out for being a mother to a preemie? **Mindfulness:** When working at the bedside as a NICU nurse, your patient's mother arrives, and you greet her warmly to make her feel comfortable in a setting that is very likely intimating to her.

Adapted from "Combating Implicit Bias and Stereotypes," U.S. Department of Health and Human Services.

Do You Radically Accept Yourself?

There is another type of bias that is important to speak about; it is called *negativity bias.*

Negativity has a more substantial influence on our behavior and survival, which dates back to human evolution, as it is more critical for survival to avoid harmful stimuli than focusing on a positive one (Norris, 2021). *Negativity bias* is our tendency to register negative stimuli more readily, noticing more things when we have a negative interaction and remembering the details more vividly (Cherry, 2023). Most people brush off compliments and forget about them over their day, yet an insult can bother us for days (Struiksma et al., 2022). Negative biases can leave us anxious and full of self-doubt (Vermani, 2023). If we cannot accept ourselves for who we are, it will be difficult, if not impossible, to accept others. Identifying patterns of negative self-talk is critical to your ability to shift them toward healthier, more constructive thoughts through journaling and seeking the help of a therapist or professional counselor (Mosunic, n.d.).

Asking Others to Dance

*Diversity is being invited to the party. Inclusion is being asked
to dance.*

(Meyers, 2024).

Verna Meyers' (2024) words are often quoted as they relate to DEI. It is essential to recognize that diversity and inclusion are not synonymous (Sherbin & Rahsid, 2017). *Diversity* refers to the representation or composition of various social identity groups in a workgroup, an organization, or a community. At the same time, *inclusion* creates an environment that offers affirmation and appreciation of various approaches, styles, perspectives, and experiences (American Psychological Association, 2021). When interviewing with a potential employer, it is essential to ask about which policies and practices are in place to support a diverse and inclusive workplace. In order for us to contribute to our positive work environments, we, too, need to take an active role in our personal and professional development to ask not only more people to the party but also for them to dance with us in our lives.

What More Can I Do?

While the issues raised in this chapter are longstanding and of great scope, you might be asking yourself what you can do as a new nurse entering practice to have a positive impact on our profession. Perhaps you have heard the term *allyship,* which is "an ethical duty through intentional interventions, advocacy, and support to eliminate harmful acts, words, and deeds and creating space to amplify voices that are not traditionally heard, recognized or welcomed" (NCEMNA, 2022). An individual does not define authentic allyship but is recognized by marginalized groups (Arif et al., 2022). While I was not in the room when Janeá met her patient and set up the video interpreter device with her patient, I would like to think that her patient perceived Janeá as an ally. Ask yourself, *"Where am I when it comes to allyship in my role as a nurse?"* Figure 10.1 can help you identify where you are on the continuum of allyship in nursing and help you progress to the next zone. Allyship promotes accountability to advance the culture of inclusion through intentional, positive, conscious efforts and actions (Noone et al., 2022). Some people tend to ignore inequities because they do not know what to do, are afraid to cause friction with others, or, perhaps, are afraid to act because the situation is uncomfortable (Arif et al., 2022).

One other concept that affects our patients and colleagues can be *racial microaggressions,* which are the insults, invalidations, and offensive behaviors that people of color experience in daily interactions with generally well-intentioned individuals who may be unaware that they have behaved in racially demeaning ways toward targeted groups (Sue et al., 2019). For example, did you consider the images that you see in your nursing textbooks? A recent study by Pusey-Reid et al. (2023) analyzed 14,192 photo images and drawn graphics depicting skin tones completed across 15 foundational and clinical nursing textbooks and found that 12.3% of photo images and 2.4% of drawn graphics depicted dark skin tones in these textbooks, compared with 60.9% of photo images and 82.8% of drawn graphics that displayed light skin tones. Many faculty members wish to show more diverse images in their teaching,

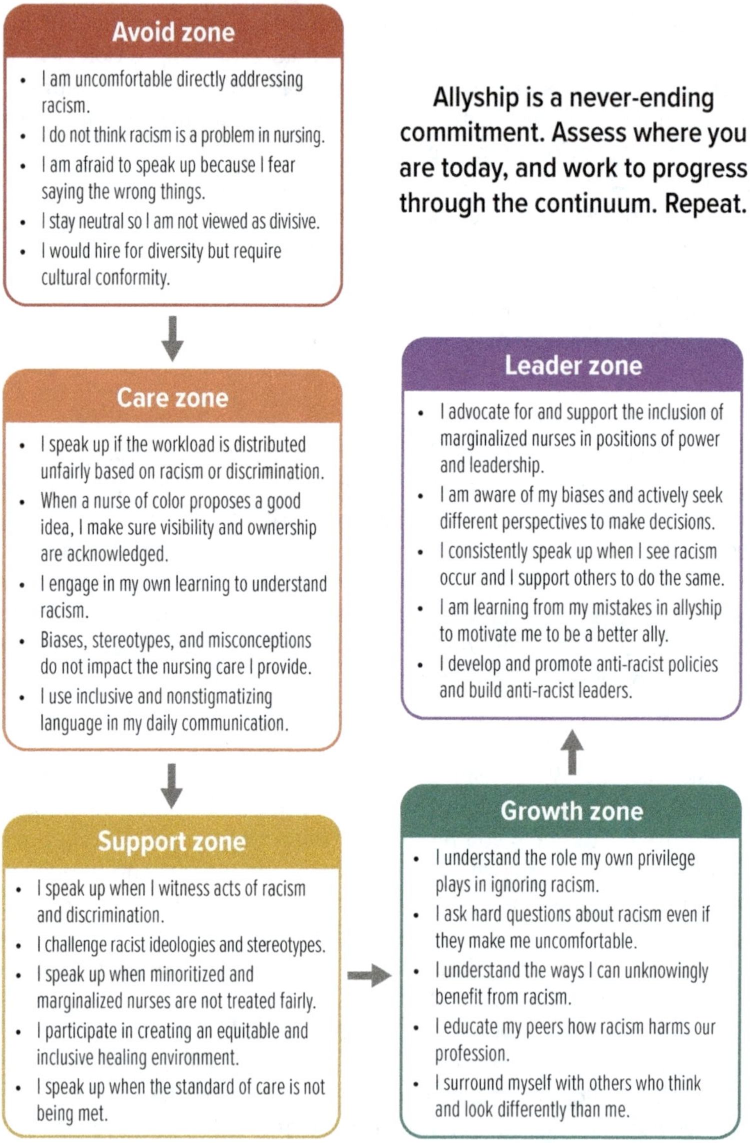

FIGURE 10.1 Allyship in Nursing (Copyright © by National Commission to Address Racism in Nursing. Reprinted with permission.)

but there is not much accessible information. Brown Skin Matters (https://www.instagram.com/brownskinmatters), an Instagram account, is helping address the challenge of the lack of reference photos of dermatological conditions on skin of color by sharing digital images as well as encouraging user submissions to add to the library of photos.

Additionally, racial microaggressions can come out in nursing practice and catch us off guard when they are said during a moment when we are in the middle of a task with a heavy cognitive load or when we are stressed. We

TABLE 10.3 **Responses Nurses Can Use to Disarm Microaggressions in the Healthcare Setting**

Example of Microaggression/ Scenario	What to Say
A colleague states to a coworker that the new manager received their position because they are a person of color.	The co-worker can say: • "I don't agree with what you said." • "That's not how I view it." • "While I understand you have the right to say what you want, I'm asking you to show a little more respect for me by not making offensive comments."
A new nurse is hired on the unit, and her manager informs the charge nurse that the new nurse will need brief coverage three times during her 12-hour shift. The charge nurse is heard telling one of her colleagues in the breakroom, *"Maybe I should become Muslim, too, so I can walk out of the surgical ICU [SICU] and have someone else cover my patients whenever I want."*	The colleague can say: • "I know you didn't realize this but the comment you made about our new coworker is demeaning and violates her privacy." • "I know that you really care about the SICU and the members of our team, but saying that really undermines our unit's values to be welcoming and inclusive." The colleague can also: • Report the incident to the nurse manager/ unit leadership or through the critical event reporting processes at the organization to pursue opportunities for improvement.
A new nurse is caring for a 18-year-old following an appendectomy. The patient was an assigned female at birth and is a trans male. The nurse walks into the patient's room to find the patient tearful and very upset. They state, *"The housekeeper just asked me if I went to prom. I said no, and they told me not to worry because I am a very pretty girl and will find a date next time."*	The nurse can: • Thank the patient for bringing this to their attention and ask them how they would like to handle this situation. • Take time to listen to the patient. Ask for their preferred name and pronouns. Ensure that this information is added to the EHR. The nurse can also: • Report the incident to the nurse manager/ unit leadership or through the critical event reporting processes at the organization to pursue opportunities for improvement.

Source: Adapted/modified for relevance to nursing practice from Sue et al., 2019, and Anderson, 2022.

all have varying speed and comfort with responding to something shocking that is said, so considering examples and reflecting on difficult situations in advance might help us feel more comfortable as we develop these skills. Sue et al. (2019) offer specific tactics and examples for responding to racial microaggressions that might be helpful to consider as you develop your toolkit of responses to address injustice in the workplace and beyond. The following content has been adapted to consider your role as a new nurse encountering microaggressions in health care.

Continuing to invest in your knowledge base of how you can be an inclusive and welcoming nurse and teammate is a long-term investment. It is also important to remember that even with an open mind and a commitment to this goal, you will have missteps and make mistakes. Just like everything in our nursing careers, taking the time to reflect and process our experiences and continuously strive to do better each time we encounter a new challenge can only help us contribute to the inclusive environments we hope to be part of throughout our careers. Following are a few online resources. Please feel free to discover more through your professional and social networks.

TABLE 10.4 Additional Online Resources to Help You Develop Allyship in Nursing

Resource	Website
American Organization for Nurse Leaders (AONL): *AONL Guiding Principles: Diversity, Equity, Inclusion, and Belonging Toolkit* (2024)	https://www.aonl.org/resources/DEIB-Toolkit
Guide to Allyship (2021)	https://guidetoallyship.com/
AARP Center for Health Equity Through Nursing (Campaign for Action, n.d.)	https://campaignforaction.org/about/center-for-health-equity-through-nursing/
American Hospital Association: *Building the Team: Diversity, Equity and Inclusion* (2024a)	https://www.aha.org/workforce-strategies/diversity-equity-inclusion
National Equity Project: Implicit Bias, Structural Racialization, and Equity	https://www.nationalequityproject.org/

YOU MATTER: SPEAKING UP AND TAKING ACTION

When you feel unsure of yourself or others make you feel as if your opinion does not matter, it is easy to feel silenced. Many nurses feel frustrated when they feel that a situation is heading in the wrong direction and others do not share the same mental model. Hierarchical structures and closed communication among those who do not know one another well can challenge nurses working as part of an interdisciplinary team. Focusing on using evidence-based communication and leadership strategies, such as the tools from Team STEPPS (AHA, 2024b), and committing to a growth mindset will support you in taking action for a safer, more inclusive work environment.

Book Club Questions

1. Have you seen marginalization and/or racism toward patients and colleagues in health care? Using Table 10.3, can you describe responses you could use if you reencountered the same situation?
2. What does being an ally for patients, families, and colleagues mean to you?
3. In speaking with a patient, you say something you immediately regret and can sense that you have offended them. What should you do?

About This Chapter's Authors

Janeá Butler, MSN, RN

Janeá was born and raised in Bridgeport, Connecticut. She attended Fairfield University's Marion Peckham Egan School of Nursing and Health Studies from 2016 to 2020. She moved to North Carolina, where she continued her education and obtained her master's degree in nurse leadership and management. Her nursing career started in medical-surgical, where she discovered she had a passion for preoperative/postoperative patient care. Janeá started teaching clinical rotations in 2023 at a local college in North Carolina. Janeá has a passion for patient-centered care and education. Janeá is currently enrolled in a Doctor of Nursing Practice (DNP) program. Outside of work, Janeá enjoys talking with friends and family, going to church, and traveling the world.

Laura A. Conklin, MSN, RN

Laura has been an RN at VA (Veterans Affairs) Connecticut (VACT) for 33 years. After spending many years in the ICU and teaching basic life support (BLS) and advanced cardiac life support (ACLS), she wanted to transfer her skills to nursing education. She spent 10 years as the critical care educator, BLS/ACLS program director, and simulation coordinator at VACT before taking on the role of clinical instructor/faculty for Fairfield University with the partnership with VACT, combining the best of educating students, and still being able to be at the bedside caring for veterans. In this role, she teaches clinical for medical-surgical, mental health, population health, and geriatrics; she also teaches lab for fundamentals and health assessment and theory for "Professional Nursing Leadership and Fundamentals." She is passionate about nursing and proud to be the mother of three RN daughters. She enjoys running, cooking, and spending time with her family, who include two dogs.

Danielle Hall, DNP, MSN, RN

Danielle is an experienced RN with 28 years of clinical practice. She earned her Bachelor of Science in Nursing from the University of Scranton and has worked in various high-acuity settings, including medical-surgical, emergency, and cardiac intensive care at Yale New Haven Hospital in Connecticut.

After receiving her Master of Science in Nursing from Yale University, Danielle pursued her DNP from Case Western Reserve University. As she advanced in her career, Danielle transitioned into nursing education, focusing on acute care settings. For more than 10 years, she served as a clinical nurse educator, specializing in transition-to-practice programs that supported onboarding NGNs at both Greenwich Hospital and St. Vincent's Medical Center in Connecticut.

Currently, Danielle is an assistant professor of the practice of nursing at Fairfield University, where she has taught for the past eight years. She teaches a variety of undergraduate courses, including on health assessment, fundamentals of nursing, medical-surgical nursing, and nursing leadership. In addition to her professional work, Danielle is a dedicated mother of three high school–aged children and enjoys spending time with her two dogs.

References

Alharbi, H. F., & Alzahrani, J. (2023). The experiences of newly graduated nurses during their first year of practice. *Healthcare (Basel)*, *11*(14).

American Association of Colleges of Nursing. (2021). *The essentials: Core competencies for professional nursing education*. https://www.aacnnursing.org/Portals/0/PDFs/Publications/Essentials-2021.pdf

American Association of Colleges of Nursing. (2023). *Data spotlight: Men in nursing: Five-year trends show no growth*. https://www.aacnnursing.org/news-data/all-news/data-spotlight-men-in-nursing-five-year-trends-show-no-growth

American Hospital Association. (2024a). *Building the team: Diversity, equity, and inclusion*. https://www.aha.org/workforce-strategies/diversity-equity-inclusion

American Hospital Association. (2024b). *TeamSTEPPS® video toolkit*. AHA Center for Health Innovation. https://www.aha.org/center/project-firstline/teamstepps-video-toolkit

American Nurses Association. (2015). *Code of ethics for nurses with interpretive statements.* http://www.nursingworld.org/MainMenuCategories/EthicsStandards/CodeofEthics-forNurses/Code-of-Ethics-For-Nurses.htm

American Nurses Association. (2022). *Racial reckoning statement.* https://www.nursingworld.org/practice-policy/workforce/racism-in-nursing/RacialReckoningStatement/

American Organization for Nurse Leaders. (2024). *AONL guiding principles: Diversity, equity, inclusion, and belonging toolkit.* https://www.aonl.org/resources/DEIB-Toolkit

American Psychological Association. (2021). *Equity, diversity, and inclusion framework.* https://www.apa.org/about/apa/equity-diversity-inclusion/framework

Anderson. (2022). A transition to find herself. *American Association of Critical Care Nurses.* Nursing Excellence. https://www.aacn.org/nursing-excellence/nurse-stories/a-transition-to-find-herself

Arif, S., Afolabi, T., Mitrzyk, B. M., Thomas, T. F., Borja-Hart, N., Wade, L., & Henson, B. (2022). Engaging in authentic allyship as part of our professional development. *American Journal of Pharmaceutical Education, 86*(5), 8690. https://doi.org/10.5688/ajpe8690

Armstrong, G. (2019). Quality and safety education for nurses teamwork and collaboration competency: Empowering nurses. *Journal of Continuing Education in Nursing, 50*(6), 252–255. https://doi.org/10.3928/00220124-20190516-04

Brach, T. (2004). *Radical acceptance: Embracing your life with the heart of a Buddha.* Bantam Books.

Campaign for Action. (n.d.). *AARP Center for Health Equity Through Nursing.* https://campaignforaction.org/about/center-for-health-equity-through-nursing/

Centers for Disease Control and Prevention. (2022). *Principle 1: Embrace cultural humility and community engagement.* https://www.cdc.gov/globalhealth/equity/guide/cultural-humility.html

Cherry, K. (2023). *What is the negativity bias?* Verywell Mind. https://www.verywellmind.com/ negative-bias-4589618

Etchegaray, J. M., Ottosen, M. J., Dancsak, T., & Thomas, E. J. (2020). *Barriers to speaking up about patient safety concerns. Journal of Patient Safety, 16*(4), e230–e234.

Galanti, G. A. (2000). An introduction to cultural differences. *Western Journal of Medicine, 172*(5), 335–336. https://doi.org/10.1136/ewjm.172.5.335

Gill, R. (2021). Being watched and feeling judged on social media. *Feminist Media Studies, 21*(8), 1387–1392. https://doi.org/10.1080/14680777.2021.1996427

Gomez, L. E., & Bernet, P. (2019). Diversity improves performance and outcomes. *Journal of the National Medical Association, 111*(4), 383–392. https://doi.org/10.1016/j.jnma.2019.01.006

Grant, R. (2022, November 8). *How do I radically accept others who are different at work?* LinkedIn. https://www.linkedin.com/pulse/how-do-i-radically-accept-others-who-different-work-risha-grant/

Guttman, O. T., Lazzara, E. H., Keebler, J. R., Webster, K. L., Gisick, L. M., & Baker, A. L. (2021). Dissecting communication barriers in healthcare: A path to enhancing communication resiliency, reliability, and patient safety. *Journal of Patient Safety, 17*(8), 465–471.

Jensen, E. (2023, October 11). *The chance that two randomly chosen people of different race or ethnicity groups has increased since 2010.* Census.gov. https://www.census.gov/library/ stories/2021/08/2020-united-states-population-more-racially-ethnically-diverse-than-2010.html

Jones, J. (2022). *LGBT identification in U.S. ticks up to 7.1%.* Gallup. https://news.gallup.com/poll/389792/lgbt-identification-ticks-up.aspx

Kimhi, S., Marciano, H., Eshel, Y., & Adini, B. (2022). Do we cope similarly with different adversities? COVID-19 versus armed conflict. *BMC Public Health, 22*(1), 2151. https://doi.org/10.1186/s12889-022-14572-0

Minority Nurse. (2025). *Nursing statistics.* https://minoritynurse.com/nursing-statistics/

Mosunic, C. (n.d.). *Negative self-talk: 8 ways to quiet your inner critic.* Calm Blog. https://www.calm.com/blog/negative-self-talk

Murphy, M., Engel, J. R., McGugan, L., McKenzie, R., Thompson, J. A., & Turner, K.M. (2022). Implementing a standardized communication tool in an intensive care unit. *Critical Care Nurse, 42*(3), 56–64. https://doi.org/10.4037/ccn2022154

Nakatani, K., Nakagami-Yamaguchi, E., Hagawa, N., Tokuwame, A., Ehara, S., Nishimura, T., & Mizobata, Y. (2024). Evaluation of a new patient safety educational programme to reduce adverse events by encouraging staff to speak up: application of the trigger tool methodology. *BMJ open quality, 13*(1), e002162. https://doi.org/10.1136/bmjoq-2022-002162

National Commission to Address Racism in Nursing. (2022, June 3). *Resources for change.* American Nurses Association. https://www.nursingworld.org/practice-policy/workforce/racism-in-nursing/resources-for-change/

Noone, D., Robinson, L., Niles, C., & Narang, I. (2022). Unlocking the power of allyship: Giving health care workers the tools to take action against inequities and racism. *NEJM Catalyst.* https://catalyst.nejm.org/doi/full/10.1056/CAT.21.0358

Norris, C. J. (2021). The negativity bias revisited: Evidence from neuroscience measures and an individual differences approach. *Social Neuroscience, 16*(1), 68–82. https://doi.org/10.1080/17470919.2019.1696225

Office of Minority Health. (n.d.). *Combating implicit bias and stereotypes.* Think Cultural Health Education. U.S. Department of Health and Human Services. https://thinkculturalhealth.hhs.gov/maternal-health-care/assets/ pdfs/Combating_ implicit_ bias_and_stereotypes.pdf

Osta, K., & Vasquez, H. (n.d.). *Implicit bias and structural racialization.* National Equity Project. https://www.nationalequityproject.org/frameworks/implicit-bias-structural-racialization?gad_source=1&gclid=CjwKCAjw57exBhAsEiwAaIxaZhHBnmwD-Kvd-cCbgwDU4tykHSIYTc14751EXLHI1iVhNh2FQg9HhVRoCBiQQAvD_BwE

Pusey-Reid, E., Quinn, L. W., Wong, J., & Wucherpfennig, A. (2023). Representation of dark skin tones in foundational nursing textbooks: An image analysis. *Nurse Education Today, 130,* 105927. https://doi.org/10.1016/j.nedt.2023.105927

Schwappach, D., & Richard, A. (2018). *Speak up-related climate and its association with healthcare workers' speaking up and withholding voice behaviours: A cross-sectional survey in Switzerland. BMJ Quality Satisfaction, 10,* 827–835.

Shaikh, U. (2020, January 29). *Improving patient safety and team communication through daily huddles*. Patient Safety Network. https://psnet.ahrq.gov/primer/improving-patient-safety-and-team-communication-through-daily-huddles

Sherbin, L., & Rashid, R. (2017). Diversity doesn't stick without inclusion. *Harvard Business Review*. https://hbr.org/2017/02/diversity-doesnt-stick-without-inclusion

Stanford, F. C. (2020). The importance of diversity and inclusion in the healthcare workforce. *Journal of the National Medical Association, 112*(3), 247–249. https://doi.org/10.1016/j.jnma.2020.03.014

Stevens, J. P. (2022). *Rapid response systems*. UpToDate. https://www.uptodate.com/contents/16280

Stavropoulou, A., Rovithis, M., Kelesi, M., Vasilopoulos, G., Sigala, E., Papageorgiou, D., Moudatsou, M., & Koukouli, S. (2022). What quality of care means? Exploring clinical nurses' perceptions on the concept of quality care: A qualitative study. *Clinics and Practice, 12*(4), 468–481. https://doi.org/10.3390/clinpract12040051

Struiksma, M. E., DeMulder, H. N., & Van Berkum, J. A. (2022). Do people get used to insulting language? *Frontiers in Communication, 7*. https://doi.org/10.3389/fcomm.2022.910023

Sue, D. W., Alsaidi, S., Awad, M. N., Glaeser, E., Calle, C. Z., & Mendez, N. (2019). Disarming racial microaggressions: Microintervention strategies for targets, White allies, and bystanders. *The American Psychologist, 74*(1), 128–142. https://doi.org/10.1037/amp0000296

The Joint Commission. (2016). Implicit bias in healthcare. *Quick Safety, 23*. https://www.jointcommission.org/resources/news-and-multimedia/newsletters/newsletters/quick-safety/quick-safety-issue-23-implicit-bias-in-health-care/implicit-bias-in-health-care/

The Joint Commission. (2023, October 18). *New sentinel event data available for first 6 months of 2023*. https://www.jointcommission.org/resources/news-and-multimedia/newsletters/newsletters/joint-commission-online/oct-18-2023/se-data/

Theard, M. A., Marr, M. C., & Harrison, R. (2021). *The growth mindset for changing medical education culture. eClinicalMedicine, 37*, 100972. https://doi.org/10.1016/j.eclinm.2021.100972

Ursery, S. (2019). *Mindbugs: The ordinary origins of implicit bias*. National Apartment Association. https://naahq.org/mindbugs-ordinary-origins-implicit-bias

U.S. Census Bureau. (2025, January 8). Data. Census.gov. https://www.census.gov/data.html

U.S. Department of Justice. (2021). *Understanding bias: A resource guide*. Community Relations Services Toolkit for Policing. https://www.justice.gov/d9/fieldable-panel-panes/basic-panes/attachments/2021/09/29/understanding_bias_content.pdf

Vazquez, A. (2022). *How to mitigate your unconscious bias*. Gladstone Institute. https://gladstone.org/news/how-mitigate-your-unconscious-bias?gad_source=1&gclid=CjwKCAjw57exBhAsEiwAaIxaZt-nvyUcVhyRyE1ZmELU_AlXHm2APv5NE4GR-F9o8O-PYj-7S06tMuBoCvmgQAvD_BwE

Vela, M. B., Erondu, A. I., Smith, N. A., Peek, M. E., Woodruff, J. N., & Chin, M. H. (2022). Eliminating explicit and implicit biases in health care: Evidence and research needs. *Annual Review of Public Health, 43,* 477–501. https://doi.org/10.1146/annurev-publhealth-052620-103528

Vermani, M. (2023). *Why our negative thoughts are so powerful?* Psychology Today. https://www.psychologytoday.com/us/blog/a-deeper-wellness/202309/why-our-negative-thoughts-are-so-powerful

Verna Meyers. (2024). *About Verna Meyers.* https://www.vernamyers.com/about-verna/

Zauderer, S. (2023). *41 nursing statistics & demographics: How many are there?* Cross River Therapy. https://www.crossrivertherapy.com/research/nursing-statistics-and-Demographics.

CHAPTER 11

Compassion in Action

Leadership at the Bedside

Grace Rankin, BSN, RN, CCRN; Kevin Traille, CRNA, DNP; and Linda Roney, EdD, RN-BC, CPEN, CNE, FAAN

Learning Goals

1. Describe Grace's successes and challenges in caring for critically ill patients as a new-graduate nurse in a critical care setting.
2. Understand the vital role of situational awareness and leadership in challenging patient care situations.
3. Plan your approach to new situations in clinical practice using the situational awareness model.
4. Reflect on your beliefs and attitudes that affect influence as a situational leader.

Charlie's Last Call

By Grace Rankin, BSN, RN, CCRN

As a new-grad nurse, my first job was in a surgical intensive care unit (SICU). My unit primarily specialized in liver and bowel transplants. When I first began at my position, I was lucky enough to have an amazing mentor who taught me the ins and outs of bedside nursing. My four months of orientation were a whirlwind; as part of my training, we had the highest-acuity patients, which helped broaden my experience. By the time I was on my own, the unit had had a large shift in acuity. We were dealing with a second wave of COVID-19, and transplants had slowed down. For roughly six months, our unit was primarily an overflow step-down unit. The transplants that occurred went smoothly, and most of our patients did not require ICU-level care after just a few days postop. During this time, I rarely took care of an intensive care unit (ICU) patient unless I was floating to assist in the COVID-19 ICUs.

By the time I had been at this facility for about a year, our acuity in the SICU started picking up. During this time, we also experienced a large exodus in our staff, causing much of our staff in the SICU to have under three years of experience. This led to me getting trained on equipment and moving into leadership roles faster than initially anticipated. I was becoming a preceptor and charge nurse as well as being trained to care for patients who require continuous renal replacement therapy (CRRT). CRRT is a form of dialysis used on critically ill patients who are hemodynamically unstable. Typically, dialysis will run more than two to four hours, which causes large amounts of fluid shifts in a patient over a short period of time. With CRRT, we run the dialysis treatment 24/7 to split the fluid shifts over a longer time period as these patients require intravenous (IV) medication to maintain a stable blood pressure. Initially, this was exciting as I was getting to expand my knowledge and nursing practices, but as I began to be assigned these roles regularly, I experienced higher levels of stress and anxiety due to the minimal resources and assistance on my unit. Charlie was a patient for whom I primarily cared during this time on my unit, and my experiences working with him changed how I practiced nursing and, ultimately, were the beginning of my end on this unit.

Charlie first arrived at my unit in September after receiving an ABO-incompatible liver. An ABO-incompatible liver transplant means that the patient is receiving an organ from a donor who has an incompatible blood type with theirs. These transplants are performed in urgent situations when no other option is available, and their success is still being investigated. Due to receiving a blood type mismatch, that patient must undergo aggressive therapies to mitigate their body's rejection to the incompatible organ. Charlie initially had a rocky start fresh out of surgery, requiring massive transfusion protocol (MTP) activation due to hemorrhaging from his coagulopathy. However, after a couple of weeks, he had stabilized and could be transferred to the floor. The majority of liver transplants I saw coming through our unit went very similarly to Charlie's start and did not leave a lasting memory on most of us. Despite this, there were also many patients who were stuck in the ICU with long-term complications leading to monthslong stays and occasionally their death. Because of this, many of my coworkers and I rarely saw liver transplant patients in a bright light. Charlie ultimately returned to us a few weeks later in rejection, renal failure, fluid overload, and respiratory failure. He became a patient I never forgot and opened my eyes to many issues in our unit.

Charlie was my first patient whom I cared for on CRRT. Due to a shift toward online education instead of having a typical in-person class to discuss how to run CRRT and care for a patient while on treatment, I was sent a two-hour–long video to watch on how to set up a cartridge and then was given an open-book quiz about the video. I was also provided one shift during which I was precepted by a trained CRRT nurse. At the beginning of a stretch of four shifts, I trained on Charlie my first day and then was expected to care for him the next three days on my own. I brought up my concerns to my educator about my ability to care for Charlie appropriately on my own. In response, I was told that I could call the resource nurse (who was one nurse for the entire hospital) or my charge nurse if I needed any assistance. This did not calm my anxiety as I arrived for my first shift alone with Charlie.

On this first shift, I was not only caring for Charlie and his CRRT machine but was also assigned a new-graduate nurse to precept on only her third week. All of a sudden, I was one of the nurses with the most responsibility on the unit and had not even been off orientation myself for a year. To make things worse, seven hours into the shift, the new-graduate nurse and I had to admit a fresh kidney transplant from the postanesthesia care unit. Previously, patients on CRRT were singled (meaning that there was one patient assignment for the nurse), but due to short staffing, they were often paired with another stable patient. Pairing a fresh kidney transplant who required hourly fluid checks with a CRRT patient who needed hourly machine pressure checks was unheard of. As I spoke up to the charge nurse about my concerns with this admission and offered to take a stabler patient from another nurse so that they would be open to admit, I was told that I shouldn't take away the opportunity for my new grad to care for a fresh kidney transplant patient. I felt immediately silenced and as though my voice had been taken away. Not only did I feel as though my concerns were dismissed, but I also felt that my new grad was actually neglected in this case. Because of her minimal time on the floor, I did not feel comfortable with having her do an admission or care for a brand-new patient population without being in the room with her. I was unable to allow her to practice many of her skills as I was stretched so thin between both rooms. I clearly remember being so flustered at the end of my shift, trying to troubleshoot my CRRT cartridge, that instead of teaching her, I told her to just keep dumping the Foley catheter and adjusting the IV fluid replacement in the kidney room. Her education was stunted because my concerns were dismissed and we were given an unsafe assignment.

Charlie continued to stay on CRRT during his entire multiweek stay in the SICU due to his hemodynamic instability and need for vasopressor medications to maintain his blood pressure. Charlie was also unable to come off the ventilator and ultimately received a tracheostomy for long-term ventilator support. Charlie's mom, Donna, was his healthcare proxy and, ultimately, was making decisions regarding his care as he was unable to communicate with us. Donna was a sweet lady who lived about six hours away from the hospital. She would call for updates twice a shift and then, every Sunday, make the long drive down to the hospital with Charlie's dad to visit for only a couple of hours before making the journey back home. Over the course of Charlie's admission to our SICU, I became extremely close with Donna, as I was one of the most frequent healthcare workers to provide her with updates. Every morning, we had a long phone call, and I updated her on Charlie's stability, progress, and plans for the day. In the afternoon, Donna wanted just a quick update and then just to chat. Donna mentioned that with everything going on, it was quite overwhelming, and sometimes she just liked to have a distraction. We talked about vacations and found out we had both been to Newport, Rhode Island, at the same time years before. We created a very strong bond over those couple of months, as the only communication she could have with her son was through the nurses, and I believe that she found comfort in getting to know the people who were caring for her son. These nursing updates were commonly the only updates in condition that Donna received on a day-to-day basis. The SICU residents were able to provide small updates about current issues, such as bleeding or infection. However, under our hospital's leadership, they were unable to discuss Charlie's transplant status. This was regarding whether it meant discussing whether his initial transplant was a success or failure or he was being reconsidered for a second transplant. To receive an update regarding this pertinent information, Donna had to call the nursing staff and asked us to request that someone directly from the transplant service call to provide her an update. This was due to the fact that although the patient was receiving their care in the SICU and by the SICU residents, his primary care team was still considered the transplant service during his first year postop. Any deaths or complications that occur in the first year of transplant affected the hospital's ability to be recertified as a transplant center. Thus, the team wanted total control of information and decision-making regarding the patient's care. Sadly, being far away and unable to be at Charlie's bedside, I believe that Donna was largely left in the dark about the severity of Charlie's situation because she was unable to receive in-person updates. As one of the sole people updating her about her son's condition frequently, I felt a large amount of stress and pressure in making sure that I was able to give detailed and accurate updates about his status without crossing over into discussing Charlie's transplant. I also feel that from a nursing perspective, I looked at caring for the whole person and many times found it hard to give Donna bad news about adding an additional vasopressor or needing to transfuse because I did not want to upset her. I was never trained on how to give bad news to a family member or how to distance myself from the situation emotionally. This led to me leaving most of my Charlie shifts extremely emotionally and mentally drained.

About six weeks into this SICU stay, Charlie was experiencing common complications that we saw in our unit with long-term patients: multiple clots that required a heparin drip and multiple runs of atrial fibrillation with a rapid ventricular rate, which necessitated an amiodarone drip. Charlie also struggled with hyperemesis and routinely failed in advancing his tube feeds for nutrition, so he required total parenteral nutrition. This all meant that Charlie needed continuous IV medication to prevent him from clotting, keep his heart rate at a normal nonlethal rhythm and rate, and receive nutrition. Looking at this from far away, these were just other forms of life support that we were providing Charlie to keep his body alive longer but not medications that were curing his root issues. With all these barriers, he was not considered stable enough to be evaluated for retransplantation. Despite this fact that was known by most of the nursing staff, the information had not been relayed to Donna by the physicians, and it was not in the nursing scope of practice to provide a family member with this information. I did my best to explain to Donna Charlie's barriers to leaving the SICU and hospital. I reflected on previous patients and used them as examples for Donna to help her understand the severity of his case. I remember telling Donna on one phone call that I personally had not cared for a patient who had been on two pressors, CRRT, and a ventilator for six weeks straight before with minimal improvement, as many patients in this condition do not make it this long. Sadly, my updates regarding his severity couldn't bridge to a discussion about goals of care since he had had his liver transplant only a couple of months prior; thus, comfort care, do-not-resuscitate status, and palliative care were not in discussion per protocol. Since this patient remained on the transplant service for that first year, which could affect the hospital's standing in getting recertified, all efforts were made to keep that patient alive for the first year despite a poor quality of life or no chance of survival outside the hospital. As nurses, we were able to consult with our ethics department if we felt that we were providing unethical care. This practice was rarely used on our unit, as I feel we weren't encouraged to speak out against the transplant team. Despite this fact, a consult with the ethics department had been ordered by one nurse to help urge the transplant surgeons to have a more open discussion regarding Charlie's chance of survival with his family, but these meetings never went in our favor.

The ethics department was meant to come bedside and deliver an unbiased view on whether we were ethically caring for our patient and was there to advise us on how to care in the best interest of our patient. I never once saw the ethics department go against the transplant service. As was typical on our unit, the attending transplant surgeon argued in the case of the donor, stating that we owed it to the life of the donor and the donor's family to do everything possible to save this organ that was implanted in our patient. It seemed as if they always overlooked the recipient's quality of life and death. These surgeons were on our floor for only an hour or two per day. They did not see the suffering of those who had had unsuccessful transplants. Per usual course, the ethics department sided with the surgeon's argument and told us, as nursing staff, that we could reconsult them if anything changed in the case. This felt like they were dismissing our concerns about the advancement in Charlie's care. No one asked me how this decision made me feel or if they could help support me as I morally struggled with the care I was providing. I felt as though I was doing harm to my patient by doing everything to keep him alive to assist in keeping up transplant statistics even though he was never going to make it outside of the four walls of his hospital room.

By week seven, Charlie was on our unit and about to celebrate his birthday. To make this day as enjoyable as it can be while being in the ICU, we nurses got together to decorate his room while he slept. We covered his walls with birthday signs and pictures, placed balloons at the foot of his bed, and even made him a birthday hat. I was lucky enough to be Charlie's nurse on his birthday and tried to fill the day with as many happy moments as possible. I could see that Charlie would not celebrate another birthday after this one, but I didn't want him to think about that on this day. Surprisingly, his birthday was also the first time we would trial a speaking valve on Charlie's trach. Since Charlie had arrived in our unit, we had only been able to communicate via communication boards and reading lips. I had yet to hear his voice, and more importantly, his parents hadn't heard him speak in almost two months. When we placed the speaking valve, I set up a FaceTime with his mother, who was currently at work six hours away. Charlie did not tolerate the speaking valve as well as we hoped, but in the short time he had it on, the only three words he was able to say were "*I love you*" to his mother via FaceTime. I was able to hold back tears while witnessing this in the room, but I found myself crying on the phone with Donna later that afternoon. Donna exclaimed how happy she was to hear her "baby's" voice finally. Donna and I also made plans for her visit this upcoming Sunday when I would be working, and as always, she planned on bringing a treat for the staff, which, this time, would be birthday cupcakes. I told Donna that I would bring the plates and napkins and help with anything she needed. I left that day feeling like I was able to create some good amid so much sadness.

When Sunday rolled around, I was back with Charlie and came in ready to get all my care front-loaded before Donna arrived. Over the course of the morning, Charlie's condition deteriorated as he required an increased pressure load as well as a large increase in lactate. A computed tomography (CT) scan of the abdomen/pelvis was ordered, and I was just about to head off the unit when Donna arrived. I let her say hello and told her that she could wait in the room while we were gone. By the time we were at CT, Charlie had gotten notably paler, and when we pulled him over to the scanner, about a liter of blood came out of his rectum. By the time I got back to the unit only 20 minutes later, Charlie was still profusely bleeding, and additional pressors were added while an MTP was being activated. The room was about to become very busy as gastroenterology (GI) was coming bedside for a scope, and multiple nurses were in the room helping me titrate medications and transfuse via the Belmont. I brought Donna and Charlie's dad in the room to say goodbye as their visit was now being cut short due to Charlie's instability. Donna and Charlie's dad waited outside our room for two hours before deciding to make the trek back home. During Charlie's scope, the GI fellow stated that he had never seen someone's bowel look so necrotic. It was never mentioned to Charlie or his parents that he now had a dead bowel and next to no chance of survival. This was one of the busiest shifts I had ever had in my career. I don't believe that I ever left Charlie's room after 10 a.m. Charlie remained unstable for the next couple of days, bleeding from multiple spots in his GI tract, which required a numerable number of interventions.

I came back that Wednesday, and Charlie was slightly stabler, requiring fewer transfusions per shift and not having large derangements in labs. Despite Charlie objectively looking better, I thought that he looked off. For the first time in weeks, Charlie had a vacant gaze, rarely tracking me across the room and unable to muster up the strength to smile. I sensed that his end was near, and I voiced my concern to the transplant physician assistant on his case. I urged them to call Donna and tell her to make the drive down to the hospital, but they told me that he appeared stable and that maybe he was just tired. They refused to address my concerns even though I had intimately cared for Charlie over the past two months and they had been in his room for possibly a total of a few hours during that time. My opinions and judgment were ignored, and by the end of my shift, Donna had not been called by anyone from the transplant service, and our 6 p.m. afternoon call was arriving soon. I gave her the update on the minimal changes in medication and labs, but I felt it was my duty to tell her that personally, based on my opinion, Charlie had a look of impending doom. I told her that if I were her, I would get in the car and come to the hospital as soon as possible because being nearby couldn't hurt. Donna agreed, and I left that shift expecting to see Donna in the morning.

I woke up to my coworker calling me at 2 a.m. She gave me the news that Charlie had decompensated rapidly after I left and had just coded and passed. She told me that Donna had made it there just in time to see her son for an hour before he coded. Donna had asked me to call her the next day when I was available. I spoke with Donna that afternoon, and she thanked me for calling her the night before to come and be with Charlie as she had not ever received a phone call from someone on the transplant service. I stayed on the phone with her for a while and let her talk and cry. When I went back to work, Charlie's name was never mentioned by the transplant physicians, his death was overlooked, and the care that we ICU nurses had provided was overlooked. We had worked for months trying to save Charlie and watching him suffer only for him to pass. It was a mess the transplant physicians did not have to witness and an unfortunate picture that they refused to see.

After caring for Charlie, I came to the realization that I was at a facility where my concerns, opinions, and knowledge were dismissed. There was no respect or collaboration between different disciplines, and if I spoke about my disgruntlement regarding this to a manager, it was brushed off. As nurses, our voices were not being heard and supported when we brought up concerns regarding patient care. We were overlooked and underused when it came to any discussion of the management of care for a critical patient, and there was no one willing to back us up when we were concerned. With Charlie, I realized that I was left caring for everyone, but no one cared *about me*. I chose then to begin looking into the future to find a new job, one where I felt supported and heard. I stayed at my first position for about eight more months, during which time I had similar situations to that which I had encountered with Charlie. Our staffing had worsened, and I soon became one of the most senior nurses even with only two years' experience. When I interviewed for my new positions, I asked questions regarding interdisciplinary rounds, the variety of experience on staff, and the usage of palliative care. I ended up finding a job that was a wonderful fit. Although Charlie's case brought me so much moral distress, I believe that I truly learned from him and grew as a nurse, learning to advocate for my patients and care for all one's needs, whether when titrating medication or decorating their room for their birthday. Looking back, I hope that I provided Charlie and Donna some comfort during his final weeks.

When Your Patients' Triumphs Become Your Triumphs and Their Setbacks Become Extremely Personal

By Kevin Traille, CRNA, DNP

> I solemnly pledge myself before God and in the presence of this assembly, to pass my life in purity and to practice my profession faithfully. I will abstain from whatever is deleterious and mischievous, and will not take or knowingly administer any harmful drug. I will do all in my power to maintain and elevate the standard of my profession, and will hold in confidence all personal matters committed to my keeping and all family affairs coming to my knowledge in the practice of my calling. With loyalty will I endeavor to aid the physician in his work, and devote myself to the welfare of those committed to my care. (Gretter, 1893, p. 1)

The Florence Nightingale oath has been a staple in guiding new nurses along their path in this journey called Nursing. It is a basic tenet for registered nurses (RNs) to adhere to when there is uncertainty. At its core, this oath should have been a guiding light for Grace during her time of need. At this point, this principle has failed to consider the evolution of nursing as a whole. The role and scope of an RN have grown throughout the years, and the advent of the advanced practice RN has only compounded the inadequacy of the creed. If we look closely into Grace's experience, it is evident that her "loyalties" between physician and patient are ultimately tested.

Safe staffing ratios have plagued hospitals across the country for years. This issue predated the COVID-19 pandemic. The effects of disproportionate staffing ratios can be felt throughout the spectrum of nursing. Staffing ratios can directly correlate with nurse satisfaction, attrition, and burnout (Shah et al., 2021). Grace had an inadequate orientation process that benefitted neither her nor the care that she could render to her patients. New-graduate nurses have the daunting task of implementing theoretical concepts into clinical practice. They require adequate training with all necessary equipment under the direct supervision of a senior colleague to optimize their under-standing of various treatment modalities. This daily interaction between a preceptor and a new-graduate nurse is a foundation for that nurse's future practice. They are acquiring the tools necessary to be a vital portion of the interdisciplinary team.

Grace shares a story of how a lack of preparation created a stress-filled environment, resulting in an unwavering visceral response. The stressors of COVID-19 only enhanced this feeling for anyone involved in direct patient care. Roles were altered during this period of uncertainty. Fear of the unknown, amongst other variables, led to a mass exodus of many healthcare providers, including RNs. The effects of this acute high-volume transition have yet to be fully understood (Cole et al., 2021). Those who continue to work in the hospital setting can see and feel the immediate aftermath, and stories similar to Grace's echo through healthcare institu-tions nationwide. It is important to highlight that Grace used her education to take on a preceptor role about which she had doubts. She continued to persevere and be an advocate for her orientee and her patients. As you read this, *imagine yourself in Grace's scenario*. You may one day be faced with similar situations, and you may not feel ready for the responsibility. Understand that this feeling is normal, and your drive to be a compas-sionate advocate can be enough to get you through. This feeling of unease represents a healthy fear because you understand the magnitude of your role in your patients' well-being. This feeling doesn't depend on the practice environment, resources, or years of service. This feeling isn't crippling as much as it is humbling. In the right dosage, it serves as an autonomous check-and-balance system. It allows you to keep your patient at the fore-front of your decisions.

Grace's ascension through the nursing ranks on her unit resulted from necessity due to high nursing turnover and inadequate replacement of lost staff. This cycle prematurely catapults relatively new nurses to the forefront of leadership positions because they become the most tenured by default. The nurse isn't at fault for this situation; instead, it is a direct result of sys-temic institutional failures. Taking on new roles in any line of work can be exhilarating in the beginning, especially when these positions are achieved organically. In instances in which you are thrust into a position, it is easy to feel loneliness, resentment, and anxiety. There is something to be said about learning on the job, but it is not always beneficial for your growth and development. Becoming a charge nurse can usually entail making assignments for the unit, facilitating coordination of interdisciplinary teams, managing care team family conflicts, and rendering care to your specific patient assignment. This job can be difficult and require a wealth of knowledge to be done effectively. For these reasons, it is understandable why Grace felt this rush of emotions when asked to take on these challenges continuously. It opened up a great deal of newfound knowledge but, at the same time, offered up a plethora of critical thinking issues requiring remedies on a daily basis. Grace handled this new role with poise, and although it was initially met with uncertainty, it helped shape her into the RN whom she is today.

In any hospital unit, it is possible to find Charlie. My saying this refers to patients who are relegated to lengthy admissions or are in your care for extended periods of time. The relationship has the potential to evolve from a nurse-patient dynamic to that of genuine friendship. Their triumphs become our triumphs, and their setbacks become extremely personal. It is commonplace for nurses to request ongoing assignments and, ultimately, become their patients' primary nurse. Roles such as these should never be undertaken lightly, as the emotional burden can be exhausting. This sentiment pales in comparison to being able to witness your Charlie conquer an insurmountable obstacle and graduate from your care. As we can see in Grace's experience, the road to recovery may never be actualized, but it doesn't diminish the roles you played as a caregiver and an advocate for your patient.

Grace found herself in a difficult position when having to receive a new graduate, a complex patient, and a fresh transplant patient all in one shift. The voicing of her concerns was absolutely appropriate, and in some institutions, you can go as far as filling out a protest form documenting the risk to patient safety. It is important to note that this does not absolve you of your patient care responsibilities; however, it chronicles the deficiencies in the institution's practices. It would have been an amazing learning experience for the new-graduate nurse had they been assigned an individual assignment that allowed Grace to explain and demonstrate at a reasonable pace. It would have also been beneficial to have a designated preceptor for the new graduate so a sense of familiarity could be built between preceptor and orientee. Grace was being stretched thin, and the charge nurse's role in this situation is to handle all aforementioned responsibilities but also to protect the staff from potentially harmful events. Recognize that your nurse expresses genuine concern and facilitate an assignment where everyone can succeed. Situations such as these can contribute to premature burnout and apathy towards the nursing profession.

When we graduate and enter the nursing profession, our instinctual goal is to help patients survive their acute health episodes. It is difficult to encounter situations in which, against our best efforts, we are unable to accomplish a positive outcome. This burden is further compounded when you witness your patient's fight for an extended period. Grace and her fellow nurses became advocates for Charlie when they expressed concern to the ethics committee. The committee should act as an independent body that allows staff to voice concerns without fear of retaliation. If their purpose is skewed by their inability to govern impartially, they fail to serve any useful purpose.

Education is key to empowering your patient and their families. Although it may be difficult to deliver news that may be speculative about a patient's prognosis, it may be easier to educate them on what normal timelines usually resemble. In addition, take the time to let them know what medications they are receiving and their purpose in health promotion. Make them aware of dosage changes and let them know how this correlates to their overall plan. When you arm your patients and their families with knowledge, that is also a form of advocacy. This education allows them to ask appropriate questions during rounds and take a more proactive approach to interacting with their care team.

Grace became an extended family member for Donna and Charlie. The memories that Grace facilitated will stay with that family forever. Moments such as Charlie uttering *"I love you"* represent instances that cannot be quantified in terms of how impactful they are to families. Although Grace felt like she wasn't seen by leadership, she was seen by Charlie's family. The part of Grace's testimony that resonated the most with me was allowing Charlie to speak to Donna over the phone. As a certified registered nurse anesthetist (CRNA), I had an opportunity to manage airways on a COVID-19 team during the height of the pandemic. As a result, I found myself tasked with intubating compromised patients on an almost hourly basis. As I began to do this task at a higher frequency, I inquired with patients about whether there was anyone they would like to call before we started the procedure. In almost every case, there was a grateful family member receiving this all-too-important phone call. For some people, this would be the last phone call they would ever have with their loved ones. As a person who had the opportunity to witness these phone calls, I was honored to have been a part of these moments. I will never know what it meant to the person on the other end of the phone, but I knew that in that moment, my patient was extremely thankful.

Understand that everything Grace went through made her who she is today. This experience has allowed her to identify what she is looking for from an organization and enlightened her about what she wants in her professional career. As she continues along her journey, she can stay true to her values and effect change in any environment. Given the changes in roles as an RN across the healthcare and advanced practice spectrum, it is necessary for an update to our creed, with my suggestions for an emphasis on the final portion:

> With loyalty will I hold physicians and interdisciplinary teams accountable to optimal patient-centered care. I will devote myself to the welfare of those committed to my care, utilizing all acquired knowledge and my full scope of practice. I will ensure that all patients in my care are seen, have a voice, and are advocated for at all times.

By Dr. Kevin Traille

'Why Didn't You Tell Me It Was Going to Be This Hard?'

By Linda Roney, EdD, RN-BC, FAAN

We open this casebook with Grace's story as a new-graduate nurse in a SICU specializing in organ transplants. As a nursing professor who remains in contact with many of her former students, I have been asked on more than a few occasions, usually when someone faces an unexpected challenge at work, "*Why didn't you tell me it was going to be this hard?*" Although the patient acuity on the unit was challenging, there were other significant issues that also challenged Grace as a newer nurse. In addition to being a nursing professor, I have continued to work as a bedside nurse and often bring back stories from my clinical practice to class. Most often, the cases I have presented speak to the challenges that the patient faced to help reinforce the patient's clinical diagnosis and nursing care with the hope that a piece of the story might help my students remember something for the National Council Licensure Examination.

Until now, I did not think to share my experiences of how I dealt with my reactions to caring for a child who had life-threatening injuries from physical abuse; I focused my story on the actual nursing care of this patient. I have described the care of critically ill patients to my students but never shared my experiences of feeling helpless when, despite the precise and perfect actions of our entire team, we are unable to restart the child's failed heart. I never shared that there is nothing to prepare you for one of the worst meetings you can have in your life when you meet in a tiny room with the attending physician and social worker as we share the devastating news with the child's grieving parents: "*Your child has died.*" No one tells you in nursing school what you are supposed to do at the end of the shift like this when you are mentally and physically exhausted, and you come home and your partner or family does not understand what is wrong with you. In our day-to-day work, we commonly encounter extremes of human lived experience, substantially more so than the average person may witness—if they see any at all—throughout their lifetime (Roney & Acri, 2018). We hope that through our collective voice and transparency, we will share stories in this casebook that empower you with examples to amplify your impact in your nursing practice and your work-life integration.

I absolutely *love* our nursing profession and want new nurses to feel empowered to be leaders, which is required in today's practice. Your commitment to learning to be a nurse requires tremendous commitment and dedication to your studies and to your patients, which can, at times, make it challenging to consistently see the big picture of how critical your role as a leader is outside the day-to-day tasks that you were striving to master as a student.

Prelicensure nursing curricula are required to prepare graduates to "develop a capacity for leadership" (American Association of Colleges of Nursing, 2021, p. 54), and nursing programs across the country are innovating ways best to support our students and graduates in this goal. New nurses often hear the term *nurse leader* and think of a nurse manager or an administrator. Perhaps this is incredibly challenging because, throughout nursing school, you were challenged to pick the best answer to a question that sometimes had only one answer. The American Nurses Association (2023) defines a nurse leader by "their actions and not always a position of authority." Throughout this book, we will be sharing examples of new nurses developing leadership skills by taking action. Sometimes these examples of leadership are highly visible, or, in the cases of Grace and her care of Charlie and Kevin in facilitating calls to family members before intubating their patients who had COVID-19, only those who are directly involved in the situation are aware but exemplify nursing leadership at its best. Table 2.1 outlines Grace's specific actions to demonstrate competency in the American Association of Colleges of Nursing (AACN) essentials' (2021) domains 2 and 10 competencies and subcompetencies.

TABLE 11.1 **Examples of Domain 2: Person-Centered Care and Domain 10: Personal, Professional, and Leadership Development in This Exemplar**

Domain 2: Person-Centered Care	
2.1 Engage with the individual in establishing a caring relationship.	Grace demonstrated qualities of empathy, compassion, and mutual respect with Charlie and his mother. She saw her patient as an individual and was thoughtful about making memories for him and his family.
2.2 Communicate effectively with individuals.	Grace demonstrated relationship-centered care with Charlie and his family. She considered their values as individuals and as a family to give them the information in a timely way when it counted the most using multiple communication modes. While she noted that she did not receive formal training in conducting sensitive conversations, she was successful in doing so, leading with emotional intelligence

(Continued)

TABLE 11.1 (Continued)

Domain 10: Personal, Professional, and Leadership Development	
10.2 Demonstrate a spirit of inquiry that fosters flexibility and pro-fessional maturity.	Grace identified a mentor to support her professional growth. She reflected on the situation of caring for Charlie for several months and considered multiple perspectives. Despite it being sooner than had she expected, Grace expanded her knowledge in the roles of charge nurse and preceptor.
10.3 Develop capacity for leadership.	Grace demonstrated leadership behaviors in all the challenges she faced while working with Charlie. She demonstrated self-efficacy in her roles as charge nurse and preceptor and tried as often as she could to use available resources when encountering new and challenging situations. Grace verbalized her leadership role in several practice issues, including the ethical challenges.

Grace's first position presented her with challenges in many different dimensions.

She describes so many changes in her first two years of practice—four months of orientation on her unit with the highest-acuity patients to "broaden her experience," a patient population change due to the second wave of the COVID-19 pandemic, and then the return of critically ill transplant patients with less experienced staff to care for the patients as many of the experienced staff leaving their position in the ICU. These changes could not have been anticipated, yet Grace worked as hard as she could to be flexible, adaptable, and open to continuously learning while still making decisions to provide holistic, family-centered care. I had the opportunity to ask Grace about what experiences prepared her to care for Charlie. Grace was at the end of her junior year of nursing school in March 2020 at the start of the COVID-19 shutdown, when she returned home to continue her nursing studies remotely and work as a nursing assistant:

> I feel that I was able to practice my empathetic communication with the family members who were separated from their loved ones while working in dementia care. In April 2020, we had our first resident test positive (for COVID-19) and immediately locked down our floor. Most of our residents ended up passing, and we transitioned to being an end-of-life COVID facility. I had to talk with families through windows and help them FaceTime during their loved one's final moments. Going through all that taught me always to consider the family perspective during a health crisis and involve them in all health discussions. (Grace Rankin personal communication, April 20, 2024)

New Nurses as Leaders

One of the first skills that new nurses need to develop is situational leadership, which is the ability to take the lead in patient care as appropriate to their scope and role and demonstrate their ability to be a leader and follower on a team (AACN, 2024). This aligns well with being patient- and family-centered when working on a multidisciplinary team. As we have read in the stories Grace and Kevin describe, they were challenged to deploy authentic leadership in challenging situations and rose to the occasion. As a new nurse, Grace was a leader on her team and an advocate for Charlie. Many nurses emerging into practice worry about knowing all the psychomotor (hands-on) skills of being a nurse in the unit where they will practice, sometimes thinking that the interpersonal reactions will be easier than the hands-on care of your patients. Your clinical education foundation has prepared you to use some of the equipment and complete some of the tasks that you may encounter in your first position, but not all of them. For example, it is not possible to know how to use every possible IV or enteral feeding pump that is being used at every medical center in the United States, but having learned one or several types throughout your nursing program empowers you with the tools to learn how to use a new one if needed. You understand there is an "on" button somewhere; there is a process for programming the device and administering the medication or feeding. I am not minimizing the technology we use in our everyday practice of caring for patients, but rather, I am sharing with you an understanding that you have the foundation to learn how to use new equipment at work.

As a new grad, Grace quickly learned to use life-saving technology such as specialized IV pumps to administer lifesaving medications, ventilators, and CRRT. There are written protocols for using this equipment that you can access, and hopefully, each person on the unit uses them uniformly. Many of these things are very complex, but the situations are also challenging because you usually use them in stressful conditions in which your patient is very sick. When the pressure is high, the potential that the emotional temperature of the multidisciplinary team may elevate is significantly increased, causing a greater chance for miscommunication. Later, in Chapter 5, you will learn about best practices for creating positive team communication and dynamics that will positively affect your influence as a leader and, ultimately, your patients' care.

PRN (PLEASE READ NOW)

"More experienced nurses must take the time to show those who are new and less experienced the most effective ways of being an exceptional nurse at the bedside, in the boardroom, and everywhere in between. Leadership skills must be learned and mastered over time" (Institute of Medicine, 2011, p. 228).

To develop skills in situational leadership, emerging and new nurses must first develop *situational awareness*, which can be easily defined as "anticipating needs by "knowing what is going on, why it is occurring, and what is likely to happen next" (Swift, 2023, para. 1). Situational awareness contributes to excellent nursing care by detecting patient safety threats, preventing medical errors, and ensuring patient well-being (Avalos et al., 2021). It also helps to practice mindfulness to decrease stress and increase attention, empathy, and presence with patients and families (Penque, 2019). Grace had excellent situational awareness while at work, yet her concerns were minimized by more experienced nurses in leadership roles. When she expressed concern that she received one day of training to use CRRT and then was responsible for the patient's care for the next three days, she was offered the support of a resource nurse who might be available to answer questions. When she shared her concerns with the educator that she would be taking this on while precepting a new nurse on her third week of orientation, and then they were given a second patient (a fresh kidney transplant), the educator did not want to change the assignment. They felt that the second patient was a great learning experience for the orienting nurse, yet they lacked the situational awareness that this placed Grace under unnecessary stress and potentially put Charlie and the new patient at risk. Additionally, a nurse caring for Charlie brought concerns to the ethics board, but their concerns were not addressed to her satisfaction.

Despite having others who did not share her mental model in all the challenges she described to us, she persisted in putting her patients first and displayed tremendous, meaningful leadership. Grace excelled in her situational leadership in caring for Charlie and his mother, ensuring family-centered care for their holistic needs. The nursing team planned Charlie's birthday celebration on the unit, and Grace gave his mother the best possible gift: She facilitated a video call during which Charlie used the speaking valve on his trach for the first time and said, *"I love you."* There was no order in the patient's chart to do this. At the height of the COVID-19 pandemic, Kevin shared with us that he would ask patients whether there was anyone they would like to call before he intubated them, knowing there was likely an uncertain outcome for them. There was no protocol for this. Grace and Kevin used their intellect, experience, and compassionate heart to assess the situation, knowing what would happen next for these patients and their families. These are examples of situational leadership and clinical leadership at its best. They observed environmental cues, understood what they meant, predicted how the situation may evolve (Weller et al., 2024), and then took patient- and family-centered action. We all manifest our leadership differently in practice, but bringing ourselves to these situations with authenticity and compassion makes us nursing leaders.

YOU MATTER: LEADERSHIP IN THE MOMENT

Grace and Kevin provide excellent examples of situational leadership in new, uncharted situations. While Grace's advocacy was not always met with the response for which she had hoped, she preserved and kept speaking up for what she knew was right. Her voice matters; as we have seen in this case, her leadership immeasurably affected Charlie and his mother's life.

Book Club Questions

1. Have you observed nurses providing situational leadership in the clinical setting? What was the situation and its outcome?
2. What are some barriers to situational awareness, especially in busy clinical situations?
3. What role does technology have in supporting or distracting nurses from situational awareness?
4. How can communication and teamwork among the interdisciplinary team support situational awareness?

About This Chapter's Authors

Grace Rankin, BSN, RN, CCRN

Grace was born and raised in a suburb of Boston. She graduated from Fairfield University's Marion Peckham Egan School of Nursing and Health Studies in 2021. Her nursing experience began as an emergency room tech in spring 2020, during the height of COVID-19. Since graduation, Grace has worked in a transplant-surgical ICU and medical ICU in Washington, D.C., and Boston. She has taken on charge and preceptor roles and taught her facility's CRRT class. On the side, Grace also works as a home health nurse for at-home ventilator patients. When she is not working, she loves to travel, run marathons, and find new restaurants.

Kevin Traille, CRNA, DNP, APRN

With a 14-year career in health care, including the past seven as a CRNA, Dr. Kevin Traille has found his true calling. His journey began in finance, but a desire for more meaningful work led him to nursing. This career change has allowed him to positively affect countless lives and balance his professional aspirations with his children's basketball and dance commitments. Kevin's passion for travel and cultural exploration has deepened his empathy for patients from diverse backgrounds. He hopes his experiences resonate with the reader and inspire them on their own nursing journey.

References

American Association of Colleges of Nursing. (2024). *Leadership concept.* https://www.aacnnursing.org/developing-nurse-well-being-and-leadership-tool-kit/tool-kit/leadership-concept

American Association of Colleges of Nursing. (2021). *The essentials: Core competencies for professional nursing education.* https://www.aacnnursing.org/Portals/0/PDFs/Publications/Essentials-2021.pdf

American Nurses Association. (2023). *Leadership in nursing: Qualities and why it matters. ANA Nursing Resource Hub.* https://www.nursingworld.org/content-hub/resources/nursing-leadership/leadership-in-nursing/

Avalos, J., Roy, D., Asan, O., & Zhang, Y. (2021). *The influential factors on nurses' situational awareness in inpatient settings: A literature review. Human Factors in Healthcare, 1,* 1–9. https://doi.org/10.1016/j.hfh.2022.100006

Cole, A., Ali, H., Ahmed, A., Hamasha, M., & Jordan, S. (2021). Identifying patterns of turnover intention among Alabama frontline nurses in hospital settings during the COVID-19 pandemic. *Journal of Multidisciplinary Healthcare, 14,* 1783–1794. https://doi.org/10.2147/JMDH.S308397

Gretter, L. E. (1893). *Florence Nightingale pledge.* American Nurses Association. https://s3.amazonaws.com/nursing-network/production/attachments/28811/original/FlorenceNightingalePledge-2015.pdf?2015

Penque, S. (2019). Mindfulness to promote nurses' well-being. *Nursing Management, 50*(5), 38–44. https://doi.org/10.1097/01.NUMA.0000557621.42684.c4

Rankin, G. (personal communication, April 20, 2024).

Roney, L. N., & Acri, M. C. (2018). The cost of caring: An exploration of compassion fatigue, compassion satisfaction, and job satisfaction in pediatric nurses. *Journal of Pediatric Nursing, 40,* 74–80. https://doi.org/10.1016/j.pedn.2018.01.016

Shah, M. K., Gandrakota, N., Cimiotti, J. P., Ghose, N., Moore, M., & Ali, M. K. (2021). Prevalence of and factors associated with nurse burnout in the US. *JAMA Network Open, 4*(2), e2036469. https://doi.org/10.1001/jamanetworkopen.2020.36469

Swift, H. (2023, October). Encouraging situational awareness in nursing students. Wolters Kluwer. https://www.wolterskluwer.com/en/expert-insights/encouraging-situational-awareness-in-nursing-students

Weller, J. M., Mahajan, R., Fahey-Williams, K., & Webster, C. S. (2024). Teamwork matters: Team situation awareness to build high-performing healthcare teams, a narrative review. *British Journal of Anaesthesia, 132*(4), 771–778. https://doi.org/10.1016/j.bja.2023.12.035

CHAPTER 12

The Power of Self-Care

Kayla Beckman, BSN, RN; Teresa Fuller, MSN, RN, NEA-BC, CPXP; and Linda Roney, EdD, RN-BC, CPEN, CNE, FAAN

Learning Goals

1. Identify and describe common barriers to effective self-care for nurses during a shift.
2. Understand the value of the chief nursing officer's (CNO) role in caring for those who care for patients.
3. Analyze the concept of self-care in nursing and design three personalized, evidence-based strategies to incorporate into your daily routine to enhance well-being.
4. Apply the Next-Generation Care Plan to create your nurses' wellness strategy.

Sleeping During the Day and Working During the Night

By Kayla Beckman, BSN, RN

The time was 1 p.m., the middle of the afternoon, a time when most people were halfway through their workday, counting down the hours until they could call it a day and head home. I, however, was trying to adjust to this new routine that night-shift nurses called "normal," altering my circadian rhythm to something that was extremely far from ordinary and considered unhealthy. However, as I quickly learned, this was the expected routine of a night-shift nurse: sleeping during the day and working during the night.

Rewind to three months prior: my graduation day. I vividly remember that day and its excitement. It was a celebration and recognition of the effort and hard work I had put in for the past four years. Walking across that stage and being handed my diploma was something that seemed impossible when I was in the thick of nursing school. I was extremely fortunate for the education I received, the professors who believed in and educated me, and the clinical opportunities I had at world-renowned hospitals and facilities. Those early-morning drives to clinical, late nights spent studying, and endless care plans were all worth it. To have the letters *BSN* next to my name was something that I was and always will be extremely proud of, and I was excited for the opportunities ahead. Words alone are not enough to describe the feelings associated with the 48 hours after taking the National Council Licensure Examination (NCLEX) and waiting for the results. Having graduated from a rigorous nursing program and having spent endless hours studying, I was more than prepared, but the pit in my stomach was an unmatched feeling. After seeing the word *PASS* on my screen, I finally breathed a sigh of relief.

Although I had just passed the boards and was a licensed nurse, there was still a large amount of fear and anxiety associated with the start of my first nursing job. In the spring of my senior year of nursing school, I accepted a job on a cardiovascular stepdown unit at a level one trauma center. Now, some people would have thought I would not have these jittery first-job feelings since I had worked on the unit as a patient care associate (PCA). Arguments were that I knew the unit, the people who worked there, the values of the hospital, and even my manager. However, the roles of PCA and registered nurse (RN) are entirely different, and the thoughts of the unknown and transition scared me. With the help of the new-graduate RN program, my coworkers, nursing manager and educator, and unit orientation, I had an extremely supportive transition.

Fast-forward to being several weeks into my nursing career and journey. I was hopeful that the anxiety and worrying would lessen. Soon, I learned that I was naive to think this. What I did not understand was that the worrying and anxiety would present in different ways and situations as compared to my past experiences. I was quickly introduced to the term *preshift anxiety*. *Preshift anxiety* can be described as anticipatory fear and worries that nurses experience in the lead-up to their shift. It ranges in severity and affects everyone—both new and seasoned nurses—in different ways. As a new nurse, my preshift anxiety was at an all-time high. I had so many worries and fears when I set foot in the hospital. A lot of self-doubt and many negative thoughts ran through my head. Unfortunately, as my orientation progressed and I was exposed to different experiences and situations on my unit, my preshift anxiety seemed to worsen, leading to my questioning my career choice and dreading going to work.

It was 2 a.m., and all was calm in the unit as patients were sleeping and nurses were charting. I took a sip of my water for what I believed was the first time that night when the telemetry monitor alarmed. Upon turning my eyes, I saw a red alarm and rushed over to see an asystole alarm on my patient. I and several other nurses rushed into the room to find the patient unresponsive to my voice and touch; however, not more than five seconds later, he came to spontaneously, and his heart rate was back in the 60s. My heart was racing as the patient was looking at us with a confused look as to why so many people were in his room in the middle of the night. I returned to the desk, and just as I was about to sit down, a bed alarm started going off. I rushed down to my other patient's room to find him trying to escape out of bed, ripping all his wires off, and attempting to pull his intravenous line out. He was extremely confused and disoriented.

Several hours later in the morning, I received a call from an angry and frustrated family member of a patient. They were mad about the provider's plan of care and the team's lack of communication. I provided empathetic listening to the family while taking the brunt of it simultaneously. Unfortunately, this was not the first phone call with verbal abuse I had dealt with. I wanted the call to end just like I wanted the clock to hit 7 a.m. with the day shift coming in. Suddenly, I realized I was awake and in my bed with the clock reading 5 p.m. Two hours, and I would be getting report for the night. The horrible shift was over, but it never really happened; *it was all a dream*. At that moment, I realized a pattern: The majority of dreams that I had while sleeping were work-related and reliving all the bad situations that had happened to me or scenarios I fear could happen. Dreams of making a medication error, forgetting to complete my charting, having patients who do not like me, fear of being verbally or even physically abused while working—and the list went on. My love for nursing and the career I had just started dwindling quickly. But I was just a new nurse; how could I make this preshift anxiety go away?

As a new graduate, my preshift anxiety was already at an all-time high due to many factors, including being new to the field and having very little to no experience at all. In general, preshift anxiety leads to many things going through RNs' mind, including second-guessing their identity as nurses, their career choices, and even becoming resentful regarding work. Unaddressed preshift anxiety leads to an increase in burnout and compassion fatigue. For these reasons, healthcare professionals must be aware of ways to combat this issue to create and foster a positive work environment and career.

It took several months and many restless sleeps before realizing how I would start to combat this awful feeling. The trick—which sounds simple but is extremely effective—is self-care. I quickly saw a correlation between incorporating self-care into my routine and a decrease in preshift anxiety. When I learned to focus on myself on my days off or when doing minor things before a shift, I was less anxious and worried. I now have many tools in my self-care toolbox that address my physical, emotional, and social well-being. On my days off, I find myself regularly exercising as it releases my "happy hormones," leading to an elevated mood and reduced anxiety. I enjoy cooking and baking, which I have always found joy in; however, it also serves as a way to meal-prep for a stretch of shifts. I also try to meet up with friends often and discuss topics unrelated to work. Most importantly, I surround myself with the people I love the most: my family. Whether we have board game nights or family dinners or simply watch a movie at home, I am filled with happiness and reminded of how fortunate I am for my family.

It is just as important that I partake in self-care activities on days when I work to get into the right mindset. Journaling has been an extremely effective means of self-care for me. I have found that reflecting on my feelings before and after a shift has led to less personal and professional stress, improved my understanding of myself, and helped me gain control of my emotions. Meditating and listening to my favorite playlist on my way to work have also been effective.

Why is taking care of you so important? Is it not my job to care for others? As new nurses, it is easy to get caught up in our main role—caring for others. Throughout nursing school, we are taught ways of caring for others. However, it is equally important to care for ourselves. What new nurses need to understand is that caring for ourselves is directly related to the care we provide to patients. When partaking in self-care, nurses report feeling enhanced job satisfaction, feeling better about themselves, and being better equipped to handle the challenges and demands of the job. This, in turn, leads to reduced absenteeism and callouts, more compassionate and effective care, and decreased burnout rates. It also improves the quality of care and promotes patient safety.

Now, almost two years into my nursing practice, an essential aspect that I learned that I clearly needed to understand upon graduating and beginning my career is that you can help others only if you help yourself first. Self-care is essential to maintaining the ability to care for others effectively, especially during the first few years of practice. Making time to care for yourself is critical to a job that requires caring for others. Without self-care, preshift anxiety is hard to combat and leads to burnout, causing nurses to feel mental fatigue and emotionally drained, which result in their moving away from the bedside.

'Stepping Out!'

By Teresa Fuller, MSN, RN, NEA-BC, CPXP

When I read Kayla's story, I was reminded of my novice nurse journey. I was fortunate to complete my undergraduate nursing degree at the University of Pennsylvania (Penn). My parents developed and implemented what they called "the One-Third Plan" to afford what was, in 1994, the most prestigious and rigorous, number one–ranked nursing school in the country. This meant that my parents would pay for one-third, one-third

I would pay for through loans, and one-third would be paid for by scholarship. I applied for many scholarships, and after many phone calls, Penn offered me an extraordinary scholarship that paid for two years at the Ivy League university. Rita Hillman, the donor for the endowed scholarship I received, was a patient cared for by Penn nurses while recovering at a New York City (NYC) medical center. She envisioned creating an ongoing program that requires Penn nursing graduates to work in NYC hospitals after graduation.

As part of the conditions of my scholarship, I did my senior year clinical rotation in the surgical intensive care unit (ICU) in NYC, traveling back and forth between classes in Philadelphia and clinicals in NYC each week. My clinical group would sleep over in the medical dorms—we had our own suite! After two days of intense clinical experiences and usually some fun in Manhattan, we were on the train back to Philadelphia in time for classes on Monday. I was fortunate to love the surgical ICU and the clinical team and was hired for my first nursing job, directly into the unit—very much like Kayla. I went through a nurse residency program and learned more about being a critical care nurse. With the help of some senior nurses, I was able to successfully come off orientation and start my career as a novice ICU nurse.

I vividly remember feeling butterflies in my stomach each morning and feeling a little bit like an imposter: *Did everyone really think that I could do this?* To get past those feelings of dread, I became so focused on my work that I did not participate in the camaraderie with the other nurses and interns around me. It was well into my second year as a nurse when I finally realized that there existed culture, friendships, and teamwork in my environment. I remember one intern saying hello to me and saying, *"Oh, you are so nice now."* I remember looking at him, puzzled. *Was I not nice before?* He mentioned that I was so intent on caring for my patients that he had never seen me smile, laugh, or talk to anyone. Yikes! The intensity of the work caused others to perceive me as unfriendly and unhappy. I was not myself at all. Rather, I was, for a brief time, someone else. Trying to get through the day and keep my patients safe made me so intent and intense that I was not my true, outgoing self. Not knowing everything I needed to know in the clinical space made me unsure of myself and focused and unfriendly rather than open and accepting.

Beyond the technical aspects of ICU nursing and the checklist of daily care items for my patients, there was a level of intensity that, to me, required a focus beyond what had been required or developed in my training in nursing school. At the beginning of my career, to ensure that I was doing everything I could to take care of my patients, I found that I couldn't do it all. I was stressed about the interactions occurring with difficult patients and families. Especially difficult for me at the beginning of my career was supporting those family members who acted out or behaved badly while still providing intensive care to their loved ones. I needed help with the social support that was expected of me for the patients' family. I quickly found my resources in our Patient Advocacy Team, and they lovingly did that supportive work so that I could continue caring for my patients.

Equally stressful were the emotional aspects of the job; caring for patients who were dying was not what I thought my strong suit would be, rather this part came easily to me. Reflecting on this ease, I realize how each of us is a different nurse. We have different ways of knowing and finding ease or difficulty in certain parts of our work. I was able to easily transition from performing critical care for a patient to performing palliative, supportive care for the patient and their family. Ensuring a peaceful, comfortable death, one in which the patient was the center of care, was even more natural for me than the technical critical care that I provided to my patients.

In one circumstance, a patient named Lynn decided she wanted to turn off her automatic defibrillator and say goodbye to her family. She was awake and alert, making that decision for herself. I was amazed by her calm demeanor and her careful but insistent decision. Her family disagreed but acquiesced. I ensured that everyone was notified, and the family descended on the unit to say goodbye. Lynn's strength was incredible. She waited for her last niece to come in and then looked up at her family and me and said goodbye. It was an amazing tribute to her life. Her family meant everything to her, and they were all around her as she died. Albeit difficult and sad, these moments shaped my early learning as a nurse.

We have ways of knowing that go beyond acquiring knowledge. Those deeper ways of knowing help us to help others. The domains of nursing practice describe the nurse in a helping role, stating that "nurses are often trained to believe that they are most effective when doing for a patient." Several nurses noted, however, the essential importance of "just being with a patient" (Benner, 1984, p. 57). In fact, Benner found through interviews with nurses that they "need to allow patients to ventilate their feelings, often without speaking at all themselves" (Benner, 1984, p. 58). Nurses have an innate understanding that to know what is best for their patients is to help them figure it out for themselves. By keeping their minds open, being present, and listening to their patients, nurses can assist their patients in gaining an understanding of what is happening to them and support the healing process. You can learn and grow together by taking that leap, trusting in your more profound knowing, and sharing stories with your patients. Through these experiences in which I was open and, at times, vulnerable, I grew as both a nurse and a person.

As I developed my knowledge in nursing, similar to Kayla, I suffered through some long shifts (including night shifts) when I seemed to take care of everyone except myself. I remember agonizing about this with my mother, telling her that I barely had time to use the bathroom, never mind eat a healthy meal. I worked 12 hours straight to complete my two-patient critical care assignment. Things were so crazy that even stopping to use the bathroom was not an option. My mother, ever the problem-solver, set out to solve this problem for me. She suggested that I pack a healthy snack in a plastic baggie and put the baggie in the pocket of my scrubs. Then she suggested that I keep a bottle of water handy in the unit with me and take frequent swigs from it (this was the start of the water bottle age; it was a new thing to walk around with a bottle of water all the time back in the late '90s). In doing so, I would need to use the bathroom more frequently (not a bad thing), and I could eat my snack quickly while walking back from the bathroom. So, I did as she suggested. We used to shout, *"Stepping out!"* when we left the unit, alerting the other nurses that we were headed out and would be momentarily leaving our patients. It was my cue for wellness. That was the only thing I did for myself for those 12 hours for those first few years of my career. That equated to wellness during my novice early nursing career.

Later, as the butterflies went away and I became more confident, I joined a gym and would run the two blocks to the gym on my lunch break (we could get an hour for lunch—shocking!). I did a quick workout, showered, and ate my healthy snack while walking back to the hospital. My unit and its nurses supported each other to allow for this well-being. We would cover for each other to ensure that everyone, when able, received time away from their patient assignment to eat, relax, or exercise. We held each other accountable, ensuring that not only did we take the break but also that each other's patient assignments were covered so that we could have an uninterrupted break. Most likely, we were ahead of our time in this regard, but it happened because of a great team that cared deeply for each other.

On the days I was off from work, I would seek out tiny bits of nature in the cement city. I would find little nooks with green spaces between two skyscrapers and sit outside, sip a coffee, read a book, and meditate. In those moments of exercise, meditation, and nature, I could relax and destress from the physical and emotional drain of critical care nursing.

My career turned toward leadership when I finally moved out of the city. I realized that I wanted something more out of my job: to care for the people taking care of our patients. I started as an ICU manager and, from there, continued to find additional opportunities, which culminated in a chief nursing officer position (CNO). Now, I truly get to care for those who take such good care of our patients. As a CNO, my perspective and lens have shifted toward caring for caregivers. This can sometimes be more stressful and harder than taking care of patients.

Caring for those who care for patients can be overwhelming. Not only are the colleagues under your care, professionally and in terms of their well-being, but you are also directly responsible for all the care they provide to our patients. This level of responsibility is very daunting and, at times, stressful. As a CNO, I deal with multiple layers of leadership. I must navigate the waters of operations and finance to ensure that nurses have the physical supplies and human capital they need to get the job done. Bringing forward arguments for what nurses need at the bedside can be challenging, given that there is an immense need for more understanding of what nurses do for our patients. Explaining that nurses provide the utmost safety, quality, and experience for our patients and their families is one of the most important things I do every day. While the nurses may realize the effect they have on their patients and their safety, they may not realize or be aware of the intensity with which their nurse leaders fight for them on a daily basis. Ensuring the nurses' voice is heard at the executive table is extremely important to me. I do this work to support the nurses and the care they provide to their patients every day.

While I bring nurses' voices forward, I also must ensure a healthy work environment for our nurses to work in. I am always looking for ways to get more care back to the bedside, whether advocating for shorter documentation or more human resources to assist with direct patient care. I make sure that the nurses' voice is heard by directly communicating and hearing their voice through town hall meetings, rounding, and shadowing experiences. This level of visibility is rewarding but can be as exhausting as a 12-hour shift in an ICU. I know that everyone is watching me and listening to what I say. That level of vulnerability and transparency leaves me open and exposed. I am also in a prime position to let the nurses know that I care about them and am their voice at the executive table.

I find myself perfectly placed in the CNO role to ensure the well-being and wellness of myself and the nurses in my care. Supporting the nurses in caring for themselves is as important as leading by example. I advocate for nurses to be able to take lunch breaks, knowing how important mine were when I was at the bedside. I advocate for them to have the schedule they want that matches their lifestyle. I advocate for them to check in with themselves daily, monitor their stress level before they leave, and make sure that they transition healthily to home.

To take care of others, you first need to take care of yourself. As Kayla described in her story, as a new nurse, two years into her career, she realized that *"self-care is an essential aspect of maintaining the ability to care for others effectively."* Some acknowledge this fundamental truth about wellness, and Florence Nightingale herself worked to uphold this truth with her nursing students. Nightingale, in her letter to the nurses of the Nightingale School at St. Thomas Hospital on May 23, 1873, describes a similar vein of the importance of self-care when she details the school's new plan to give *"more time and leisure to less tired bodies"* (Nightingale, 2009, p. 18). The school incorporated two afternoons off from work and school for rest and relaxation. Nightingale continued to describe self-care time as essential to caring for our patients. If the nurse *"wishes to do this, she must keep up a sort of divine calm and high sense of duty in her own mind"* (Nightingale, 2009, p. 19). Essential in caring for others is practicing self-care techniques that work to calm you, and what works for you may not work for others. And what works for you at one time may not work at another time.

In her letter to the nursing students, Nightingale (2009, p. 19) further suggests that:

> *quiet in our own rooms; a few minutes of calm thought to offer up the day … . How indispensable it is, in this ever-increasing hurry of life! When we live so fast, do we not require breathing time, a moment or two daily, to think where we are going? At this time, especially when we are laying the foundation of our afterlife, it is, in reality, the most important time of all.*

Even in the 1870s, in an age before the internet, cell phones, and social media, Nightingale noticed that the fast, hurried pace of life was disrupting her students' ability to relax and take care of themselves. The lack of wellness of her nursing students, in turn, affected the patients' care. Remember how I needed a little help finding a daily source of wellness in my early days in the ICU? The cue *"Stepping out!"* meant taking a moment for yourself, using the bathroom, and having some water and food. All were necessary for me to continue to take care of my patients. My wellness needed to come first; my mom helped me incorporate it into my busy day. Nightingale also tried to instill wellness by allowing for unhurried time for the nurses to relax, read, and sleep.

Self-care is "deliberate decisions made and actions taken by individuals to address their own health and well-being" (Ashcraft & Gatto, 2018, p. 140). New and early-career nurses are at a higher risk of burnout, anxiety, and stress related to ill health (Cleary et al., 2012). New nurses also may have unmet expectations in their work environment as their workloads shift between school preparation and the heavy workloads of a potentially unsupportive environment (Cleary et al., 2012).

New nurses may have barriers to self-care as well. The nurses and self-care survey found that self-care barriers include not having time, feeling overworked, consistently lacking adequate resources, feeling fatigued, lacking sleep, having outside commitments, and living with an unhealthy food culture (Ross et al., 2019). Researchers have also found that others influence nurses in their environment and have discovered barriers that include unsupportive individuals and negative role models (Ross et al., 2019). Some nurses have even indicated that they themselves are the barrier to their wellness, meaning that their willpower and motivation drive them to have unhealthy behaviors (Ross et al., 2019). They have described a norm of self-sacrifice in their new workplaces, stating that *"working to the point of exhaustion is respected and self-care is considered selfish"* (Ross et al., 2019, p. 371).

In my experience, even nurse leaders feel guilty about not asking for or taking the time they need for self-care. My nursing director team at my current organization suffers from feelings of needing to be constantly available to our colleagues, coinciding with guilt surrounding their self-care. To combat these real feelings, as a nursing leadership team, we are working on a modified workweek schedule to allow for protected self-care time for each of them. We are currently on a journey to study and publish this work so that other nurse leaders can benefit from the work-life balance and intentional well-being model we are creating.

Well-being and wellness is a lifelong journey. The first step on your health and well-being journey as a new nurse is determining which area of life you must focus on. The wellness dimensions are physical, mental, emotional, spiritual, intellectual, social, financial, and environmental (Fontaine et al., 2021). Determining which sphere needs your most attention is a great place to start. Essential to continued well-being and wellness are creating habits and reassessing how the tactics influence your health journey.

We can use the nursing care-planning process to create a personalized action plan for wellness. A model that fits well with wellness is the

TABLE 12.1 Application of the Next-Generation Care Plan to a Nurse's Wellness Strategy

Noticing	Interpreting	Responding	Reflecting
Begin noticing what is happening with your health and wellness. What is important to your self-care? What kinds of activities make you feel healthy and happy? What is going well? What is not going well? Which wellness dimension do you feel you need to fous on? • Physical • Mental • Emotional • Spiritual • Intellectual • Social • Financial • Environmental	*Begin thinking about how you can address your health and wellness concerns.* What problems with your wellness can you identify? What are outcomes that would address the problems? What interventions could assist in achieving the outcomes? What wellness interventions feel right to you?	*Begin prioritizing your wellness.* What are you going to work on? List the wellness areas with specific interventions you want to try to address each. Who can assist you on your journey? Having a buddy or social group can help build healthy habits. Where can you go for help? Do you need medical advice for some of your wellness concerns? What resources do you need?	*Begin reflecting on your journey so far.* What demonstrates that your outcomes were met? Are your wellness and well-being improving? What's next on your wellness journey? Activities: Journaling during this stage is helpful for future planning.

Source: Application of Derr, 2022.

Next-Generation Care Plan (NGCP), described in an article by Rachel Derr (Derr, 2022). This new nursing care-planning model combines the nursing process (assessing, diagnosing/analyzing, planning, implementing, and evaluating) with the Clinical Judgment Measurement Model to create a four-step care-planning model that promotes nurses doing what they can to provide care for their patients based on what they know at the time (Derr, 2022). Upon review, this model promotes more introspection and becomes

TABLE 12.2 Application of the Next-Generation Care Plan to a Nurse's Wellness Strategy Using Kayla's Story

Noticing	Interpreting	Responding	Reflecting
Kayla noticed that her sleep was disrupted and occurring at different hours of the day from others working the night shift. Kayla noticed that her dreams seemed to be related to the stress and anxiety of being a nurse. Kayla noticed that she was particularly stressed right before her shift (preshift anxiety).	Kayla interpreted her current situation and identified the problems associated with her wellness: • Sleep • Anxiety/worry (preshift anxiety) Outcomes: • Better, more rejuvenating sleep • Less preshift anxiety	Kayla chose the wellness dimensions that respond to her current problems, as follows: **Physical:** Prioritize sleep. • Prioritize sleeping at normal times when off from work. • Rest as much as possible on worknights. • Exercise to promote rest. **Emotional:** Decrease preshift anxiety by incorporating stress-reduction activities, such as: • Journaling • Listening to music • Spending time with family and friends • Cooking and baking to prepare healthy meals	Kayla reflected that the promotion of those activities decreased her preshift anxiety. Kayla found that regular exercise assisted in her being able to sleep better. Kayla found joy and love in connecting with friends and family. Kayla found joy in cooking and baking and preparing healthy meals for her days at work. Kayla's journaling will help determine which self-care activities are working and which may need to be adjusted. Next steps on Kayla's wellness journey may be to continually reassess her wellness and the wellness dimensions and adjust the interventions as needed to continue better outcomes.

more enriched and personalized as care is provided. This is ideal for a self-care journey. This care-planning model may be used to model a wellness routine and can be continuously adjusted as we experience the wellness journey based on the outcomes we achieve.

Adapted from Derr's model for the NGCP (Derr, 2022), I have incorporated the four steps and focused the model on the wellness perspective. This care-planning model may guide you in creating your wellness and well-being journey.

Let's work through an example of Kayla's wellness journey using this model.

Enjoy working through the model to determine the best wellness routine to support your transition to practice and journey from novice to expert. Remember, if you do not care for yourself, you will not be able to care for others. Our calling to be nurses is a lofty one. We must remember that deep caring for ourselves through wellness and self-care is essential to caring for others, including for our friends, families, and patients. Please take care of yourself. You are so important.

Self-Care Is Not Selfish

By Linda Roney, EdD, RN-BC, FAAN

Through Kayla's story and Teresa's response, we hear the impact of caring on the lives of two nurses. Most nurses can help patients feel more relaxed and confident in their care by considering situations from their perspective. However, we must develop skills that prevent us from being drained by work situations where we help others (Ethan Allen Workforce Solutions, 2023). Most nurses view serving patients as their duty and give of themselves endlessly despite how they feel on any given day (Williams et al., 2022). Sometimes, this also spills into how nurses approach relationships in their personal lives. Nursing practice has inherent emotional burdens, time pressures, and physical demands that challenge one's ability to engage in self-care (Wood et al., 2022). Nursing is stressful since it is associated with complex job demands and needs, high expectations, and excessive responsibility (Babapour et al., 2022). As Kayla and Teresa both describe, developing strategies to help care for yourself is essential. The effects of prolonged, unmanaged stress can hurt nurses' personal or professional lives, causing physical and psychological changes, such as job stress, anger, anxiety, dissatisfaction, and frustration (Lan et al., 2014). The American Nurses Association's (ANA) *Code of Ethics for Nurses With Interpretive Statements* (2015) states that nurses need to practice self-care to apply the moral respect that they carry for others to themselves, including activities that preserve their wholeness of character and continue personal growth. Let's explore how Kayla demonstrated the American Association of Colleges of Nursing (AACN) essentials' (2021) competency in Domain 10.

TABLE 12.3 Examples of Domain 10: Personal, Professional, and Leadership Development in This Exemplar

Domain 10: Personal, Professional, and Leadership Development	
10.1 Demonstrate a commitment to personal health and well-being.	Kayla developed strategies to promote her wellness regarding preshift anxiety and work-life imbalance. She developed strategies to manage the stress that she experienced from work when she was home (and sleeping).

Source: Adopted from AACN, 2021.

Time Pressures of Caring

Time pressure is more than a lack of measurable time; it also describes nurses' high workloads and inadequate nursing staffing levels, which may affect patient outcomes and experiences (Vinckx et al., 2018). It can lead to nurses avoiding actively exploring patients' feelings; telling patients that they have to postpone conversations to a quieter moment in their shift; giving non-verbal signals that they do not have enough time, including walking in a rushed manner; making less eye contact; and moving away from patients while they are still talking (Vinckx et al., 2018). Time pressure is inversely proportional to the nursing quality and satisfaction perceived by patients and the decision-making ability of nurses (Shi et al., 2023).

Whereas some nurses reported increased motivation under time pressure, others reported anxiety and a high level of mental stress (Shi et al., 2023).

Strong time management skills are essential to your overall health and well-being and can help you manage work stress (ANA, 2023). Nurses have different personalities and diverse ways of thinking and working and, therefore, different perceptions of time pressure (Shi et al., 2023). Nurses have identified that their mood at work as well as their work experience and work schedule could affect their work efficiency (Shi et al., 2023). You need to manage your time at work intentionally when you are not at work.

Planning and Managing Your Time at Work

Plan on arriving for your shift about 10 minutes before it starts (ANA, 2023). It is easy to get distracted before you leave and leave later than anticipated. Preparing meals in advance, laying out work clothes the night before, and keeping your work items together in a location near the door can help facilitate a smooth exit, especially when you are on a stretch of shifts in a row. Traffic, unexpected delays, and other obstacles can add to your time to get to your unit, and giving yourself a time buffer can help should something happen. Beginning your day in a rush will have a snowball effect and add to your stress throughout your shift (INSCOL, 2022).

Identifying your most important tasks and creating a plan to get those things done is critical (ANA, 2023). When starting a clinical shift, take a few minutes before you receive a report to review the electronic health records of your assigned patients for highlights (e.g., diagnosis, medications, tests, labs, and current orders; Leis & Anderson, 2020). Use a system to keep track of your workload and patient assignment tasks that makes you feel organized but adheres to your institution's policies for securing patient information. When appropriate to your work setting, bedside report helps ensure safer environments, refocus patient-centered care, and aid your shift in starting more smoothly (McAllen et al., 2019). Bedside report also provides an excellent opportunity for an environmental scan, ensuring that emergency equipment is readily available and immediate patient needs are met.

Be aware of which tasks need to be completed by you as the RN and which tasks you can delegate. Delegate where and when you can (ANA, 2023). Taking the time to teach patients and families about routine tasks, such as ordering their meals, can save you a lot of time. Organize your tasks so that you do not create a gridlock of team members for the patient. For example, if you know that your patient has speech, physical, and occupational therapy, coordinating times and organizing your assignment around those appointments and other patient tasks can help your shift go smoother.

For the most part, focus on one task at a time throughout your day because multitasking slows you down by dividing your attention and draining your cognitive resources which slows you down (ANA, 2023). As you grow in your skills and nursing practice, there will be times when you can multitask—for example, while doing a dressing change and simultaneously offering distraction and active listening. If you are focused on an essential task (e.g., medication preparation or administration), politely tell coworkers not to interrupt you unless they have a pressing matter (ANA, 2023).

Shi et al. (2023) found that in the face of intermittent pressure, nurses may have the energy left to take steps to ensure that all patient care is completed; however, when faced with constant stress, nurses have no opportunity to replenish their resources and might be exhausted. It is typical for nurses to skip their breaks to prioritize wrapping up tasks or patient care; however, this leaves them exhausted and less effective for the rest of their shift (ANA, 2023). Breaks help you feel refreshed, reduce fatigue, and improve time management skills and teamwork (Leis & Anderson, 2020).

Planning and Managing Your Time Away From Work

Although it is good occasionally, passive rest is less effective in helping you recover from the stress of your work days (Giurge & Bohns, 2021). Having plans for your days off is associated with time spent pursuing social activities and greater happiness (Giurge & Bohns, 2021). Finding a hobby or activity outside of work that has nothing to do with nursing gives you something to look forward to and helps you establish your identity outside of work (*Scrubs Mag*, 2023). Planning an important trip in the future affects how you feel; 97% of survey respondents reported that doing so made them happier (Institute for Applied Positive Research, 2020).

Mitigating the Physical Demands of Caring

Imagine this scene: You start your shift at 7 p.m. and hit the ground running after report. Nothing is going as planned, and it is 2 a.m. by the time you think about quickly eating something. As you put your leftovers in the microwave for precisely two minutes, you scroll through TikTok. With dopamine hit after dopamine hit from the funny videos, you suddenly feel better than before. The microwave's beep interrupts your scrolling, and you take out your hot container. Two bites into your leftovers, the unit secretary comes into the breakroom and while apologizing for interrupting your lunch, she tells you that after waiting all evening, patient transport is here to take your patient to radiology. However, the patient requests to use the restroom before they get on the transport stretcher, and the nursing assistant is not available because they are relieving the sitter for their break. You tell yourself that you will get back to your meal right after you complete this task, but after you send your patient off the unit, one of your other patients puts their call light on and requests an as-needed pain medicine. At 4 a.m., a coffee list goes around among the staff, and you give in. You are exhausted, and drinking half of an iced coffee might be the only thing to help you through this seemingly never-ending shift. The rest of the night slips from your grasp, and at the end of your shift, you see your cold leftovers in the same place that you left them as you never had a chance to finish eating.

You go home to your apartment, and after opening your fridge only to see it is empty, you decide to go straight to bed. As you roll on your side, the roar of a lawnmower startles you, and you realize there is no chance of falling asleep until they are done. You begin to think about your patient who went for MRI during your shift. The radiologist's report was not dictated before the end of your shift, so you do not know the result. You wonder whether her cancer is back. You grab your phone and start scrolling through the Instagram stories of friends who documented their fun and exciting weekends while you were on three 12-hour overnight shifts on Friday, Saturday, and Sunday. A group trip among friends to Nashville that you did not know about until seeing the photos—front-row seats to your favorite performer's concert—and a marriage proposal are a little more than you can take after another sleepless night.

Still feeling the effects of the 4 a.m. iced coffee, you switch to swiping through Instagram reels, after which watching videos of strangers telling you to go to the gym and meal-prep for the week and that you can quit your hospital-based job in exchange for a work-from-home job after signing up for the free webinar has you feeling even worse than before. Looking at the clock, you see that it is already 11 a.m., and in just seven hours, you have to leave your house to commute to work for the overtime shift you picked up. You decide to take a nighttime sleep aid with diphenhydramine, even though it is in the middle of the day—you are desperate for sleep. If you could get a better routine, maybe you could get on track and feel better. Before you know it, your alarm blares—it is 5:15 p.m. and time to get into the shower for work. You crawl out of bed and head to the kitchen. Your stomach is rumbling. Opening your fridge, you forget that it is empty and curse under your breath. You walk over to your coffee pot and turn it on. A cup of coffee at home, as you prepare for your fourth 12-hour–long night shift, might help you take the edge off your exhaustion until you can pick up your mobile order at your favorite coffee shop. While you wait for your coffee to finish brewing, you check your phone again only to see a text from the coworker to whom you gave report this morning: "Hope you got sleep today. It is a zoo here—see you soon." You throw your phone down on the counter, and your eyes tear up. *I am so tired; I cannot even think. I cannot do this again.*

What is wrong with this story? The protagonist—the nurse (you)—gave everything and had nothing for themselves. Working 48 hours at night in four days with limited sleep and food, no personal time, and no meaningful contact with the outside world left them depleted.

- Can you identify what went wrong for the nurse in this story?
- What could the nurse have done better to address their needs?

Since nursing work is expected to be performed rapidly and accurately, the physical demands on the nurse can be very high (Chang & Cho, 2022). Some of the physical activities of nurses during their shifts include standing, walking, lifting objectives, moving items, changing patient positions, supporting patient ambulation, pushing wheelchairs, providing support for patients' activities of daily living, and changing bed linens (Chang & Cho, 2022). Let's focus on practical strategies to promote self-care and work-life integration in our own lives.

Sleep

This story has many problems; however, key is the nurse's lack of sleep, which demonstrates a foundational challenge. Forty percent of adults in the general population have difficulty falling asleep (Scullin et al., 2018). Of all types of workers, protective services and military jobs have the highest prevalence of short sleep duration (less than seven hours a night) across the years of working, followed by a high prevalence of short sleep duration in healthcare workers (Khubchandani & Price, 2020). Nurses regularly report experiencing poor sleep quality, sleeping fewer than the seven to nine hours recommended for optimal health and safety, and difficulty prioritizing their health and self-care over others (Hittle et al., 2023). Sleep is critical to your work as a nurse; it is not selfish or decadent. Research shows that the chance of having a workplace injury or making a medical error increase by 2.43 when a shift worker's sleep is impaired compared with workers without sleep issues (Booker et al., 2024).

Prioritize Sleep

Maintain a regular sleep schedule to the extent possible on both work-days and off-work days, with a goal of seven to nine hours per 24 hours. Most night-shift nurses want to resume a daytime schedule on their days off to align with their families and friends and sleep at night in the dark. However, adjusting your sleep one or more times a week can tire you even more (Centers for Disease Control and Prevention [CDC], 2020). It is recommended that on the nights you work, you go to sleep as soon as you get home for as long as you can. On your days off, try to stay up until the middle of the night (e.g., 3 to 4 a.m.) and sleep until noon to 1 p.m. so that your body has some hours of sleep that are always the same in every 24 hours (e.g., 8 a.m. to noon is always a sleep time on both work-days and days off; CDC, 2020). Day-shift nurses may also encounter sleep problems due to early start times and wanting to stay up late even if they have to get up early in the morning (CDC, 2020). Prioritizing sleep also includes taking naps and sleeping longer than you usually would when you need to catch up on sleep when you have the chance (ANA, 2020). Coffee (107 milligrams [mg] per 250 milliliters) should be consumed at least 8.8 hours prior to bedtime, and a standard serving of preworkout energy drink (217.5 mg) should be consumed at least 13.2 hours prior to bedtime (Gardnier et al., 2023).

Using Light to Promote Wake-Up Time and Sleepiness at the End of Your Day

When you wake up, whether in the morning or the evening, exposure to bright light can help you throughout your day. If you have slept at night, in the morning, your eyes sense the sunlight, and the suprachiasmatic nucleus in your brain (which controls your sleep-wake cycle) triggers the release of cortisol to help your body wake up (Johns Hopkins Medicine [JHM], 2024). When darkness arrives at night, the suprachiasmatic nucleus sends messages to the pineal gland for the release of melatonin to make you fall asleep (JHM, 2024). Future research should explore active light manipulations in night-shift employees; bright light in the evening/early night delays the circadian rhythm and causes an immediate, increased alertness (Grønli et al., 2018). Getting bright light before and in the early part of the night shift can help you feel more awake (Bostock, 2022).

Two hours before bedtime, dim the lights to avoid shifting the circadian rhythms to later bedtimes and wakeup times (CDC, 2020). If you work at night in dim lights and the day staff comes, flipping on all the light switches for a bright glow, you know what kind of a jolt this feels like for your body. Negotiate with the day staff to transition to bright lights on the unit after the night staff leave. Night-shift nurses should reduce their light exposure as much as possible after leaving work to facilitate getting to sleep when they get home (Salamon, 2023). Blackout curtains and a sleep-eye mask can help keep your bedroom as dark as possible; ear plugs or a noise machine can help you avoid or distract you from daytime noises (Bostock, 2022). Stay off your smartphone at least one hour before bedtime as it can affect your sleep by keeping your mind engaged, you may encounter content that causes intense emotion, and the light from your screen can throw off your circadian rhythm and make it harder to fall asleep (Cleveland Clinic, 2022).

Pre-Bedtime To-Do List

Do you feel like you come from work and your mind is racing with worry for all you must do when you get up or on your upcoming days off? Spend five minutes writing your to-do list. Scullin et al. (2018) found that those who spent five minutes before bed writing their specific list of tasks that needed to be completed in the upcoming days fell asleep faster than those who spent five minutes journaling about completed activities.

Leave Work at Work

Do your best to leave the job behind when your shift ends (ANA, 2023). At the end of your shift, acknowledge any challenge you faced, take a deep breath, and let it go by saying a mantra such as "I am leaving work" (American Nurses Foundation [ANF], n.d.). Acknowledge three positive things from your shift and, if you choose to, process your day during your commute home. Before you walk inside your home, acknowledge the transition by saying something positive that notes your transition to being off from work, such as "I am home now, and it feels good" (ANF, n.d.).

Intrusive Thoughts While Trying to Sleep

In Kayla's story, which opens this chapter, the stress of her workdays carried over into her dreams. Research supports that burnout and some sleep disturbances are closely related to the type of work performed by nurses in terms of the work environment; for example, working with dying patients, dealing with the psychological demands of the job, and receiving a lack of support from colleagues all directly affect sleep (Membrive-Jiménez et al., 2022). Some experts believe that dreaming is part of the mind's way of processing emotions and consolidating memories, but more research is needed in this area (Center for Victims of Torture [CVT], 2021). Garcia et al. (2021) found that days with greater stress for nurses were associated with a higher chance of experiencing a nightmare and more severe nightmares that night, and nights during which at least one nightmare was reported were associated with greater next-day stress severity. Targeting stress is one critical way to promote restful sleep and lessen nightmares for nurses (Garcia et al., 2021).

Worrying about patients when you are not at work does not help solve problems and leaves you depleted and inattentive to loved ones (ANA, 2023). If your thoughts about work or someone you have cared for are affecting the way you work, live, or spend your free time; are interrupting or complicating your relationships; or influencing your use (or overuse) of alcohol or other substances, please seek the help of a mental health professional (CVT, 2021). Since the COVID-19 pandemic, nurses have endured a dramatic increase in stressful experiences and a simultaneous rise in professional demands, leaving us uniquely vulnerable to the emergence of maladaptive coping strategies (Arble et al., 2023). Proactively advocating for your mental health needs is critical to your happiness.

Nurturing Interpersonal Connections

In Chapter 1 of this casebook, we presented the concept of mattering and how important it is for the new nurse. Rosenberg and McCullough (1981) introduced *mattering*, which is defined as a person's need to believe that they are significant to others. Over time, the definition of *mattering* evolved to include seven components: attention, importance, dependence, ego extension, noted absence, and appreciation (Flett, 2021). All these parts are important for your interpersonal connection inside and out of work. Developing trusting and enjoyable work relationships helps create a caring environment and reduce work-related stress (Wei et al., 2020). Social connectedness includes the frequency of social contact and the perception that available social contacts can meet emotional and relational needs (Wood et al., 2022). Social support is critical to nurses coping with work stressors and mitigating burnout (Wood et al., 2022). Working antisocial hours and the impact of cumulative fatigue affect nurses' social lives and ability to be present even when you are physically present at an event (Booker et al., 2024). Wood et al. (2022) found that social support is at least moderately and inversely correlated with burnout and critical to coping with work stressors. Find ways to build social connections, especially outside of work, to help you decompress when you are not at work. This can include joining a social or service group, taking a class, trying a new hobby, or joining a gym (Madaus, 2023). Do not mistake mindlessly scrolling through your phone on your time off from work as nurturing social connections.

Wirtz et al. (2020) found that people turn to social media more when they are feeling lonely. This might be for you when you are up in the middle of the night on your day off while your friends are sleeping. In the study, they found that people felt worse after spending time on social media, which made them feel lonelier due to social comparison. The more study participants compared themselves with others while using social media, the less happy they felt (Wirtz et al., 2020).

Mindfulness and Movement

Mindfulness and movement are two strategies for stress reduction. Nurses experiencing a stressful or traumatic situation become immersed in feelings of stress that can lead to anger, sorrow, discomfort, tension, and illness; mindfulness programs help redirect negative thinking and reframe difficult situations (Penque, 2019). Mindfulness-based stress reduction programs have been researched as a holistic intervention for reducing stress and burnout in nurses by cultivating present awareness, emotional regulation, and positive thinking (Green & Kinchen, 2021). Practicing mindfulness regularly helps you access the skill more easily when needed.

Be aware of your mindset. Warning yourself that you are going to have an awful week because you are on four 12-hour shifts in a row sounds like you are setting yourself up for a self-fulfilling prophecy. Instead, invest time and energy into how you can make the next four shifts better for you. Maybe you can save a couple of episodes of your favorite podcast for the commute to work each day. Perhaps you can treat yourself to your favorite hot beverage on your way to work each night. Schedule a dinner date with a friend at your favorite restaurant to celebrate that your stretch of shifts is over. Whatever you do, force yourself out of the scarcity mindset, which is a pattern of thinking that focuses on what you do not have (Burdick, 2023), and create a more positive mindset that will make you feel better about things in the upcoming days.

Movement increases overall well-being. Aerobic activities, such as tennis and power walking, increase the production of endorphins, which can help you feel better and improve your mood (Mayo Clinic, 2024). Regular yoga practice can effectively reduce stress levels (Zok et al., 2024). We are often too tired on our days off, either from workload, shift rotation, or stress, and set ourselves up for failure with unrealistic expectations for movement on our days off. Health and wellness with movement does not need to be all or nothing. Small incremental changes, such as going for a 10-minute walk during your lunch break and then doing a 20-minute stretching video on YouTube after work, may make movement more accessible. Consider habit stacking, which is doing something you might find challenging (e.g., riding a stationary bike) while watching your favorite new series on Netflix. It will help you enjoy movement while reaping the positive benefits.

Nutrition and Hydration

It is very easy for nurses to put off eating and drinking water while caring for patients, but this will leave you feeling terrible throughout your shift. Some nurses find it helpful to meal-prep for the entire week to ensure that they have balanced meals at work. Consider bringing snacks that you can eat on the go. Not having a plan for meals can mean that by the time you finally make it to the cafeteria during your shift, it might be closed. If you do not eat all day but consume a large meal at night, you may not feel your best. Bringing a refillable water bottle can help you meet your hydration goal of drinking 72 to 104 ounces per day (Harvard T. H. Chan School of Public Health, 2024).

Humor (Light to Dark)

Humor is a coping strategy that allows people to distance themselves from stress, which increases positive emotions and eases tension (Dionigi et al., 2023). Some types of humor can be an effective coping strategy in clinical settings to release stress, recover from compassion fatigue, and develop better team cohesion (Aultman & Meyers, 2020). Nurses and other healthcare providers sometimes use dark humor, which is a comic style that makes light of typically taboo subjects that are usually considered painful to discuss (Dionigi et al., 2020). Dark humor can be a common mechanism, especially for those who work in trauma and crisis-related fields, to cope with sadness, hurt, frustration, and grief (Potter, 2023). Humor enables the development of relationships among colleagues in tense and sometimes unimaginable situations, provides anxiety relief, and affords an outlet for anger using socially acceptable means but also avoidance or denial of hurt (Ghaffari et al., 2015). An anonymous emergency department nurse (2020) wrote about their experience with humor while working the front line of the COVID-19 pandemic:

> The emergency department attracts a certain personality type. Whether a physician, nurse, or tech, we all have the ability to laugh when most would cry. How else could we come back to work after doing CPR on a 2-year-old or having comforted a family who lost their 90-year-old grandfather? We don't disrespect the deceased; we just cope with the reality of life with humor. We save our sadness and tears for home. (Anonymous, 2020, para 2).

Although using dark humor can help some nurses get through the worst situations, it is more prone to misunderstanding (Proyer & Rodden, 2020). While, on the surface, it helps the healthcare provider get out of the stress of a challenging clinical shift, it can also be a sign of something greater. Dionigi et al. (2023) investigated how specific categories of humor related to depression, anxiety, and stress as well as nonsense, irony, and cynicism were primarily associated with emotional distress. With reference to darker styles, irony was observed as the best predictor of anxiety and stress, and cynicism was a positive predictor of depression (Dionigi et al., 2023). If you and your team consistently use dark humor to get through the painful situations that you encounter at work, speak with your manager about resources available to support you through challenging situations. One team leadership strategy for support would be debriefing, an opportunity for an after-action review of key events, an analysis of why the event occurred, what worked, and what did not, and any lessons learned for future care (American Hospital Association [AHA], 2024). Debriefing allows for emotional processing and reflection on areas for possible improvement following critical and high-stakes incidents, such as patient codes, and is one way to improve overall performance, reduce equipment-related problems, and improve communication and teamwork (Przednowek et al., 2021). Your supervisor can also connect you with employee assistance resources to help you navigate the issues you encounter during your shift.

TeamSTEPPS TIP

It is important to reinforce what went well and avoid assigning blame or failure to any individual regarding what did not go well (AHA, 2024).

Emotional Wellness

Gawlick et al. (2024) describe *emotional wellness* as having the knowledge and skills to identify personal feelings and the ability to regulate those emotions. They suggest strategies to implement in the clinical setting to handle life stresses, including using breathing exercises, practicing gratitude, and using positive reframing. Let's talk more about each of these strategies now.

Box Breathing

Combat tactical breathing, also known as *box breathing*, is an evidence-based strategy adopted by the U.S. Navy SEALs to address anxiety and stress in even the most intense situations (Navy Medicine, n.d.). It is taught widely to first responders and others who must remain calm during intense situations.

PRN (PLEASE READ NOW)

Relax by taking three to five breaths, as described below. Visualize each number as you count.

- Breathe in, counting 1, 2, 3, 4. Stop and hold your breath, counting 1, 2, 3, 4.
- Exhale, counting 1, 2, 3, 4.
- Breathe in, counting 1, 2, 3, 4. Pause and hold your breath, counting 1, 2, 3, 4.
- Exhale, counting 1, 2, 3, 4.
- Repeat as many times as you need to calm down.

Practicing Gratitude

Practicing gratitude is a way of shifting your thoughts to notice the good things in your life. Keeping a gratitude journal allows you to remind yourself by writing about the good things you enjoy each day; these can be associated with ordinary events, your personal attributes, or people whom you value (Mindful.org, 2025). Placing visual reminders around your home and work can also serve as cues to trigger thoughts of gratitude (Mindful.org, 2025).

While much literature focuses on practicing gratitude by acknowledging the people and things we are grateful for in our lives, I suggest you start by expressing gratitude for things within *you*. We all engage in self-talk, which includes statements we say to ourselves that might be said automatically or strategically, either silently or out loud, and either positively or negatively and have a motivational purpose (Santos-Rosa et al., 2022). Because the path to becoming a nurse is challenging and we want the best for our patients, when something adverse happens after work, that self-talk becomes increasingly hostile as it is compounded by any personal challenges we might have experienced. Like a tiny snowball that grows gigantic as each negative thought is added, we eventually have something in the way of not only our happiness but also our ability to function. One tool to take action against this giant snowball is cognitive reframing.

Cognitive Reframing

Cognitive reframing is a helpful tool to use to view experiences in a more constructive light. It involves three steps (Williams, 2022). First, recognize that what your mind tells you may or may not be a fact. Next, question the thought and any cognitive distortions by asking, "*What evidence do I have to support this thought?*" Finally, replace negative thoughts with more realistic ones (Williams, 2022). An example of this might include when you walk onto the unit for your night shift and you do not see two of the nurses who are scheduled to work with you. You see a nurse who floated to your unit from another floor to cover one of the sick calls; however, it seems like you are down a nurse for the shift. You begin to tell yourself that you are about to have an awful night.

Then you decide to try cognitive reframing. First, you tell yourself that both outcomes are possible at this point in time: The night might be OK, or it might be not very good. Next, you ask yourself for evidence to support this idea. Other than your two coworkers calling out only to be replaced by one person instead of two, you do not have any other information. You have yet to meet this nurse who was floated to help your team, so you do not know anything about their ability to handle a full assignment on your unit. When you look at the bed board for your unit, you see that there were five discharges during the day, so you have the appropriate number of nurses on tonight, even though you are down one nurse. You decide that the nurse will probably be fine, and you introduce yourself and thank the nurse who floated to your unit.

Boundaries and Self-Care: You Have Heard It Before, but What Does It Mean?

Boundaries

You have heard that nurses must maintain professional boundaries. Perhaps you have heard that it is important to maintain boundaries in your personal life. Let's consider what boundaries are within the context of how you feel about your work as a nurse and how you feel about yourself as a person. *Boundaries* are about what we expect or our limits, communicated through actions or communication (Sanok, 2022). Living within the boundaries you create can help you lower your stress, increase your life satisfaction, and limit the anxiety and stress that some develop when they take on the responsibility for others' emotions (Oswald, 2023). Having boundaries at work means that sometimes you need to say no. It takes courage to advocate for yourself so that you can have the energy to work consistently (CVT, 2021). This includes saying no to additional work or duties that will overload you (CVT, 2021). Nurses often have to learn to set boundaries with their workers when they are already experiencing stress and feeling overwhelmed. Your time is precious, and you should guard it to ensure that others do not take too much of it (Fahkry, 2021). Time is finite, so if you are saying yes to something above your expected responsibility, you are saying no to something else because there is not enough time to do everything (Fahkry, 2021). There are many times that you will be able to say yes to take on extra work, help the unit, or help others, but if you are already feeling signs of stress and burnout, think twice about extending yourself beyond what you are expected to do. The following is an example.

Jeff is a new nurse on the unit; he has been off orientation for one month when one of his coworkers asks if he can switch upcoming winter holidays with her. The coworker is assigned to work day shifts on Christmas Eve and Christmas Day, and Jeff is assigned to work overnights on New Year's Eve and New Year's Day. The coworker asks Jeff for the switch, saying that she has little children at home, really wants to be home Christmas morning to watch them open their gifts, is willing to "give him the night off to celebrate New Year's," and states, *"Christmas probably doesn't matter to you anyways since you do not have kids, right?"* Her comment upsets him; Jeff already has plans to go skiing with his partner over Christmas and does not want to make the switch. Jeff caught off guard by the request, says, "I am not sure, so *let me check.*" While at work, Jeff tries to avoid the coworker as much as possible so that she does not have the chance to follow up with him. Finally, a few days later, she texts him on his day off and asks, *"Well, did you figure out if we can switch yet? My husband wants to know if we are going to have Christmas this year."*

Jeff is upset that his coworker is texting him on his day off. He does not want to make the switch but feels that as a new nurse on the unit, he needs to make as many friends as possible. If he does her this favor, then maybe people will like him more. Jeff has been very stressed about his transition off orientation; he feels like it takes him much longer to get things done than his coworkers. He has not been sleeping well because of his stress and has been staying late most nights to help because they have been short. Then he wonders, *will other people get mad at him if he switches with her?* There are probably other people who would like to have Christmas off and might be mad if he agrees to this switch. His partner walks into the room and notices that Jeff is upset. Jeff tells him about the situation and the latest text from his coworker, and his partner reminds him that they already have plans and that he just needs to say no. While many people have a hard time saying *no* to others, remember that *"no"* is a complete sentence (Benjamin, 2022). Jeff can choose not to respond to the text since this is a work issue and he is off today, and then he can respond to the coworker in person the next time he sees her. He texts her back today and says, *"I would love to, but I am going away."* The coworker texts back, *"OK."*

Jeff is at work a few days later, and he hears his coworker telling a colleague, *"Yeah, can you believe he did not want to do this for me? It is not like he has kids or anything."* She then makes eye contact with Jeff and walks away from the nurses' station. This was exactly what Jeff did not want to have happen. He wonders whether he should apologize and tell her that he can do the switch now. His partner will be upset, but they can reschedule their trip. Jeff cares deeply about other people and feels bad that the coworker will miss the experience of seeing her children open their gifts on Christmas morning. Lost in his thoughts, Jeff's fellow new nurse, Rick, comes up to him and asks him what's wrong. Jeff tells him the story about the switch, and Rick tells him to stop thinking about it; he already said no. Rick reminds Jeff that he is not responsible for his coworker's happiness or schedule.

Consider the following:

- If you were in Jeff's position, what would you have done?
- Should Jeff have a follow-up conversation with his coworker after hearing part of a conversation he believes might have been about him? Why or why not?

Jeff can deploy any of the tools we discussed so far in this chapter to deal with his emotions in this situation, but let's apply cognitive reframing to it.

In the example of Jeff and the winter holiday switch, he feared that his coworker was mad at him, and he considered changing his plans to appease her. If he applied cognitive reframing to the situation, he would first recognize that his coworker might not, in fact, be angry at him. He then asks himself if he has evidence to support that she is upset with him. He notes that he heard her tell the coworker, "*Yeah, can you believe he did not want to do this for me? It is not like he has kids or anything.*" Is he certain that this comment was about him? It was not a pleasant comment if it was about him, but nothing in the words she said states that she is angry at him. Finally, he decides to replace his negative thoughts with realistic ones. He decides that while she is probably disappointed that he cannot make the switch with her, she will move on, and their relationship will go back to baseline at some point soon. Until then, he can enjoy spending time with his other coworkers and staying out of her way.

Boundaries With Patients and Families

In *A Nurse's Guide to Professional Boundaries*, the National Council of State Boards of Nursing (NCBSN) (2018) offers nurses guidance in navigating patient relationships within professional boundaries. *Patient boundaries* are the spaces between the nurse's power and the patient's vulnerability; the nurse's power comes from their professional position and access to the patient's sensitive personal information (NCBSN, 2018). This difference in power can cause an imbalance in the nurse-patient relationship, threatening patient-centered care. Brief excursions across professional lines of behavior by the nurse are called *boundary crossings* and occur when nurses share excessive personal information, keep secrets with or for a patient, speak poorly about colleagues with a patient or their family, show favoritism, or meet patients in places outside of the care setting when they are not at work (NCBSN, 2018). Inexperienced and young nurses are at particular risk for committing boundary violations because of their lack of experience or understanding. Emotional life events can also put nurses at risk for crossing professional boundaries with patients when they seek compassionate feedback and seek to connect with others who can empathize with them (Nurses Service Organization, 2024).

Social Media Risks for Nurses Related to Boundaries

You and your patient really bonded last night. You believe you have a lot in common because of your conversations: cooking meals that are five ingredients or less, shopping online to find designer lookalike clothing, and watching cute puppy videos. That night, when you get home from work, you go onto your Instagram account and see a follow request from a name that sounds familiar. You look at the profile image, and it is your patient whom you had the connection.

- Do you hit "Accept?" She will be discharged before you go back to work.

In a recent survey of U.S. nurses regarding their social media practices, 87% of participants reported using a social media account (Lefebvre et al., 2020). Wang et al. (2019) found that 67.2% of nurses with social media accounts disclosed that they "often" communicate work-related information to colleagues via social media, with half having received friend requests from patients and 32.5% reporting witnessing colleagues disclose identifiable information. Most employers have social media guidelines for employees that provide instructions for social media use even outside of work hours for employees of an organization. Frequently, these policies remind employees that policies such as the Health Insurance Portability and Accountability Act of 1996 and nondiscrimination, even if the patient is deidentified, still apply to their personal social media accounts (JHM, 2024).

Two high-risk areas for nurses related to their nursing role and social media are violations of patient privacy/confidentiality breaches and unprofessional behavior (Healthcare Providers Service Organization [HPSO], 2024). Patient privacy violations can be intentional or inadvertent with inappropriate posts that include patient photos, negative comments about patients, or details that might identify patients (HPSO, 2024).

Nurses and healthcare professionals are held to ethical conduct standards that require professional and moral behavior. Violations of these standards include posting photos or comments about alcohol or drug use; profane, sexually explicit, or racially derogatory comments; negative comments about coworkers or employers; or threatening or harassing comments (HPSO, 2024). For example, four labor and delivery nurses in Atlanta were fired from their jobs for making a TikTok video about their perceptions of the irritating habits of the patients and families for whom they care as part of their jobs (Algar, 2022). The video went viral, and after an investigation by the hospital, the nurses were fired because the video did not represent the values and standards that their organization expects all team members to uphold (Belvins, 2023). In general, you should not record any videos or take photos at work, and if there is some specific reason that you need to do so, do not do it without your supervisor's permission because even the most well-intended posts can be determined by others as inappropriate (Belvins, 2023). Failing to comply with your employer's social media standards and the profession's expectations for responsible use can result in loss of job and complaints to professional governing boards, resulting in disciplinary action ranging from a reprimand and fine to temporary or permanent loss of licensure. If federal or state laws are broken, there also is the potential for civil and criminal penalties (HPSO, 2024).

YOU MATTER: TAKING TIME TO CARE FOR YOURSELF

As you search for your first job or strive to integrate your work and life after starting the position, you must determine your top priorities in work and life (Sanok, 2022). Perhaps now more than ever, you need to have a clear plan for integrating self-care into your life. If you are at work for 12.5 hours, you need to sleep for seven hours when you get home, and your commute with parking is 30 minutes each way, that leaves only 3.5 hours in your day if you return to work. Intentionally claiming some of that time for you is important to feel restored. Without this time, you will feel depleted and worse than when you started.

Book Club Questions

1. What self-care practices do you incorporate into your daily routine, and how consistently do you implement them? Reflect on the impact these practices have on your sense of well-being.
2. Do you follow coworkers on social media? If so, do you follow supervisors and your organization? What could be the potential positive and negative implications of both?
3. Are specific scheduling requests among coworkers more important than others? How can multiple requests for the same dates and times off be fairly addressed?

About This Chapter's Authors

Kayla Beckman, BSN, RN

Kayla was born and raised in Central Massachusetts. Growing up, she always wanted to enter the medical field and has a passion for helping others. She obtained her Bachelor of Science in Nursing (BSN) in 2022 from Fairfield University's Marion Peckham Egan School of Nursing and Health Studies. Her nursing career began while she was in school, working as a patient care associate in a stepdown unit, where she fell in love with the patient population and the challenges that came with it. Upon graduating, Kayla returned to Massachusetts and accepted a job in a new-graduate nurse residency program on a cardiovascular stepdown unit. Kayla continues to work in this role with added responsibilities, including precepting new graduates and charge nurses. Additionally, she is enrolled in a Doctor of Nursing Practice program and looks forward to furthering her education and advancing her career. Outside of work, Kayla enjoys spending time with family and friends, working out, cooking and baking, and taking trips to the beach.

Teresa Fuller, MSN, RN, NEA-BC, CPXP

Teresa is honored to be the vice president of patient care services and chief nursing officer at St. Vincent's Medical Center in the Fairfield region of Hartford Healthcare in Connecticut. She is a compassionate nursing leader with more than 25 years of experience, including 15 ycars of leadership experience. She graduated from the University of Pennsylvania with a BSN and from the University of Hartford with a Master of Science in Nursing. She is certified in patient experience and studying for her nursing leadership certification (Nurse Executive Advanced). She enjoys mentoring others, investing time in developing teams, promoting and encouraging interdisciplinary collaboration and communication, and promoting continued professional development. She is highly passionate about advancing the patient experience, encouraging the nursing leaders' and nursing staff's wellness and well-being, and creating healthy work environments for all colleagues.

She lives on a small organic farm in Northwest Connecticut with her husband and daughter, six baby-doll sheep, two dogs, and 12 chickens. They create products from the farm and bake extraordinary treats every weekend for their farm store.

References

Arble, E., Manning, D., Arnetz, B. B., & Arnetz, J. E. (2023). Increased substance use among nurses during the COVID-19 pandemic. *International Journal of Environmental Research and Public Health, 20*(3), 2674. https://doi.org/10.3390/ijerph20032674

Algar, S. (2022). Atlanta nurses who mocked expectant moms in TikTok video fired from Emory Healthcare hospital. *New York Post.* https://nypost.com/2022/12/13/atlanta-nurses-who-mocked-expectant-moms-in-tiktok-video-fired-from-emory-healthcare-hospital/

American Association of Colleges of Nursing. (2021). *The essentials: Core competencies for professional nursing education.* https://www.aacnnursing.org/Portals/0/PDFs/Publications/Essentials-2021.pdf

American Hospital Association. (2024). *AHA TeamSTEPPS video toolkit.* https://www.aha.org/center/project-firstline/teamstepps-video-toolkit

American Nurses Association. (2023, May 1). *Time management tips for nurses.* American Nurses Association Nursing Resource Hub. https://www.nursingworld.org/content-hub/resources/workplace/time-management-tips-for-nurses/

American Nurses Association. (2020). *Guide to sleeping better and restoring energy.* https://www.nursingworld.org/~4a4d62/globalassets/covid19/wbi-sleepguide-08252020-final-w-partner-logos.pdf

American Nurses Association. (2015). *Code of ethics for nurses with interpretive statements.* https://www.nursingworld.org/practice-policy/nursing-excellence/ethics/code-of-ethics-for-nurses/coe-view-only/

American Nurses Foundation. (n.d.). *After-work checklist.* https://www.nursingworld.org/~4ab553/globalassets/covid19/well-being-initiative_sharegraphic_checklist_-091720a.pdf

Anonymous. (2020, March 31). *The ER diaries: Dark humor gets us through – we save our tears for home.* The Guardian. https://www.theguardian.com/us-news/2020/mar/31/the-er-diaries-dark-humor-gets-us-through-we-save-our-tears-for-home

Ashcraft, P. F., & Gatto, S. L. (2018). *Curricular interventions to promote self-care in pre-licensure nursing students. Nurse Educator, 43*(3), 140–144. https//doi.org/10.1097/NNE.0000000000000450

Aultman, J., & Meyers, E. (2020). Does using humor to cope with stress justify making fun of patients? *AMA Journal of Ethics.* https://journalofethics.ama-assn.org/article/does-using-humor-cope-stress-justify-making-fun-patients/2020-07

Babapour, A. R., Gahassab-Mozaffari, N., & Fathnezhad-Kazemi, A. (2022). Nurses' job stress and its impact on quality of life and caring behaviors: A cross-sectional study. *BMC Nursing, 21*(1), 75. https://doi.org/10.1186/s12912-022-00852-y

Benjamin, A. (2022). *How to set boundaries at work as a nurse.* Nurse.org. https://nurse.org/articles/nurse-boundaries-at-work/

Benner, P. (1984). *From novice to expert: Excellence and power in clinical nursing practice.* Prentice Hall Health.

Belvins, J. L. (2023, February 1). Nurses fired after posting TikTok video disparaging patients. *Healthcare Risk Management.* https://www.reliasmedia.com/articles/nurses-fired-after-posting-tiktok-video disparaging-patients.

Booker, L. A., Fitzgerald, J., Mills, J., Bish, M., Spong, J., Deacon-Crouch, M., & Skinner, T. C. (2024). Sleep and fatigue management strategies: How nurses, midwives and paramedics cope with their shift work schedules: A qualitative study. *Nursing Open, 11*(1), e2099. https://doi.org/10.1002/nop2.2099

Booker, L. A., Barnes, M., Alvaro, P., Collins, A., Chai-Coetzer, C. L., McMahon, M., Lockley, S. W., Rajaratnam, S. W., Howard, M. E., & Sletten, T. L. (2020). *The role of sleep hygiene in the risk of shift work disorder in nurses. Sleep, 43*(2), zsz228. https://doi.org/10.1093/sleep/zsz228

Bostock, S. (2022, June 22). *How to sleep well as a night shift worker.* The Sleep Scientist. https://www.thesleepscientist.com/post/how-to-sleep-well-as-a-night-shift-worker

Burdick, E. (2023, October 23). *There will always be more: Overcoming scarcity mindset.* Headspace. https://www.headspace.com/mindfulness/there-will-always-be-more-overcoming-scarcitymindset#:~:text=Scarcity%20Mindset%20can%20be%20defined,%2C%20housing%2C%20income%2C%20etc.

Center for Victims of Torture. (2021). *Boundaries. Professional Quality of Life.* https://proqol.org/boundaries

Centers for Disease Control and Prevention. (2020). *The National Institute for Occupational Safety and Health* (NIOSH) *training for nurses on shift work and long work hours.* https://www.cdc.gov/niosh/work-hour-training-for-nurses/default.html

Chang, H. E., & Cho, S. H. (2022). Nurses' steps, distance traveled, and perceived physical demands in a three-shift schedule. *Human Resources for Health, 20*(1), 72. https://doi.org/10.1186/s12960-022-00768-3

Cleary, M., Horsfall, J., Baines, J., & Happell, B. (2012). Mental health behaviours among undergraduate nursing students: Issues for consideration. *Nurse Education Today, 32*(8), 951–955. https://doi.org/10.1016/j.nedt.2011.11.016

Cleveland Clinic. (2022). *Why you should ditch your phone before bed.* https://health.clevelandclinic.org/put-the-phone-away-3-reasons-why-looking-at-it-before-bed-is-a-bad-habit

Derr, R. (2022). *Rethinking the nursing care plan.* https://sites.rutgers.edu/changing-course/rethinking-the-nursing-care-plan/

Dionigi, A., Duradoni, M., & Vagnoli, L. (2023). Understanding the association between humor and emotional distress: The role of light and dark humor in predicting depression, *anxiety, and stress. Europe's Journal of Psychology, 19*(4), 358–370. https://doi.org/10.5964/ejop.10013

Ethan Allen Workforce Solutions. (2023, August 8). Six ways you can help prevent nurse burnout in your staff. Ethan Allen Workforce Solutions. https://eaworkforce.com/prevent-nurse-burnout-on-your-staff/

Fahkry, T. (2021). *How to stop giving away your personal power over your time.* LinkedIn. https://www.linkedin.com/pulse/how-stop-giving-away-your-personal-power-over-time-tony-fahkry/

Flett, G. L. (2021). An introduction, review, and conceptual analysis of mattering as an essential construct and an essential way of life. *Journal of Psychoeducational Assessment, 40*(1), 3-36. https://doi.org/10.1177/07342829211057640

Fontaine, D. K., Cunningham, T., & May, N. (2021). *Self-care for new and student nurses.* Sigma Theta Tau International.

Garcia, O., Slavish, D. C., Dietch, J. R., Messman, B. A., Contractor, A. A., Haynes, P. L., Pruiksma, K. E., Kelly, K., Ruggero, C., & Taylor, D. J. (2021). What goes around comes around: Nightmares and daily stress are bidirectionally associated in nurses. *Stress and Health, 37*(5), 1035–1042. https://doi.org/10.1002/smi.3048

Ghaffari, F., Dehghan-Nayeri, N., & Shali, M. (2015). Nurses' experiences of humour in clinical settings. *Medical Journal of The Islamic Republic of Iran, 29*(82).

Giurge, L., & Bohns, V. (2021). Be intentional about how you spend your time off. *Harvard Business Review.* https://hbr.org/2021/12/be-intentional-about-how-you-spend-your-time-off

Green, A. A., & Kinchen, E. V. (2021). The effects of mindfulness meditation on stress and burnout in nurses. *Journal of Holistic Nursing, 39*(4), 356–368. https://doi.org/10.1177/08980101211015818

Grønli, J., & Mrdalj, J. (2018). Can night shift workers benefit from light exposure? *Journal of Physiology, 596*(12), 2269–2270. https://doi.org/10.1113/JP276043

Harvard T. H. Chan School of Public Health. (2024). *Water.* https://www.hsph.harvard.edu/nutritionsource/water/

Healthcare Providers Service Organization. (2024). *Perils of social media for healthcare professionals.* https://www.hpso.com/Resources/ Privacy-and-Confidentiality/Perils-of-Social-Media-for-Healthcare-Professional

Hittle, B. M., Hils, J., Fendinger, S. L., & Wong, I. S. (2023). A scoping review of sleep education and training for nurses. *International Journal of Nursing Studies, 142,* 104468. https://doi.org/10.1016/j.ijnurstu.2023.104468

INSCOL. (2022, March 21). *Time management tips for nurses at work.* LinkedIn. https://www.linkedin.com/pulse/time-management-tips-nurses-work-inscol-healthcare-inc/

Institute for Applied Positive Research. (2020). *Planning travel creates happiness.* https://www.ustravel.org/sites/default/files/media_root/document/PlanningTravel_MichelleGielan.pdf

Johns Hopkins Medicine. (2024). *Social media guidelines.* https://www.hopkinsmedicine.org/webcenter/social-media-guidelines/highlights

Khubchandani, J., & Price, J. H. (2020). Short sleep duration in working American adults, 2010–2018. *Journal of Community Health, 45*(2), 219–227. https://doi.org/10.1007/s10900-019-00731-9

Lan, H. K., Subramanian, P., Rahmat, N., & Kar, P. C. (2014). The effects of mindfulness training program on reducing stress and promoting well-being among nurses in critical care units. *Australian Journal of Advanced Nursing, 31*(3), 22–31. https://search.informit.org/doi/10.3316/ielapa.285671898965330

Lefebvre, C., McKinney, K., Glass, C., Cline, D., Franasiak, R., Husain, I., Pariyadath, M., Roberson, A., McLean, A., & Stopyra, J. (2020). Social media usage among nurses: Perceptions and practices. *Journal of Nursing Administration, 50*(3), 135–141. https://doi.org/10.1097/NNA.0000000000000857

Leis, S. J., & Anderson, A. (2020). Time management strategies for new nurses. *American Journal of Nursing, 120*(12), 63–66. https://doi.org/10.1097/ 01.NAJ.0000724260.01363.a3

Madaus, S. (2023, October 12). *17 smart ways to make friends in a new city, according to experts.* Oprah Daily. https://www.oprahdaily.com/life/relationships-love/a45342932/how-to-make-friends-in-a-new city/?utm_source=google&utm_medium=cpc&utm_campaign=arb_ga_opr_md_dsa_hybd_org_us_21018453020&gad_source=1&gclid=C-jwKCAjw9IayBhBJEiwAVuc3fkzyohhWRs50YwFctYasYEBBI3clbLfg2QVqzV3QFBqt-KascZS_TsxoCnWUQAvD_BwE

Mayo Clinic. (2024). *Stress management.* https://www.mayoclinic.org/healthy-lifestyle/stress-management/in-depth/exercise-and-stress/art-20044469

McAllen, E. R., Stephens, K., Swanson-Biearman, B., Kerr, K., & Whiteman, K. (2018). Moving shift report to the bedside: An evidence-based quality improvement project. *Online Journal of Issues in Nursing, 23*(2).

Membrive-Jiménez, M. J., Gómez-Urquiza, J. L., Suleiman-Martos, N., Velando-Soriano, A., Ariza, T., De la Fuente-Solana, E. I., & Cañadas-De la Fuente, G. A. (2022). Relation between burnout and sleep problems in nurses: A systematic review with meta-analysis. *Healthcare (Basel, Switzerland), 10*(5), 954. https://doi.org/10.3390/healthcare10050954

National Council of State Boards of Nursing. (2018). *A nurse's guide to professional boundaries.* https://www.ncsbn.org/public-files/ProfessionalBoundaries_Complete.pdf

Navy Medicine. (n.d.). *Combat breathing.* https://www.med.navy.mil/Portals/62/Documents/NMFA/NMCPHC/root/Documents/health-promotion-wellness/psychological-emotional-wellbeing/Combat-Tactical-Breathing.pdf

Nightingale, F. (2009). *Florence Nightingale to her nurses.* Letter dated May 23, 1873. Digireads.com Publishing.

Nurses Service Organization. (2024). *Don't cross the line: Respecting professional boundaries.* https://www.nso.com/Learning/Artifacts/Articles/Don-t-cross-the-line-respecting-professional-boundaries

Oswald, R. (2023). *Map it out: Setting boundaries for your well-being.* Mayo Clinic Health System. https://www.mayoclinichealthsystem.org/hometown-health/speaking-of-health/setting-boundaries-for-well-being

Penque, S. (2019). Mindfulness to promote nurses' well-being. *Nursing Management, 50*(5), 38–44. https://doi.org/10.1097/01.NUMA.0000557621.42684.c4

Potter, Z. (2023). Laughing through the pain: An analysis of dark humor in trauma-and-crisis-centered occupations. *PDX Scholar.* https://doi.org/10.15760/honors.1335

Proyer, R., & Rodden, F. (2020). Virtuous humor in health care. *AMA Journal of Ethics.* https://journalofethics.ama-assn.org/article/virtuous-humor-health-care/2020-07

Przednowek, T., Stacey, C., Baird, K., Nolan, R., Kellar, J., & Corser, W. D. (2021). Implementation of a rapid post-code debrief quality improvement project in a community emergency department setting. *Spartan Medical Research Journal, 6*(1), 21376. https://doi.org/10.51894/001c.21376

Rosenberg, M., & McCullough, B. C. (1981). Mattering: Inferred significance and mental health among adolescents. *Research in Community & Mental Health, 2,* 163–182.

Ross, A., Touchton-Leonard, M. A., Perez, A., Wehrlen, L., Kazmi, N., & Gibbons, S. (2019). Factors that influence health-promoting self-care in registered nurses: Barriers and facilitators. *Advances in Nursing Science, 42*(4), 358–373.

Salamon, M. (2023). *Shift work can harm sleep and health: What helps?* Harvard Health Publishing. https://www.health.harvard.edu/blog/shift-work-can-harm-sleep-and-health-what-helps-202302282896

Sanok, J. (2022, April 14). A guide to setting better boundaries. *Harvard Business Review.* https://hbr.org/2022/04/a-guide-to-setting-better-boundaries

Santos-Rosa, F. J., Montero-Carretero, C., Gómez-Landero, L. A., Torregrossa, M., & Cervelló, E. (2022). Positive and negative spontaneous self-talk and performance in gymnastics: The role of contextual, personal and situational factors. *PLOS One, 17*(3), e0265809. https://doi.org/10.1371/journal.pone.0265809

Scrubs Mag. (2023, July 21). "Time off? What's that?" Nurses on what they do when they are not at the hospital. https://scrubsmag.com/time-off-whats-that-nurses-on-what-they-do-when-theyre-not-at-the-hospital/

Scullin, M. K., Krueger, M. L., Ballard, H. K., Pruett, N., & Bliwise, D. L. (2018). The effects of bedtime writing on difficulty falling asleep: A polysomnographic study comparing to-do lists and completed activity lists. *Journal of Experimental Psychology, 147*(1), 139–146. https://doi.org/10.1037/xge0000374

Shi, F., Li, Y., & Zhao, Y. (2023). How do nurses manage their work under time pressure? Occurrence of implicit rationing of nursing care in the intensive care unit: A qualitative study. *Intensive & Critical Care Nursing, 75,* 103367. https://doi.org/10.1016/j.iccn.2022.103367

Vinckx, M. A., Bossuyt, I., & Dierckx de Casterlé, B. (2018). Understanding the complexity of working under time pressure in oncology nursing: A grounded theory study. *International Journal of Nursing Studies, 87,* 60–68. https://doi.org/10.1016/j.ijnurstu.2018.07.010

Wang, Z., Wang, S., Zhang, Y., & Jiang, X. (2019). Social media usage and online professionalism among registered nurses: A cross-sectional survey. *International Journal of Nursing Studies, 98,* 19–26. https://doi.org/10.1016/j.ijnurstu.2019.06.001

Wei, H., Kifner, H., Dawes, M. E., Wei, T. L., & Boyd, J. M. (2020). Self-care strategies to combat burnout among pediatric critical care nurses and physicians. *Critical Care Nurse, 40*(2), 44–53. https://doi.org/10.4037/ccn2020621

Williams, S. G., Fruh, S., Barinas, J. L., & Graves, R. J. (2022). Self-care in nurses. *Journal of Radiology Nursing, 41*(1), 22–27. https://doi.org/10.1016/j.jradnu.2021.11.001

Wirtz, D., Tucker, A., Briggs, C. & Shoemann, A, (2021). How and why social media affect subjective well-being: Multi-site use and social comparison as predictors of change across time. *Journal of Happiness Studies, 22*, 1673–1691 https://doi.org/10.1007/s10902-020-00291-z

Wood, R. E., Brown, R. E., & Kinser, P. A. (2022). The connection between loneliness and burnout in nurses: An integrative review. *Applied Nursing Research, 66*, 151609. https://doi.org/10.1016/j.apnr.2022.151609

Zok, A., Matecka, M., Bienkowski, A., & Ciesla, M. (2024). Reduce stress and the risk of burnout by using yoga techniques. *Frontiers in Public Health, 12*, 1370399. https://doi.org/10.3389/fpubh.2024.1370399

CHAPTER 13

What's Next?

Linda Roney, EdD, RN-BC, CPEN, CNE, FAAN

At the beginning of this book, I shared all the fantastic newer nurses (*Anabelle, Anna, Bridget, Grace, Iris, Janea, Katie K., Katie M., Kayla, Lauren,* and *Moira*) who share their tremendous stories are *my former students.* After graduation, they scattered across the country and worked in different nursing specialties. As I read how these nurses addressed challenges in their year or two of practice, I was overwhelmed with many emotions. I am proud of the situational leadership they have demonstrated and shared with us in this casebook. I am devastated by the overwhelmingly complex challenges that may have broken their hearts of caring for patients who teach us to be nurses and the families who trust us with their care. I am frustrated that they bear witness to patients and families who hold hope for miracles when their loved one's bodies are failing and they know that there is no hope.

I am angry that they have witnessed racism, judgment, and moments of powerlessness despite reaching out for support. I am frustrated that many of the themes of their challenges are not new but are amplified in today's healthcare setting. *Why haven't we fixed this as a profession?* I fear that the healthcare system expects way too much from these intelligent and compassionate nurses, stretching them past the limits of reasonable expectations of any healthcare profession daily. They put their all into their nursing education, and I am sure they do the same as nurses. I do fear that, as a nation, we are at a tipping point, and large numbers of this next generation of new nurses will want to leave patient care. We don't want you to leave—you matter!

As I mentioned at the start of this casebook, my motivation to write this book was after reading the results of the 2022 National Workforce Survey (Smiley et al., 2023) that noted that more than one-quarter of all nurses in the study reported planning to leave nursing or retire in the next five years (Smiley et al., 2023). The nurse leaders whom I asked to join me in this casebook project represent the best and brightest in healthcare leadership. *Aaron, Danielle, Eileen, Erin, Kevin, Laura, Laurie, Maria, Michelle, Sarah, Sean,* and *Teresa* all represent different vantage points in nursing leadership. Our paths have crossed at various times in my nursing career, and none of them hesitated at the invitation to join me in this work. Like me, they believe in you and the future of our profession. We hope that by sharing our stories and strategies for overcoming workplace challenges, you will feel supported and gain valuable insights into navigating some of the challenges you might encounter as a new nurse.

So, you may ask, what's next? That part is up to you. Within one book, we cannot possibly address every situation you might encounter, but we hope that the stories and tactical, evidence-based advice can help you through a situation or two as you begin your nursing practice. Hopefully, we have given you a framework to pair with your educational background from which to start. You have read examples of demonstrating person-centered care (Domain 2) and personal, professional, and leadership development (Domain 10) (American Association of Colleges of Nursing, 2021). Choose one strategy from each chapter to implement into your nursing practice each month—this will take you through your first year of nursing practice.

Commit to a spirit of natural curiosity and be open to learning from new experiences. The things you will witness and participate in your first days, months, and year of practice are scary. I have found success in labeling what I am feeling and asking for help when I need it. *"This feels new. Do you mind watching me the first time I do it?" "I am afraid of going into the room after the provider tells my patient their diagnosis. How would you handle it?"* Labeling your emotions and then refocusing on what you need has been helpful to me in countless situations. Be sure to take good care of yourself. It can be in small, manageable baby steps.

Assume the best in people. When you call the surgery resident and they do not immediately return your call, don't automatically get angry. Try to come at it from a place of understanding. Maybe they are assisting in a challenging case from which they can't break away. Is the unit secretary always snippy with you? Perhaps they don't have a "sparking personality," as someone else in this book is known for; perhaps it is because they are a single parent holding two jobs to support their two children. I am not saying you should make excuses for people when they do not act in the way we expect in the professional setting—instead, come to work with an open mind and a place of understanding for everyone you encounter. This should be reciprocal and manifested as mutual respect. If it isn't, then see Chapter 4.

Give yourself grace and space with your own reactions to caring. Do not overschedule yourself when you are going through a challenging time, either personally, professionally, or, unfortunately, when they happen at the same time. Spend time with *your people*, whether it's your favorite people at work or off the clock. Participate in new traditions at work and in your postnursing school life. You have earned this.

While we may receive support from our employer, I have found the most incredible opportunities for development from professional organizations related to my nursing role. If you cannot decide which organizations are most relevant to you, ask your nurse educator or manager for suggestions. If you are nervous about the commitment of membership, joining the organizations' social media pages is a great way to be exposed to issues they are addressing. Most professional organizations have a presence on Facebook, Instagram, LinkedIn, and X.

Finally, know that you are never alone in your nursing journey. Seek out mentors, colleagues, and friends. Something doesn't feel right? Ask trusted mentors for advice and speak up. Is your first job not the right fit for you? Switch—but this time, when you pick your first position, know your priorities and be open to finding the right fit. Most of all, know you are appreciated, valued, and matter in OUR nursing community.

Dr. Linda Roney
@drlindaroney.com

References

American Association of Colleges of Nursing. (2021). *The essentials: Core competencies for professional nursing education.* https://www.aacnnursing.org/Portals/0/PDFs/Publications/Essentials-2021.pdf

Smiley, R. A., Allgeyer, R. L., Shobo, Y., Lyons, K. C., Letourneau, R., Zhong, E., Kaminski-Ozturk, N., & Alexander, M. (2023). The 2022 national nursing workforce survey. *Journal of Nursing Regulation*, 14(1), S1–S90. https://doi.org/10.1016/s2155-8256(23)00047-9

INDEX

ABOUT THE EDITOR

Linda Roney, EdD, RN-BC, CPEN, CNE, FAAN is committed to nursing education in both academic and clinical settings. As an professor of nursing at the Egan School of Nursing & Health Studies (Fairfield University), she has received state and national awards recognizing her excellence in teaching. As an advocate, educator, and nationally recognized expert in pediatric trauma nursing, Dr. Roney's impact includes research, clinical practice, service, testimony to state and federal agencies, and leadership for improving nursing care for injured children. She continues to work as a bedside nurse at Yale New Haven Children's Hospital. Dr. Roney earned her BSN from Villanova University and her MSN and EdD degrees from Southern Connecticut State University.

Linda is married to her husband, John, a physician's assistant. They have two children, Natalie and Michael, and a sleepy cat, Georgia. Most mornings start at the gym with her favorite workout friends and, hopefully, a walk along the Connecticut shoreline to watch a beautiful sunrise. Her favorite place is at the beach, reading a good book with family nearby.